Alcohol: No Ordinary Commodity

Oxford Medical Publications

Alcohol: No Ordinary Commodity

Research and public policy

Thomas Babor

Raul Caetano

Sally Casswell

Griffith Edwards

Norman Giesbrecht

Kathryn Graham

Joel Grube

Paul Gruenewald

Linda Hill

Harold Holder

Ross Homel

Esa Österberg

Jürgen Rehm

Robin Room

Ingeborg Rossow

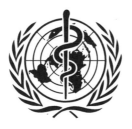

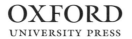

OXFORD

UNIVERSITY PRESS

OXFORD
UNIVERSITY PRESS

Great Clarendon Street, Oxford OX2 6DP

Oxford University Press is a department of the University of Oxford.
It furthers the University's objective of excellence in research,
scholarship, and education by publishing worldwide in

Oxford New York

Auckland Bangkok Buenos Aires Cape Town Chennai
Dar es Salaam Delhi Hong Kong Istanbul Karachi Kolkata
Kuala Lumpur Madrid Melbourne Mexico City Mumbai Nairobi
São Paulo Shanghai Taipei Tokyo Toronto

Oxford is a registered trade mark of Oxford University Press
in the UK and in certain other countries

Published in the United States
by Oxford University Press Inc., New York

© Oxford University Press, 2003

A catalogue record for this book is available from the British Library

Library of Congress Cataloging in Publication Data
(Data available)

ISBN 0 19 263261 2 (Pbk)

10 9 8 7 6 5 4

Typeset by Newgen Imaging Systems (P) Ltd., Chennai, India
Printed in Great Britain
On acid-free paper by Biddles Ltd, King's Lynn, Norfolk

Foreword

From its inception in 1948, the World Health Organization (WHO) has recognized the importance of alcohol policy as an instrument of public health. Whether it came from the resolutions of the World Health Assembly or the recommendations of WHO Expert Committees, WHO has been actively involved not only in documenting the global and regional dimensions of alcohol related problems, but also in the exploration of policy responses for their prevention. Although leadership of this effort has come from both WHO Headquarters in Geneva and from the WHO Regional Offices, it should be no surprise that the WHO Regional Office for Europe has taken a special interest in alcohol. The European nations produce and consume a disproportionate share of the world's alcohol, and they experience a disproportionate share of the illness, death and disability that alcohol is responsible for.

To inform its work in the alcohol area, in 1973 the European Office of WHO initiated a collaborative project with the Addiction Research Foundation of Ontario and the Finnish Foundation for Alcohol Studies that explored the impact of population-level policies on alcohol-related problems. The product of that collaboration was *Alcohol Control Policies in Public Health Perspective*, a book that has been cited repeatedly as a landmark contribution to the search for scientifically-based approaches to the prevention of alcohol-related problems (Bruun *et al.*, 1975). Inspired in part by the concepts, findings, and recommendations of that report, there has been a tremendous growth in both the study and the practice of alcohol policy, enough to generate periodic updates of the evidence and recommendations as they apply to nations and communities. One such update was *Alcohol Policy and the Public Good* (Edwards *et al.*, 1994), a collaborative effort between the WHO Regional Office for Europe and an international group of alcohol experts. The Alcohol and Public Policy group first convened in 1992 under the leadership of Cees Goos, then Coordinator of the Alcohol, Drugs, and Tobacco unit of the Regional Office, and Professor Griffith Edwards, then Director of the National Addiction Centre, London, UK. The product of that collaboration, *Alcohol Policy and the Public Good* (Edwards *et al.*, 1994), quickly became a primary source of information on effective alcohol policies worldwide, and its contents provided support for the first European Alcohol Action Plan, which set specific goals for the reduction of alcohol-related problems, and recommended policies to achieve them. Given the impressive knowledge base represented in this report, the European Regional Office also supported a ministerial resolution in 2001 concerning the promotion of alcohol to youth by commercial interests and the hospitality sector (WHO, 2001).

WHO Headquarters, Geneva, followed with a complementary collaborative study, *Alcohol in Developing Societies: A Public Health Approach* (Room *et al.*, 2002), which extends this kind of policy analysis to long-neglected areas of the world. It demonstrates that alcohol problems are likely to increase more in developing societies where there are no effective policies in place. All of these efforts are consistent with evidence-based approaches to alcohol policy advanced by WHO, where the Director-General has established an Alcohol Policy Strategy Advisory Committee to advise WHO on the development of both scientific and policy initiatives in this area internationally.

In the same tradition of collaboration established almost 30 years ago, the World Health Organization is again pleased to sponsor another timely report in this series. *Alcohol: No Ordinary Commodity: Research and Public Policy* represents more than an update of the epidemiology of alcohol problems and the promising advances in prevention policy research that have taken place during the past decade. Because of its emphasis on the economic and commercial aspects of alcohol consumption, this volume provides a valuable new perspective on the development of effective alcohol policies.

Taking a cue from the title of this book, we are pleased to contribute to the proposition that from a public health perspective, alcohol is no ordinary commodity. As the most recent chapter in what has become an ongoing international debate on the role of alcohol in modern society, we hope that this book continues to narrow the gap between alcohol science and public policy.

Dr Derek Yach
Executive Director
Noncommunicable Disease and Mental Health
World Health Organization, Geneva, Switzerland

References

Bruun K., Pan L., and Rexed I. (1975) *The gentlemen's club: International control of drugs and alcohol.* Chicago: University of Chicago Press.

Edwards G., Anderson P., Babor T.F., *et al.* (1994) *Alcohol policy and the public good.* Oxford University Press.

World Health Organization, European Office (2001) *Declaration on young people and alcohol, 2001.* Copenhagen: WHO-Euro

Room R., Jernigan J., Carlini Marlatt B., *et al.* (2002) *Alcohol in developing societies: a public health approach.* Helsinki: Finnish Foundation for Alcohol Studies.

Preface

From a public health perspective, alcohol consumption plays a major role in morbidity and mortality on a global scale. In the past fifty years, considerable progress has been made in the scientific understanding of the relationship between alcohol and health. Ideally, the cumulative research evidence should provide a scientific basis for public debate and governmental policymaking. However, much of the scientific evidence is reported in academic publications in a way that has little apparent relevance to prevention or treatment policy. To address this need for a policy-relevant review of the literature, a small group of experts, under the leadership of Professor Griffith Edwards, established in 1992 the Alcohol and Public Policy Project (APPP). The group recruited an international team of research scientists, consulted with experts throughout the world, and in the course of less than two years, critically evaluated the accumulated knowledge on how to deal with alcohol problems in the public policy arena (Edwards *et al.* 1994; Holder and Edwards 1995).

The process used by the APPP was established twenty years earlier under the leadership of Dr Kettil Bruun, who at that time gathered the best analysts of alcohol policy and research to produce a report, *Alcohol control policies in public health perspective*, published in collaboration with the European Office of the World Health Organization (WHO) (Bruun *et al.* 1975). As noted by WHO Regional Director J.E. Asvall (Edwards *et al.* 1994, p. vi): 'Few books have had so much influence on the thinking and actual policy-making in this area. Its great impact was due to the authority of the group, to the very thorough way in which they did their work, and to the practical form in which they packaged their conclusions.' The same has been said for its successor, *Alcohol policy and the public good* (Edwards *et al.* 1994). It not only established a scientific basis for the European Alcohol Action Plan, but also provided an objective analysis on which to build relevant policies globally. It represented, in a comprehensive and readily accessible way, the accumulated scientific knowledge on this subject up to 1992.

At a 1998 alcohol policy conference in Chicago, IL, USA, a small group of the APPP authors unanimously agreed to begin plans for another volume, based on the increasing knowledge base, the changing climate of alcohol policy, and international trends in drinking problems. The text of the present volume has evolved through the development of background papers, many stages of drafting, the discussion of this material at plenary meetings held in Copenhagen, London, and Berkeley, and the contributions of a small editorial group, which held additional meetings in Stockholm and London. This is a written rather than an edited volume, built on the joint input of all those involved. This participatory exercise has resulted in a text that represents the consensus view of its 15 authors, who have contributed as individual scientists rather than as representatives of any organization.

The WHO (Copenhagen regional office and Geneva headquarters) and the Society for the Study of Addiction provided a small amount of base funding to cover the organizational costs of the project. No fees were paid for any of the writing, consulting work, or background papers connected with the project. All authors provided WHO Conflict of Interest assurances, which are available from the first author upon request. Most of the support for travel costs and manuscript preparation came from the participants' own centres and universities, as well as time donated by them to the project.

The purpose of this volume is to describe recent advances in alcohol research that have direct relevance to the development of alcohol policy on the local, national, and international levels. Although the intended audience includes researchers, addiction service providers, clinicians, and prevention planners, this book above all is written to inform and empower policy-makers who have direct responsibility for public health and social welfare.

References

Bruun K., Edwards G., Lumio M., *et al.* (1975) *Alcohol control policies in public health perspective.* Helsinki: The Finnish Foundation for Alcohol Studies.

Edwards G., Anderson P., Babor T.F., *et al.* (1994) *Alcohol policy and the public good.* Oxford University Press.

Holder H.D. and Edwards G. (eds.) (1995) *Alcohol and public policy: evidence and issues.* Oxford University Press.

Acknowledgements

The preparation of this book has depended on the generous support of a large number of individuals, organizations, and academic institutions. The project benefited greatly from the financial support of the Society for the Study of Addiction and both the Copenhagen and Geneva offices of the World Health Organization (WHO). Special recognition is due Mr Cees Goos (former Co-ordinator, Alcohol, Drugs, Tobacco Unit, WHO Regional Office for Europe, Copenhagen), a member of the project's initial planning group who gave valuable input at many later points. At various times during the project, expert consultation was provided by Carol Cunradi, PhD, Prevention Research Center, Pacific Institute for Research and Evaluation, Berkeley, CA, USA; Christine Godfrey, PhD, Centre for Health Economics, University of York, York, UK; Barbara Leigh, PhD, University of Washington, Seattle, WA, USA; Paul Lemmens, PhD, University of Maastricht, Maastricht, The Netherlands; Shekhar Saxena, MD, World Health Organization, Geneva, Switzerland; and Tim Stockwell, PhD, National Drug Research Institute, Perth, Western Australia. An important initial contribution to the project was provided by the authors of commissioned papers that were subsequently published in a special issue of *Contemporary Drug Problems* (Fall 2000): Maggie Brady, PhD, Therese Reitan, PhD, and Jacek Moskalewicz, PhD.

Invaluable support was also provided by the academic and scientific organizations with which the authors were affiliated during the time of the project. These institutions not only allowed the collaborating investigators to give time to this project, but also provided travel money in most instances. The full project team and the editorial group held meetings at: WHO (Copenhagen, Denmark); National Addiction Centre (London, UK); Prevention Research Center, Pacific Institute for Research and Evaluation (Berkeley, CA, USA); and Stockholm University (Stockholm, Sweden). We are grateful to these organizations for hosting the meetings. Sally Casswell and Linda Hill were supported by core funding to the Alcohol and Public Health Research Unit from the Health Research Council of New Zealand and the Alcohol Advisory Council of New Zealand. Jürgen Rehm was supported by a grant from the Swiss Federal Office of Public Health (01.000046). The epidemiological data on exposure and alcohol-related disease burden were estimated in the framework of the Global Burden of Disease Study, Comparative Risk Analysis, Alcohol (PI, J. Rehm). This project was supported by various grants from the World Health

Organization, the Swiss Federal Office of Public Health, and the Swiss National Science Foundation. Raul Caetano was supported in part by grant R37-AA10908 from the US National Institute on Alcohol Abuse and Alcoholism (NIAAA) to the University of Texas School of Public Health. During the time of the project, Robin Room was supported as a Visiting Scientist for six months at the National Institute for Alcohol and Drug Research, Oslo, Norway. His position at Stockholm University is supported by the Swedish Council for Working Life and Social Research.

Norman Giesbrecht and Kathryn Graham were supported by the Centre for Addiction and Mental Health, Toronto, Ontario, Canada. Special thanks are due to the University of Connecticut Alcohol Research Center (NIAAA grant no. P50-AA03510), which, with the help of Deborah Talamini and Dominique Morisano, provided logistical support and coordination to the project. Finally, we are grateful for the advice and comments provided by present and former WHO officials Marestela Monteiro, Leanne Riley, Philip Lazarov, and Peter Anderson.

Contents

*Terms and phrases printed in **bold** are defined in the glossary at the end of the book.*

Section V **Conclusion**

Contributors

Thomas Babor, PhD, MPH,
Professor and Chairman,
Department of Community Medicine
and Health Care,
University of Connecticut School of
Medicine,
Farmington, Connecticut, USA.

Raul Caetano, MD, MPH, PhD,
Professor of Epidemiology and
Assistant Dean,
The University of Texas School of
Public Health,
Dallas Regional Campus, Dallas,
Texas, USA.

Sally Casswell, PhD, Professor of
Social and Health Research,
Director, Centre for Social and
Health Outcomes Research and
Evaluation, Massey University,
Auckland, New Zealand.

Griffith Edwards, DM,
Emeritus Professor of Addiction
Behaviour,
National Addiction Centre,
London, UK.

Norman Giesbrecht, PhD,
Senior Scientist,
Social, Prevention and Health Policy
Research Department, Centre for
Addiction and Mental Health,
Toronto,
Ontario, Canada.

Kathryn Graham, PhD,
Senior Scientist, Head, Social Factors
and Prevention Initiatives,
Centre for Addiction and Mental
Health, and Professor (adjunct),
Department of Psychology,
University of Western Ontario,
London, Ontario, Canada.

Joel Grube, PhD, Director and
Senior Research Scientist,
Prevention Research Center,
Pacific Institute for Research and
Evaluation,
Berkeley, California, USA.

Paul Gruenewald, PhD, Scientific
Director and Senior Research
Scientist,
Prevention Research Center,
Pacific Institute for Research and
Evaluation,
Berkeley, California, USA.

Linda Hill, PhD, Researcher,
Alcohol and Public Health Research
Unit, University of Auckland;
New Zealand Drug Foundation,
Wellington, New Zealand.

Harold Holder, PhD,
Senior Research Scientist,
Prevention Research Center,
Pacific Institute for Research and
Evaluation,
Berkeley, California, USA.

Ross Homel, PhD,
Professor and Head,
School of Criminology and Criminal
Justice, Deputy Director,
Key Centre for Ethics, Law, Justice
and Governance.
Mt Gravatt Campus,
Griffith University,
Queensland, Australia.

Esa Österberg, MSc,
Senior Researcher,
Alcohol and Drug Research,
National Research and Development
Centre for Welfare and Health,
Helsinki, Finland.

Jürgen Rehm, PhD,
Professor, Public Health Sciences,
University of Toronto, Canada;
Director and CEO,
Addiction Research Institute, Zurich,
Switzerland;

Senior Scientist and Co-Head,
Section on Public Health and
Regulatory Policies, Centre for
Addiction and Mental Health,
Toronto, Canada;
Chair, Addiction Policy,
University of Toronto, Canada.

Robin Room, PhD,
Professor of Social Research on
Alcohol and Drugs;
Director, Centre for Social Research
on Alcohol and Drugs,
Stockholm University,
Stockholm, Sweden.

Ingeborg Rossow, PhD,
Research Director,
Department of Youth Research,
Norwegian Social Research (NOVA);
Senior Scientist, National Institute
for Alcohol and Drug Research,
Oslo, Norway.

Section I

Introduction

Chapter 1

Setting the policy agenda

1.1 Introduction

In Pitkyäranta, Russia, Anatoly Iverianov, a 45-year-old log cutter, attributed the two heart attacks he suffered in 1998 to the fact that 'I've been drinking and smoking a lot'. Indeed, after a third heart attack ended his life soon after his news interview (Wines 2000), the autopsy results listed chronic alcoholism as the probable cause of death. As in other parts of Russia, violence, suicide, and cardiovascular disease play major roles in the precipitous decline in life expectancy observed here over the past decade. Alcohol control policies instituted in 1985 led to a reduction in drinking and an increase in life expectancy, but those policies were soon reversed.

In neighbouring Finland, just across the Russian border in North Karelia, epidemiological studies showed that people working in the timber industry once drank and smoked just as heavily as their Russian neighbours, and both regions shared the distinction of having the highest rates of cardiovascular disease in the world. Finland's response was to implement the North Karelia Project (Wines 2000), a five-year effort designed to change people's diet, exercise, smoking, and drinking habits through a combination of health promotion, disease prevention, and economic incentives. Twenty-five years after the policies were implemented, the rate of heart disease among working-age residents was significantly lower, in part because of the reduction in risk factors (Vartiainen *et al.* 2000).

In Kenya's capital of Nairobi, a home-made alcohol product fortified with methanol killed 121 people in November 2000, leaving 495 hospitalized, 20 of whom suffered blindness (Nordwall 2000). The toll was particularly pronounced in the urban slums surrounding the city, where unlicensed cafés serve illegal brews to the rural migrants seeking employment in the city. Policies restricting illicit alcohol distillation and the unlicensed sale of alcoholic beverages have been difficult to enforce.

In Tokyo, the headline of a newspaper article reads: 'Year-Ending Parties Pour Drunks onto Trains of Japan', referring to the *bonenkai* New Year's holiday season. Railway officials estimated that at least 60% of the passengers are intoxicated during this period. In response, two policies were instituted. Extra security guards were hired to minimize injuries, and 'women only' railway cars were introduced to prevent sexual assaults. The article made no mention of whether the policies had their intended effects (Zielenziger 2000).

In Tennant Creek, Australia, aboriginal groups successfully pressed restrictions on Thursday trading (payday for social security checks), sales of 4 litre cask wine, and hours of takeaway sale. The 'Thirsty Thursday' policy was associated with a reduction in alcohol-related police incidents, hospital admissions, and women's shelter presentations. During the same period, alcohol consumption decreased by 19% (Brady 2000).

What do these vignettes have in common? They all speak to the effects of alcohol consumption on individuals and populations, and draw attention to the search for policies that protect health, prevent disability, and address the social problems associated with the misuse of beverage alcohol. This book is at its core a scientific treatise on alcohol policy: what alcohol policy is, why it is needed, which interventions are effective, how policy is made, and how scientific evidence can inform the policymaking process.

1.2 Alcohol policy: a short history

The control of alcohol production, distribution, and consumption was first exercised by local authorities in the emerging urban areas of ancient Greece, Mesopotamia, Egypt, and Rome (Ghalioungui 1979). Greek statesmen of the 6th century BC introduced supervised festivities to provide an alternative to the Dionysian revelries that promoted drunkenness. In 594, Solon prescribed the death penalty for drunken magistrates and required that all wine be diluted with water before being sold. For over 2000 years, ingenious strategies like these were devised by monarchs, governments, and the clergy to prevent alcohol-related problems. But it was not until the rise of modern medicine and the emergence of the world Temperance Movement in the 19th century that alcohol policy was first seen as a potential instrument of public health.

Despite well over a century of experimentation with a full range of different policy options, the modern history of alcohol policy is often characterized in terms of the defining conflicts that took place in many countries over national and local prohibition. Between 1914 and 1921, laws prohibiting the manufacture and sale of all or most forms of beverage alcohol were adopted in the United States, Canada, Norway, Iceland, Finland, and Russia (Paulson 1973). Most of these laws were repealed during the 1920s and 1930s, and replaced by less extreme regulatory policies. To view alcohol policies through the narrowly focused perspective of prohibition, however, is to ignore the fact that most policymaking during the past century has been incremental, deliberate, and respectful of people's right to drink in moderation.

If alcohol policy has a long history, then the scientific study of alcohol policy as a public health strategy has a much more abbreviated past. The growing interest in alcohol policy represented by this book is part of a maturation process in the study of alcohol problems that dates back to 1975 with the publication of a seminal monograph entitled: *Alcohol control policies in public health perspective* (Bruun *et al.* 1975), often known as the 'purple book'. Sponsored by the World Health Organization (WHO), the monograph drew attention to the preventable nature of alcohol problems, and to the role of national governments and international agencies in the formulation of rational and effective alcohol policies. *Alcohol control policies* stimulated a heated debate not just among academics, but also among policy-makers. The most significant aspect of the book was its main thesis: the higher the average amount of alcohol consumed in a society, the greater the incidence of problems experienced by that society. Consequently, one way to prevent alcohol problems is through policies directed at the reduction of average alcohol consumption, particularly those policies that limit the availability of alcohol.

In the early 1990s, a new project was commissioned by WHO to review the development of the world literature pertaining to alcohol policy. The new study produced *Alcohol policy and the public good*, a book that proved to be as thought-provoking as its predecessor (Edwards *et al.* 1994). The book concluded that public health policies on alcohol had come of age because of the strong evidential underpinnings derived from the scientific research that had grown in breadth and sophistication since 1975. After reviewing the evidence on taxation of alcohol, restrictions on alcohol availability, drinking and driving countermeasures, school-based education, community action programs, and treatment interventions, it was concluded that:

♦ The research establishes beyond doubt that public health measures of proven effectiveness are available to serve the public good by reducing the widespread costs and pain related to alcohol use.

♦ To that end, it is appropriate to deploy responses that influence both the total amount of alcohol consumed by a population and the high-risk contexts and drinking behaviours that are so often associated with alcohol-related problems. To conceive of these intrinsically complementary approaches as contradictory alternatives would be a mistake.

Building on the tradition of collaboration between WHO and international alcohol researchers, preparation of the present volume was undertaken for three reasons.

1. The epidemiological research on the prevalence and determinants of alcohol problems has revealed new developments in the way alcohol affects the

health and social well-being of populations in different parts of the world, particularly in the emerging states of the former Soviet Union and in the developing world.

2. Because of the rapidly changing trends in alcohol problems, there has been a growing international interest in the application of health policies, including prevention programs and treatment services, as an important responsibility of national and local governments.

3. During the past decade there have been major improvements in the way alcohol problems are studied in relation to alcohol policies. With the growth of the knowledge base and the maturation of alcohol science, there is now a real opportunity to invest in evidence-based alcohol policies as an instrument of public health.

1.3 Alcohol policy defined

In 1975, Bruun and his colleagues defined alcohol control policies as all relevant strategies employed by governments to influence alcohol availability, leaving health education, attitude change, and informal social control as beyond the scope of a public health approach. In 1994, Edwards and his colleagues provided a broader view of alcohol policy, considering it as a public health response dictated in part by national and historical concerns. Though there was not an explicit definition of the nature of alcohol policy, its meaning could be inferred from the wealth of policy responses that were considered: alcohol taxation, legislative controls on alcohol availability, age restrictions on alcohol purchasing, media information campaigns, and school-based education, to name a few.

This book borrows from its predecessors in its definition of alcohol policy, but also expands the concept in keeping with nationally and internationally evolving views of public health. Public policies are authoritative decisions made by governments through laws, rules, and regulations (Longest 1998). The word 'authoritative' indicates that the decisions come from the legitimate purview of legislators and other public interest group officials, not from private industry or related advocacy groups.

When public policies pertain to the relation between alcohol, health, and social welfare, they are considered alcohol policies. Thus, drinking–driving laws designed to prevent alcohol-related accidents, rather than those merely intended to punish offenders, are considered alcohol policies. Generally, alcohol policies affect populations (such as underage drinkers or pregnant women) or organizations (such as programs and services within health systems). Based on their nature and purpose, alcohol policies can be classified into two categories: allocative and regulatory (Longest 1998). Allocative policies are intended to provide a net benefit to a distinct group or type of organization (sometimes at the expense of other groups or organizations) in order to achieve some public objective. Subsidies that support alcohol education in schools, the training of waiters and waitresses in responsible beverage service, and the provision of treatment for alcohol-dependent persons, are examples of policies that seek to reduce the harm caused by alcohol or to increase access to services for certain population groups. In contrast to allocative policies, regulatory policies seek to influence the actions, behaviours, and decisions of others through direct control of individuals or organizations. Economic regulation through price controls and taxation is often applied to alcoholic beverages to reduce demand and to generate tax revenues. Laws that impose a minimum purchasing age and limit hours of sale have long been used to restrict access to alcohol for reasons of health and safety. National and local laws pertaining to the potency, purity, and marketing of alcoholic beverages, and the times and places where they can be served or purchased, are examples of other regulatory policies.

From the perspective of this book, the central purpose of alcohol policies is to serve the interests of public health and social well-being through their impact on health and social determinants, such as drinking patterns, the drinking environment, and the health services available to treat problem drinkers. As discussed in Chapter 2 of this book, drinking patterns that lead to rapidly elevated blood alcohol levels result in problems associated with acute intoxication, such as accidents, injuries, and violence. Similarly, drinking patterns that promote frequent and heavy alcohol consumption are associated with chronic health problems such as liver cirrhosis, cardiovascular disease, and depression.

The environmental determinants of alcohol-related harm include the physical availability of the product, the social norms that define the appropriate uses of alcohol (e.g., as a beverage, as an intoxicant, as a medicine), and the economic incentives that promote its use. Health and social policies that influence the availability of alcohol, the social circumstances of its use, and its retail price are likely to reduce the harm caused by alcohol in a society.

Another important determinant of health in relation to alcohol is the availability of and access to health services, particularly those designed to deal with alcohol dependence and alcohol-related disabilities. Alcohol-related health services can be preventive, acute, and rehabilitative, and can be either voluntary or coercive. Health policies have a major impact on the alcohol treatment and preventive services available to people within a country through health care financing and the organization of the health care system.

1.4 **Public health and the public good**

The definition of alcohol policy proposed in this book relies heavily on concepts derived from public heath, a specialized field of knowledge and action that is not always understood by either the general public or the health professions. Public health is concerned with the management and prevention of diseases and injuries in human populations. Unlike clinical medicine, which focuses on the care and cure of disease in individual cases, public health deals with groups of individuals, called populations. The value of population thinking in alcohol policy is in its ability to identify health risks and suggest appropriate interventions that are most likely to benefit the greatest number of people. The concept of 'population' is based on the assumption that groups of individuals exhibit certain commonalities by virtue of their shared characteristics (e.g., gender), shared environment (e.g., village, city, nation), or shared occupations (e.g., alcoholic beverage service workers) that increase their risk of disease and disability, including alcohol-related problems (Fos and Fine 2000). Because populations defined by geographical boundaries are often not homogeneous, it is sometimes fruitful to focus on subpopulations rather than total populations. This is a major difference between the present volume and the 1975 monograph, *Alcohol control policies in public health perspective* (Bruun *et al.* 1975), which restricted its analysis of alcohol control policies to their impact on total populations.

Why are public health concepts important to the discussion of alcohol policy? During the 20th century public health measures have had a remarkable effect on the health of populations throughout the world. Life expectancy has increased dramatically world-wide during this period, thanks to the application of public health measures designed to improve sanitation, reduce environmental pollution, and prevent communicable and infectious diseases (WHO 1998). But even as epidemics of infectious and communicable diseases have receded, health risks associated with lifestyle behaviours and chronic diseases have increased in importance as major causes of mortality and morbidity. When population approaches are used instead of, or in conjunction with, individual-level medical approaches, the effects on health and disease are much more dramatic. As this book will show, public health concepts provide an important vehicle to manage the health of populations in relation to the use and misuse of alcohol. Whereas medical approaches oriented toward individual patients can be effective in treating alcohol dependence and alcohol-related disabilities (Chapter 12), population-based approaches deal with groups, communities, and nation states to improve the allocation of human and material resources to preventative and curative services. They also provide epidemiological data to monitor trends, design better interventions, and evaluate programs and services.

1.5 Alcohol, health, and public policy

By locating alcohol policy within the realm of public health and social policy, rather than economics, criminal justice, or social welfare, this book draws attention to the growing tendency for governments, both national and local, to approach alcohol as a major determinant of ill health. The pursuit of health as one of modern society's most highly cherished values accounts for the growing interest in alcohol policy. But it also creates a special challenge because public health often competes with other social values such as free trade, open markets, and individual freedom. In this book, health is viewed not only as the absence of disease and injury, but also as a state in which the biological, psychological, and social functioning of a person are maximized in everyday life (Brook and McGlynn 1991). The way in which health is defined and valued within a society has important implications for alcohol policy. If it is defined narrowly as the absence of disease, then the focus is often placed on the treatment of alcohol dependence and the clinical management of alcohol-related disabilities, such as cirrhosis of the liver and traumatic injuries. If health is defined more broadly, then alcohol policy can be directed at proactive interventions that help many more people attain optimal levels of health.

1.6 The structure of this book

Related to the concept of population thinking in public health is the science of epidemiology, which is a key tool for research, planning, prevention, and treatment. Epidemiology is the scientific study of the occurrence and causes of diseases and other health-related conditions (e.g., injuries) in human populations, and the application of this information to the control of health problems (Mausner and Kramer 1985). Part II of this book is concerned with the epidemiology of alcohol-related problems. Part III deals with approaches to the prevention of new cases (called primary prevention), early intervention with incipient cases (called secondary prevention), and the treatment and rehabilitation of active cases (called tertiary prevention).

Health is influenced by a variety of factors, including the physical, social, and economic environments that people live in, and by their genetic make-up, their personal lifestyles, and the health services that they have access to. As Part II of this book will show, alcohol-related health and social problems are influenced by the same factors. It follows that alcohol policies, to be effective instruments of public health and social welfare, must take into account, if not operate in, all of these domains, rather than be limited to a more circumscribed focus on either alcohol, the agent, or alcohol dependence, the result of chronic drinking.

Part IV of this book considers the international and national policy environment that affects the alcohol policymaking process. This part of the book provides a comprehensive framework to understand the alcohol policymaking process and how it can serve the interests of public health and social welfare. In the final chapter of the book, an attempt is made to synthesize what is known about evidence-based interventions that can be translated into policy. By comparing different intervention strategies in terms of their effectiveness, scientific support, generalizability, and cost, it becomes possible to evaluate the relative appropriateness of different strategies, both alone and in combination, to present problems and future needs. As the scientific basis for alcohol policy begins to take shape, it is becoming apparent that there is no single definitive, much less politically acceptable, approach to the prevention of alcohol problems; a combination of strategies and policies is needed. If this realization is sobering, so too is the conviction, argued in the pages of this book, that alcohol policy is an ever-changing process that needs to constantly adapt to the times if it is to serve the interests of public health.

1.7 **Extraordinary measures**

Whether it is holiday revelry in Tokyo, Japan, payday parties in Tennant Creek, Australia, or Perestroika binges in Pitkyäranta, Russia, alcohol is a product that enters into many aspects of social life in practically every part of the world. But as the pages of this book will show, alcohol is no ordinary commodity. For this reason, the public health response to the prevention of alcohol-related problems requires extraordinary measures, some of them relatively painless for a society to implement, others more demanding in terms of resources, ingenuity, and public support.

References

Brady M. (2000) Alcohol policy issues for indigenous people in the United States, Canada, Australia and New Zealand. *Contemporary Drug Problems* **27**, 435–510.

Brook R.H. and McGlynn E.A. (1991) Maintaining quality of care. In: Ginzberg E. (ed.) *Health services research: key to health policy*, pp. 784–817. Cambridge, MA: Harvard University Press.

Bruun K., Edwards G., Lumio M., *et al.* (1975) *Alcohol control policies in public health perspective.* Helsinki: The Finnish Foundation for Alcohol Studies.

Edwards G., Anderson P., Babor T.F., *et al.* (1994) *Alcohol policy and the public good.* Oxford University Press.

Fos P.J. and Fine D.J. (2000) *Designing health care for populations.* San Francisco, CA: Jossey-Bass.

Ghalioungui P. (1979) Fermented beverages in antiquity. In: Gastineau C.F., Darby W.J., and Turner T.B. (eds.) *Fermented food beverages in nutrition,* pp. 3–19. New York, NY: Academic Press.

Longest B.B. (1998) *Health policymaking in the United States.* Chicago, IL: Health Administration Press.

Mausner J.S. and Kramer S.K. (1985) *Epidemiology—an introduction text.* Philadelphia, PA: W.B. Saunders Company.

Nordwall S.P. (2000) Homemade alcohol kills 121 in Kenya. *USA Today,* Arlington, VA, November 20.

Paulson R.E. (1973) *Women's suffrage and prohibition: a comparative study of equality and social control.* Glenview, IL: Scott, Foresman and Company.

Vartiainen E., Jousilahti P., Alfthan G., *et al.* (2000) Cardiovascular risk factor changes in Finland, 1972–1997. *International Journal of Epidemiology* **29**, 49–56.

WHO. See World Health Organization.

World Health Organization (1998) *The World Health Report 1998: Life in the 21st century. A vision for all.* Geneva, Switzerland: World Health Organization.

Wines M. (2000) An ailing Russia lives a tough life that's getting shorter. *The New York Times,* New York, NY, December 3.

Zielenziger M. (2000) Year-ending parties pour drunks onto trains of Japan. *The Hartford Courant,* Hartford, CT, USA, December 28.

Section II

Epidemiology: establishing the need for alcohol policy

Chapter 2

Alcohol: no ordinary commodity

2.1 Introduction

Alcohol has multiple functions in any society. Alcoholic beverages have important cultural and symbolic meanings. They are commodities that are bought and sold in the marketplace. And alcohol is a drug with toxic effects and other intrinsic dangers such as intoxication and dependence. This chapter examines these different functions, paying special attention to the contrast between alcohol's role as a commodity and as a drug. An understanding of this contrast is essential to the book's central purpose.

In recent years, public discussion of alcohol policies has too often ignored or downplayed the need to understand both the nature of the agent and its harmful properties, with an implicit acceptance of the idea that alcohol is only an ordinary commodity like any other marketable product. The validity of this assumption is questioned by evidence showing that alcohol intoxication, alcohol dependence, and the toxic effects of alcohol on various organ systems are key mechanisms linking alcohol consumption to a wide range of adverse consequences.

2.2 Alcohol's cultural and symbolic meanings

The history of alcoholic beverages shows that drinking has served many purposes for the individual and society. As Heath (1984) has noted, alcohol can be at the same time a food, a drug, and a highly elaborated cultural artefact with important symbolic meanings. Nowadays, alcohol products are mainly used as beverages to serve with meals, as thirst quenchers, as a means of socialization and enjoyment, as instruments of hospitality, and as intoxicants.

In earlier times, alcoholic beverages were frequently used as medicine. Presently, the best example of a medicinal use of alcohol is when it is consumed to protect against heart disease. In earlier times, the nutritional value of alcoholic beverages was more important than it is now. In certain periods, alcoholic beverages were considered to be a healthy alternative to polluted drinking water (Mäkelä 1983).

Alcoholic beverages are used in many cultures in a variety of social situations, both public and private. They are frequently used to commemorate births, baptisms, and weddings. In a religious context, the consumption of alcohol may be limited by ritual expectations, as in the Catholic mass and the Jewish Seder, where only very light drinking is condoned. In other cases, higher levels of consumption, including intoxication, are accepted. For example, alcohol is used to induce trance-like states in African–Brazilian religious rituals. Alcohol is frequently used as a relaxant and as a social lubricant. In some communities, the provision of an abundance of alcohol in social situations is almost mandatory, and is seen as a sign of wealth and power by those who provide it.

Alcohol's meanings change as individuals go through different stages of life, and as societies' norms about alcohol change accordingly (Fillmore *et al.* 1991). Drinking can be a sign of rebellion or independence during adolescence, but societies across the world are concerned with the harmful consequences of drinking on youth. Epidemiological evidence reviewed in Chapters 3 and 4 indicates that there are good reasons for this concern. Motor vehicle crashes, for example, are the leading cause of death for teenagers in some industrialized countries (National Highway Traffic Safety Administration 2000). Thus, most societies, even those with very liberal policies toward alcohol consumption, agree that alcohol should not be made readily available to children and adolescents. Drinking during early adulthood is usually more frequent and heavier than in later life, although in some societies this can be modified by cultural factors and demographic characteristics of the drinker (Fillmore *et al.* 1991; Caetano 1997).

There are also important differences in the cultural meaning of drinking for men and women. Societies' normative expectations regarding the use of alcohol vary across age groups and between men and women. In some societies, drinking has been almost exclusively a province of men (Roizen 1981), and this remains true, for instance, in India (Room *et al.* 2002). Though the percentage of abstainers is generally higher among adult women everywhere, in many countries of Europe the gender difference is not great (Simpura and Karlsson 2001). Nowadays, women do one-fifth to one-third of the drinking in most industrialized countries (see Chapter 3), and in a few countries there has been even greater convergence between the sexes (Bloomfield *et al.* 2001).

In many societies, abstention rates increase in the later stages of life for both men and women (Demers *et al.* 2001). Besides ill health, this often reflects societal norms; older people are not supposed to engage in the intoxicated partying that may be more or less accepted among the young. However, as individuals in industrialized countries live longer and healthier lives, these cultural views about the propriety of drinking by older individuals may change.

Alcohol is thus a drug used widely in many social situations. Throughout the life cycle from youth to old age it is associated with many positive aspects of life. It is used in traditional social rituals in many places. In some rituals, even intoxication is seen as an acceptable and pleasurable pursuit. However, these situations can rapidly change from being 'alcohol-safe' to being 'alcohol-dangerous' as when party guests who have been drinking leave to drive their cars back home.

2.3 Alcohol as a commodity

There are four main modes of producing and distributing alcoholic beverages (Jernigan 2000; Room *et al.* 2002).

1. There is home-brewing and craft production, both of distilled spirits and traditional fermented beverages.

2. There is industrial production and distribution of commercial versions of these indigenous beverages, such as *chibuku* in southern Africa, *soju* in South Korea, and *pulque* in Mexico.

3. There is local industrial production of 'international' beverages, such as domestic whiskey in India and lager beer like Corona in Mexico.

4. There is the production of the branded international beverages, which are increasingly marketed on a global scale. In the case of beer, this is primarily done locally by or under license from multinational corporations. Branded spirits and wines are mainly exported from the producing countries. Distilled spirits in their various forms account for the greatest part of recorded global sales (Room *et al.* 2002), followed by European-style beer. About half of the recorded sales of spirits are of international brands, while multinational corporations are dominant in the European-style beer market.

In many countries, the production and sale of alcoholic beverages is an important economic activity. It generates profits for the producers, advertisers, and investors, provides employment opportunities, brings in foreign currency for exported beverages, and generates tax revenues for the government. Alcohol has become a major component of the travel industry, including airlines, hotels, and restaurants. For these reasons, there are many vested interests that support the continuation and growth of alcohol production and sales. It may take only a few hundred employees to operate a modern, large-scale brewery. But when beer is sold in grocery stores or restaurants, it becomes a significant source of retail sales, which bring profits to small business owners and employment to service and sales workers.

Alcoholic beverages, particularly wine and beer, are considered agricultural products in many developed countries. Wine plays an especially important role in the agricultural economies of France, Italy, and Spain. It is estimated than in Italy, alcohol production, mostly in the form of viniculture, provides employment for 1.5–2.0 million people. While beer and distilled spirits also have clear connections to agriculture, in many countries these activities come under the jurisdiction of the ministry of industry. In contrast to wine production, in developed countries beer and especially distilled spirits are mostly produced in large plants by large industrial enterprises.

Consumer spending on alcoholic beverages usually generates taxes, which make these products a popular source of income for local, state, and national governments. In many countries, taxes on alcohol are imposed under several headings and at several different administrative levels. Estimating the total amount of taxes collected from alcohol production and sales can therefore be difficult. Figure 2.1 gives US data as an example of an overall national analysis. In 1997, the total alcoholic beverage tax revenue amounted to over $18 billion. The federal government's share of that total was 43%, the state share 50%, and local revenues 7%. Revenues from beer and spirits represent approximately the same proportion of all alcoholic beverage taxes at the federal level. At the state and local level, revenues from beer represent an increasing proportion of all revenues from alcoholic beverages, while revenues from spirits decrease in proportion. At every level of the US government (and of most other administrations world-wide), alcohol is a commodity from which the revenue collected is of considerable importance to balancing the budget. Altogether, the total revenue contribution for every adult citizen in the US amounts to almost 100 US dollars per year.

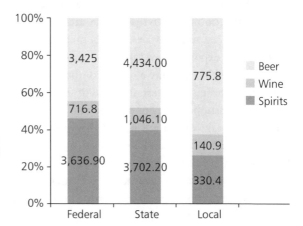

Fig. 2.1 1997 alcoholic beverage revenues in the United States (millions of dollars).
Source: Distilled Spirits Council of the United States.

In summary, alcohol is an important commodity with a complex supply chain and a considerable employment base. It must be manufactured, packaged, labelled, stored, distributed, sold, marketed, and advertised. It generates profits for the primary producers and for all sorts of middlemen and ancillary actors involved in alcohol trade. Alcohol is a commodity that is demanded, purchased, and consumed globally. Taxation of alcoholic beverages brings in revenue in larger or smaller quantities to state budgets. Alcoholic beverages are, by any reckoning, important, economically embedded commodities. But as we shall see in the remainder of this chapter, the benefits connected with the production, sale, and use of this commodity come at an enormous cost to society. Public health specialists and policy-makers who forget this fact do so only at their peril (Edwards and Holder 2000).

2.4 Mechanisms of harm: toxicity, intoxication, and dependence

Looking back at the last quarter of the 20th century, especially the past decade, it can be said that remarkable progress was made in the scientific understanding of alcohol's harmful effects, as scientists discovered biological, chemical, and psychological explanations for humans' propensity to consume what has been called 'the ambiguous molecule' (Edwards 2000). This knowledge is fundamental for an understanding of alcohol's capacity for physical toxicity, intoxication, and dependence. The remainder of this chapter will focus on recent scientific advances in the understanding of these three important *mediators* of the relation between drinking and the different kinds of harm it produces. When it is said that toxicity, intoxication, and dependence mediate alcohol consumption and drinking problems, it is implied that each of these phenomena provides a mechanism by which consumption leads to problems, and explains (at least partially) the connection between consumption and problems.

Figure 2.2 shows the relationships among alcohol consumption, the three putative mediating factors, and various types of harm. Patterns of drinking, characterized not only by the frequency of drinking and the quantity per occasion, but also by the variation between one occasion and another, represent the manner in which drinkers consume a certain volume of alcohol in a given time frame. Volume and the pattern by which alcohol is consumed can lead to different types of problems. Chronic heavy drinking is related to the toxic effects of alcohol. Sustained heavy drinking, of the type that has been common in wine drinking countries, may not lead to much evident intoxication, but can cause tissue damage and dependence. Daily drinking of even small

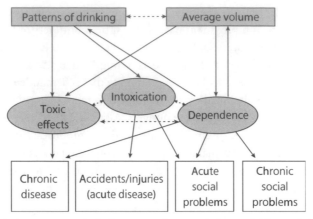

Fig. 2.2 Relations among alcohol consumption, mediating variables and short-term as well as long-term consequences.

amounts of wine per occasion over a long period of time can lead to cirrhosis because of the cumulative effects of alcohol on the liver. In contrast, a relatively low frequency of drinking together with consumption of a high number of drinks per occasion can lead, through the mechanism of acute intoxication, to a variety of medical and social problems, such as accidents, injuries, interpersonal violence, and certain types of acute tissue damage. Finally, sustained drinking may result in alcohol dependence. Once dependence is present, it can feed back to increase or sustain both the overall volume of drinking and the drinking pattern. Dependence can then lead to chronic medical problems as well as acute and chronic social problems.

2.5 **Alcohol as a toxic substance**

Alcohol is a toxic substance in terms of its direct and indirect effects on a wide range of body organs and systems. Some of alcohol's adverse health impacts can result from acute intoxication or **binge drinking**, even in a person who does not have a longstanding or persistent drinking problem. Alcohol poisoning (Poikolainen 2002), acute pancreatitis (Imrie 1997), and acute cardiac arrhythmias (Peters 1998) represent dangers of that kind. On occasion, some of these conditions may have fatal outcomes. Another category of harm can be designated as 'acute or chronic'. For example, a drinking binge in a chronic heavy drinker may turn liver impairment into liver failure, or cause the acute onset of brain damage. A third category of harm is chronic disease resulting from long-term exposure to high doses of alcohol, with cancers and cirrhosis being prime examples.

As discussed in more detail in Chapter 4, there is clear evidence for a causal role of alcohol in various cancers, including cancer of the mouth, oesophagus (gullet), larynx, and pharynx. Evidence has grown on the role of alcohol in breast cancer, and is suggestive but not conclusive on the relationship between drinking and colon cancer (WHO 1988). Some of these health risks are exacerbated by the combination of tobacco smoking with drinking (Tuyns 1983; Ström 1999). Cirrhosis of the liver is also closely associated with alcohol consumption, with research showing that the direct toxic effect of alcohol is the main cause of the condition (Lieber 1988), as well as hepatitis and fatty liver (Sherman and Williams 1994). Other conditions that can be associated with tissue damage by alcohol are disease of the heart muscle and cardiac arrhythmias (Peters 1998), pancreatitis (Searles *et al.* 1996), hypertension with consequent risk of stroke (Peters 1998), wasting of the limb muscles (Urbano-Marques and Fernandez-Sola 1996), peripheral neuritis, and brain damage of various kinds (Lishman 1998).

Heavy drinking by pregnant women can result in a range of damages to the fetus (Clarren and Smith 1978; Astley and Clarren 2000). At extreme levels of drinking, the full picture of Fetal Alcohol Syndrome (FAS) develops, which is characterized by hearing disabilities, retarded growth, and heart disorders, together with certain characteristic facial abnormalities. Children with FAS may require a lifetime of sheltered care. Lesser and often mild and recoverable types of childhood disorder can also occur. There is still uncertainty as to the intensity and timing of the alcohol exposure needed to produce any type or degree of fetal impairment.

In summary, alcoholic beverages are items of consumption with many customary uses, and are also commodities important to many people's livelihood. But social customs and economic interests should not blind us to the fact that alcohol is a toxic substance. It has the potential to adversely affect nearly every organ and system of the body. No other commodity sold for ingestion, not even tobacco, has such wide-ranging adverse physical effects. Taking account of alcohol's potential for toxicity is therefore an important task for public health policy.

2.6 **Alcohol intoxication**

There is a popular tendency to view all problems related to drinking as a part of or due to *alcoholism*. Studies of drinking practices and problems in the general population question this assumption, showing a universe of drinking problems that lie outside the bounds of alcoholism (Cahalan and Room 1974). In the mid-1970s, partly based on evidence from general population studies, a population-based vision of the broad range of problems that alcohol sets for society began to emerge (Bruun *et al.* 1975). This new approach cast off the constraints of the narrow view that made alcoholism the only salient issue. Given that alcohol-related social problems, interpersonal problems, and acute health problems are widely distributed throughout the population, the **prevention paradox** (Kreitman 1986) was put forward to draw attention to the broad range of alcohol-related problems in the drinking population at large. The main cause of alcohol-related harm in the general population is alcohol intoxication.

The term **alcohol intoxication** is defined here as a more or less short-term state of functional impairment in psychological and psychomotor performance induced by the presence of alcohol in the body. The major types of impairments (other than acute toxicity) that occur with alcohol intoxication are described in Box 2.1. The impairments that can be produced by alcohol are mostly dose related, often complex, and involve multiple body functions. Some (such as slurred speech) are evident and easily recognized, while others, such as impaired driving ability, may be subtle and picked up only on laboratory testing. Some of these effects stem directly and almost inevitably from a given blood alcohol concentration, while others depend on personal characteristics, the individual's previous experience with alcohol, and the setting and expectation of effect. Other psychoactive drugs, especially central nervous system depressants, may exacerbate the effects of alcohol when taken concomitantly.

Box 2.1 **Types of impairments that occur with alcohol intoxication**

1. **Psychomotor impairment**. Alcohol can impair balance and movement in a way that increases the risk of many types of accidents.

2. **Lengthened reaction time**. This classic dose-related impairment is of particular concern because of its causal role in traffic accidents.

3. **Impairment of judgement**. Impaired judgement can result in dangerous risk-taking, such as getting into a car and then driving in a risky and aggressive way when intoxicated.

4. **Emotional changes and decreased responsiveness to social expectations**. The factors involved in alcohol-related changes in mood, emotional state, and social responsiveness are complex and are likely to involve interaction of alcohol's physiological effects with psychological and social factors. In part because of these changes, intoxication can contribute to the risk of violence to others and intentional self-harm.

As Box 2.1 underlines, intoxication and accompanying changes in behaviour are a matter of cultural and personal expectations and understandings as well as of the concentration of alcohol in the blood. The anthropological literature has long recognized that there are striking differences between cultures in drunken comportment (Room 2001). Even within a given culture, the meaning of 'drunk' can change over time. In 1979, when US alcohol consumption levels were achieving record levels for the 20th century, adult males reported that it would take an average of 9.8 drinks (about 118 gm ethanol) for them to feel drunk, and 5.4 drinks to feel the effects of drinking. In 1995, after US consumption levels fell by 21%, men reported that it would take an average of 7.4 drinks to feel drunk and 4.6 to feel the effects (Midanik 1999). The amounts also fell for women, from 5.7 to 4.7 drinks to feel drunk and from 3.7 to 3.2 drinks to feel the effects.

Recent discussions of the prevention paradox have underlined that most alcohol-related problems are attributable to the relatively substantial portion of the population that drinks to intoxication at least occasionally. For instance, Skog (1999) found that 73% of Norwegians who reported quarrelling while under the influence of alcohol reported having drunk large amounts on their heaviest drinking occasions—at least 3.5 litres of beer, one litre of wine, or 35 cl. of spirits (about 100–120 gm ethanol). Drinking this much on their heaviest drinking occasions was not rare. Thirty-two per cent of the whole population aged 15 and older reported doing so. In a Canadian general population study, those who drank five or more drinks (about 68 gm ethanol) at least once a month were 72% more likely to report that their own drinking had harmed them in the last year in two or more life areas, after controlling for volume of drinking and demographics (Room *et al.* 1995).

These studies point to occasional intoxication as a key risk factor for the adverse consequences of drinking, but do not pin down the exact nature of the link, which might also involve dependence. In other lines of research the link between intoxication and adverse consequences is clear and strong, especially for violence (Room and Rossow 2001), traffic casualties (Hurst *et al.* 1994), and other injuries. As we shall see in Chapter 4, alcohol intoxication accounts for a substantial part of the social and health burden of alcohol in terms of years of life lost.

The following conclusions arise from these analyses:

1. Alcohol is a psychoactive substance, which can impair motor skills and judgement. The impairment from intoxication is biological, but its manifestations are affected by expectancies and cultural norms.

2. Occasional drinking to the point of intoxication is quite common among drinkers. Intoxication, even when it occurs infrequently, can result in substantial social and injury harm. In fact, the chances of harm from a single

intoxication event seem to be higher for those who drink infrequently than for those drinking more frequently (Hurst *et al.* 1994; Room *et al.* 1995).

3. Preventing alcohol intoxication is a potentially powerful strategy for preventing much of the harm from alcohol.

4. Since the link between intoxication and harm is very much affected by the social and physical context, harm can also potentially be averted by insulating the drinking behaviour. This insulation from harm can take many forms, e.g., physical (making the place of drinking safer) or temporal (separating the drinking from activities requiring vigilance).

2.7 Alcohol dependence

In 1976, Edwards and Gross (1976) put forward the concept of the *alcohol dependence syndrome.* Together with this new conceptualization of a core set of indicators, it was also noted that alcohol-related problems could occur without dependence, but that dependence was likely to carry with it many problems. The overall formulation was intrinsically two-dimensional. One dimension is that represented by the syndrome concept, which refers to a cluster of interrelated physiological and psychological symptoms in which alcohol use takes on a much higher priority than other behaviours. The second dimension, alcohol-related problems, refers to harm resulting from drinking, regardless of whether the person is alcohol dependent.

The syndrome concept has been officially recognized in the *Diagnostic and statistical manual* (DSM) of the American Psychiatric Association (American Psychiatric Association 1994), and in the *International classification of diseases*—10th edition (ICD-10, WHO 1992). The criteria for a diagnosis of alcohol dependence in this latter classification are shown in Table 2.1. Three of the six criteria must have been present in the past 12 months for a positive diagnosis of alcohol dependence.

Two factors contributing to the development of alcohol dependence are reinforcement (negative and positive) and neuroadaptation (Roberts and Koob 1997). Reinforcement occurs when a stimulus (e.g., alcohol-induced euphoria or stimulation) increases the probability of a certain response (e.g., continued drinking to maintain a rising blood alcohol level). Neuroadaptation refers to biological processes by which initial drug effects are either enhanced or attenuated by repeated drug use. Acute drug reinforcement occurs because addictive drugs interact with neurotransmitter systems, which are part of the brain reward circuitry. Alterations in this system persist after acute withdrawal and may increase vulnerability to relapse. The mesolimbic dopamine system of the brain is important in the establishment of dependence to psychomotor

Table 2.1 ICD-10 diagnostic criteria for alcohol dependence[a]

1.	Evidence of tolerance to the effects of alcohol, such that there is a need for markedly increased amounts to achieve intoxication or desired effect, or that there is a markedly diminished effect with continued use of the same amount of alcohol.
2.	A physiological withdrawal state when alcohol use is reduced or ceased, or use of a closely related substance with the intention of relieving or avoiding withdrawal symptoms.
3.	Persisting with alcohol use despite clear evidence of harmful consequences as evidenced by continued use when the person was actually aware of, or could be expected to have been aware of, the nature and extent of harm.
4.	Preoccupation with alcohol use, as manifested by important alternative pleasures or interests being given up or reduced because of alcohol use; or a great deal of time being spent in activities necessary to obtain alcohol, consume it, or recover from its effects.
5.	Impaired capacity to control drinking behaviour in terms of its onset, termination or level of use, as evidenced by: alcohol being often taken in larger amounts or over a longer period than intended, or any unsuccessful effort or persistent desire to cut down or control alcohol use.
6.	A strong desire or sense of compulsion to use alcohol.

[a] Adapted from World Health Organization (1992).

stimulants such as cocaine or amphetamine, and also plays a role in dependence to alcohol. Opioid endogenous systems (morphine-like neurotransmitters) play an important role in positive reinforcement of opiates, alcohol, and nicotine. Thus, opiate antagonists such as naltrexone reduce alcohol reinforcement in both animals and humans. Serotonin systems are also important in regulating alcohol consumption. Finally, GABA (gamma-aminobutyric acid) systems are the primary inhibitory systems in the brain. Alcohol and other sedative–hypnotic drugs (benzodiazepines) modulate receptors in this system. Changes in these neurotransmitter systems may lead to sensitization (increase in positive reinforcing effects) and counter-adaptation (increase in negative reinforcing effects), according to Roberts and Koob (1997). The remarkable advances in neurobiological research point to alcohol's psychoactive properties as a critical feature in the development of alcohol dependence.

The prevalence rate of alcohol dependence varies according to the level of drinking in the general population. Patterns of drinking and a variety of social, psychological, and biological characteristics of the population may also affect dependence rates. In the US adult population, the prevalence rate, defined by DSM-IV criteria, is about 6% for men and 2% for women (Caetano and

Cunradi 2002). Alcohol dependence rates for various regions of the world are discussed in Chapter 3.

A number of studies have examined the relationship between drinking patterns and alcohol dependence. Independent of how drinking is measured (Dawson and Archer 1993; Hall *et al.* 1993), the more a population engages in sustained or recurrent heavy alcohol consumption, the higher the rate of alcohol dependence. Both average volume of drinking and the ***pattern of drinking*** larger amounts on an occasion are related to the prevalence of dependence (Caetano *et al.* 1997), and the risk of dependence increases linearly with increased drinking. The nature and the direction of causality, however, are not clear. Dependence may perpetuate heavy drinking, or heavy drinking may contribute to the development of dependence, or these two mechanisms may operate simultaneously. As suggested in Figure 2.2, alcohol dependence is likely to have both direct and indirect effects on alcohol-related problems.

The fact that alcohol has self-reinforcing potential is of fundamental importance to understanding the dynamics of the relationship between a population and its drinking. Alcohol is not a run-of-the-mill consumer substance, but a drug with dependence potential.

Alcohol dependence was originally developed as a clinical construct that applies primarily to persons in treatment. But recent evidence strongly suggests that milder degrees of habit or dependence are widely distributed in the population and are associated with increased experience of problems. Dependence is a matter of continuities and variations with broader expression than the extreme seen in the clinic. Mild dependence is associated with a significant public health burden because it is common, and severe dependence, although less common, is likely to be associated with an intense clustering of problems.

Alcohol dependence has many different contributory causes including genetic vulnerability, but it is a condition that is contracted by exposure to alcohol. The heavier the drinking, the greater the risk. The challenge to public health is to identify policies that make it less likely that drinkers will contract dependence, and the consequent relative chronicity in behaviour patterns damaging to the individual and costly to society. The fact that alcohol dependence, once established, can become a rather chronic influence on drinking behaviour (one likely to generate more and more problems over the individual's drinking career), gives added cogency to the need for population-based strategies.

2.8 **Conclusion**

The major public health implication of the evidence reviewed in this chapter can be stated thus: The dangers in alcohol are multiple and varied in kind and degree; some but not all are dose related; they may result directly from the effect of alcohol or through interaction with other factors; intoxication is often an important mediator of harm; and dependence can significantly exacerbate the hazards and cause protracted exposure to danger. Public health responses must be matched to this complex vision of the dangers in alcohol as they seek better to respond to the population-level harm. The context for those responses should be an improved understanding of the nature of an agent that is far from being an ordinary kind of commodity.

References

American Psychiatric Association (1994) *Diagnostic and statistical manual of mental disorders*, 4th edn (DSM-IV). Washington, DC: American Psychiatric Association.

Astley S.J. and Clarren S.K. (2000) Diagnosing the full spectrum of fetal alcohol-exposed individuals: introducing the 4-Digit Diagnostic Code. *Alcohol and Alcoholism* 35, 400–10.

Bloomfield K., Gmel G., Neve R., *et al.* (2001) Investigating gender convergence in alcohol consumption in Finland, Germany, the Netherlands, and Switzerland: A repeated survey analysis. *Substance Abuse* 22, 39–54.

Bruun K., Edwards G., Lumio M., *et al.* (1975) *Alcohol control policies in public health perspective*. Helsinki: The Finnish Foundation for Alcohol Studies.

Caetano R. (1997) Prevalence, incidence and stability of drinking problems among Whites, Blacks and Hispanics: 1984–1992. *Journal of Studies on Alcohol* 58, 565–72.

Caetano R., Tam T., Greenfield T., *et al.* (1997) DSM-IV alcohol dependence and drinking in the US population: a risk analysis. *Annals of Epidemiology* 7, 542–9.

Caetano R. and Cunradi C. (2002) Alcohol dependence: A public health perspective. *Addiction* 97, 633–45.

Cahalan D. and Room R. (1974) *Problem drinking among American men*. New Brunswick, NJ: Rutgers Center of Alcohol Studies.

Clarren S.K. and Smith D.W. (1978) The fetal alcohol syndrome. *New England Journal of Medicine* 298, 1063–7.

Dawson D.A. and Archer L.D. (1993) Relative frequency of heavy drinking and the risk of alcohol dependence. *Addiction* 88, 1509–18.

Demers A., Room R., and Bourgault C. (eds.) (2001) *Surveys of drinking patterns and problems in seven developing countries*. WHO/MSD/MSB/01.2. Geneva: WHO Department of Mental Health and Substance Dependence.

Edwards G. (2000) *Alcohol: the ambiguous molecule*. Harmondsworth: Penguin.

Edwards G. and Gross M.M. (1976) Alcohol dependence: provisional description of a clinical syndrome. *British Medical Journal* 1, 1058–61.

Edwards G. and Holder H.D. (2000) The alcohol supply: its importance to public health and safety, and essential research questions. *Addiction* 95, S621–7.

Fillmore K.M., Hartka E., Johnstone B.M., *et al.* (1991) The collaborative alcohol-related longitudinal project: preliminary results from a meta-analysis of drinking behavior in multiple longitudinal studies. *British Journal of Addiction* 86, 1203–10.

Hall W., Saunders J.B., Babor T.F., *et al.* (1993) The structure and correlates of alcohol dependence: WHO collaborative project on the early detection of persons with harmful alcohol consumption: III. *Addiction* **88**, 1627–36.

Heath D.B. (1984) Cross-cultural studies of alcohol use. In: Galanter M. (ed.) *Recent developments in alcoholism*, Vol. 2, pp. 405–15. New York: Plenum.

Hurst P.M., Harte D., and Frith W.J. (1994) The Grand Rapids Dip revisited. *Accident Analysis and Prevention* **26**, 647–54.

Imrie C.W. (1997) Acute pancreatitis: overview. *European Journal of Gastroenterology and Hepatology* **9**, 103–5.

Jernigan D.H. (2000) Implications of structural changes in the global alcohol supply. *Contemporary Drug Problems* **27**, 163–87.

Kreitman N. (1986) Alcohol consumption and the preventive paradox. *British Journal of Addiction* **81**, 353–63.

Lieber C.S. (1988) Biochemical and molecular basis of alcohol-induced injury to liver tissues. *New England Journal of Medicine* **319**, 1639–50.

Lishman W.A. (1998) *Organic psychiatry: the psychological consequences of cerebral disorder.* Oxford: Blackwell Science Inc.

Mäkelä K. (1983) The uses of alcohol and their cultural regulation. *Acta Sociologica* **1**, 21–31.

Midanik L. (1999) Drunkenness, feeling the effects, and 5+ measures: meaning and predictiveness. *Addiction* **94**, 887–97.

National Highway Traffic Safety Administration (2000) *Traffic Safety Facts 2000* (DOT HS 809323). Washington, DC: US Department of Transportation, National Highway Safety Administration.

Peters T. (ed.) (1998) *Alcohol and cardiovascular diseases* (Novartis Foundation Symposium). Chichester, NY: John Wiley and Sons.

Poikolainen K. (2002) Alcohol sales and fatal alcohol poisonings. *Addiction* **97**, 1037–40.

Roberts A.J. and Koob G.F. (1997) The neurology of addiction: An overview. *Alcohol Health and Research World* **21**, 101–43.

Roizen R. (1981) *The World Health Organization study of community responses to alcohol-related problems: a review of cross-cultural findings.* Geneva: World Health Organization.

Room R. (2001) Intoxication and bad behaviour: understanding cultural differences in the link. *Social Science and Medicine* **53**, 189–98.

Room R. and Rossow I. (2001) The share of violence attributable to drinking. *Journal of Substance Use* **6**, 218–28.

Room R., Bondy S., and Ferris J. (1995) The risk of harm to oneself from drinking Canada 1989. *Addiction* **90**, 499–513.

Room R., Jernigan J., Carlini Marlatt B., *et al.* (2002) *Alcohol in developing societies: a public health approach.* Helsinki: Finnish Foundation for Alcohol Studies.

Searles H., Bernard J.P., and Johnson C.D. (1996) Alcohol and the pancreas. In: Peters T.J. (ed.) *Alcohol misuse: a European perspective*, pp. 145–62. Amsterdam: Harwood Academic Publishers.

Sherman D.J.N. and Williams R. (1994) Liver damage: mechanisms and management. *British Medical Bulletin* **50**, 124–38.

Simpura J. and Karlsson T. (2001) Trends in drinking patterns among adult population in 15 European countries, 1950 to 2000: a review. *Nordic Studies on Alcohol and Drugs* **15** (English Suppl.), 31–53.

Skog O.-J. (1999) Alcohol policy: why and roughly how? *Nordic Studies on Alcohol and Drugs* **16** (English Suppl.), 21–34.

Ström K. (1999) Alcohol, smoking and lung disease. *Addiction Biology* **4**, 17–22.

Tuyns A.J. (1983) Oesophageal cancer in non-smoking drinkers and non-drinking smokers. *International Journal of Cancer* **32**, 443–4.

Urbano-Marquez A. and Fernández-Solà J. (1996) Musculo-skeletal problems in alcohol abuse. In: Peters T.J. (ed.) *Alcohol misuse: a European perspective*, pp. 123–44. Amsterdam: Harwood Academic Publishers.

WHO. See World Health Organization

World Health Organization (1988) *IARC monographs on the evolution of carcinogenic risks to humans, alcohol drinking*, Vol. 44. Lyon: International Agency for Research on Cancer.

World Health Organization (1992) *The ICD-10 classification of mental and behavioural disorders: clinical descriptions and diagnostic guidelines*. Geneva: World Health Organization.

Chapter 3

Alcohol consumption trends and patterns of drinking

3.1 Introduction

This chapter describes alcohol consumption trends and patterns of drinking in a global perspective. The typical frequency of drinking and the amount of alcohol consumed per occasion vary enormously, not only among world regions and countries, but also over time and between different population groups. As will be shown in this chapter, variations in these 'patterns' of drinking affect rates of alcohol-related problems, and have implications for the choice of alcohol policy measures.

Two aspects of alcohol consumption are of particular importance for comparisons across populations and across time.

1. Total alcohol consumption in a population is an important indicator of the number of individuals who are exposed to high amounts of alcohol. Adult *per capita* **alcohol consumption** is, to a considerable extent, related to the prevalence of heavy use, which in turn is associated with the occurrence of negative effects.

2. The relationship between total alcohol consumption and harm is modified by the number of drinkers in a population and by the way in which alcohol is consumed.

3.2 Proportions of drinkers and levels of alcohol consumption

3.2.1 Methods of estimating and reporting alcohol consumption

The level of alcohol consumption in a population is usually expressed in litres of ethanol (100% alcohol or pure alcohol) *per capita*. An alternative procedure is to report litres of ethanol for each person aged 15 or older. The age of 15 is chosen as a lower limit to reflect the fact that children do not drink alcoholic beverages in most countries, and that drinkers in many countries, especially established market economies, typically initiate drinking within a few years of this age.

Yet another way of expressing the level of consumption is in terms of litres of ethanol per drinker, excluding from the calculation those who abstain from alcohol. This requires an estimate of the proportion of abstainers in the population, typically defined in terms of having consumed no alcoholic beverages in the last 12 months, and usually derived from interview responses to population survey questions. Expressing *per capita* consumption in litres per drinker permits a comparison of levels of drinking among drinkers in different nations, even if there are disparities in the proportion who drink at all.

Rates of abstention vary greatly between different societies. In most European countries, drinking is common in the adult population, and 80–90% currently drink at least occasionally (Simpura *et al.* 1997). The proportion of drinkers varies significantly more among countries in the Americas. Estimates for Peru (93%) and Canada (73%) are close to the European countries, whereas they are lower in the United States (65%), Mexico (54%), Costa Rica (40%), and Jamaica (32%) (WHO 1999). Very little information is available from most African countries, yet surveys (some of which were conducted decades ago) indicate that the proportion of drinkers in Namibia, Nigeria, and Zambia is around 50% (see Room *et al.* 2002). Data from surveys in Thailand (Deelertyuenyong *et al.* 1992), India (Mohan and Sharma 1995), and Sri Lanka (Hettige 1991) show that the proportion of drinkers in these countries tends to be around 30%, while the proportion seems to be higher in China (55%) and South Korea (67%) (Room *et al.* 2002). In the Western Pacific region, the proportion of drinkers varies considerably, from 87% in New Zealand and 76% in Australia to 40% in Papua New Guinea (WHO 1999). Although survey data are non-existent, it is safe to assume much lower prevalences in the Eastern Mediterranean Crescent and other regions with large Moslem populations (WHO 1999).

Consequently, when we compare the consumption per adult drinker, rather than among all adults, the consumption per drinker is higher in the US than in Denmark, although the *per capita* consumption is 36% higher in Denmark than in the US. In addition, the consumption per drinker is almost 50% higher in China than in Norway, whereas *per capita* consumption is at the same level.

In many developed societies, estimates of the annual amount of alcohol consumption are derived from statistics related to production and trade or sales. In addition to this **recorded consumption**, in most countries there is also **unrecorded consumption**, which may include alcoholic beverages from a variety of sources (e.g., home-brewing, informal or illegal production, travellers' imports), as well as consumption by the country's residents outside the country. In most established market economies, unrecorded consumption amounts to one-third or less of total consumption (Leifman 2001). But elsewhere, a much higher proportion of consumption is unrecorded. Estimates from Russia, the Baltic states, and Brazil indicate proportions of up to 60% (Shkolnikov and Nemtsov 1997; Simpura *et al.* 1999; Dunn and Laranjeira 1996), and estimates for East Africa are around 90% (Willis 2001). In such countries, estimates of overall alcohol consumption must go beyond conventional taxation and trade statistics, drawing on estimates from agricultural sources and field studies (WHO 1999, 2000a).

3.2.2 Regional estimates of drinkers and drinking around the world

Our primary focus in this chapter will be on 15 regional groupings of countries, covering the entire world. These regions have been defined as part of the World Health Organization's (WHO's) effort to estimate the Global Burden of Disease (Murray and Lopez 1996) in Africa, the Americas, the Middle East, Europe (including all successor states to the former Soviet Union), South-East Asia, and the Western Pacific. Within each general geographical area, countries are grouped in terms of adult and infant mortality (see WHO 2000b). Estimates for each of the 15 regional groupings are derived from a population-weighted averaging of country estimates. In regions like Western Europe or North America, the figures are mostly derived from country-level empirical data, but elsewhere the figures include a substantial element of extrapolation and expert judgement. The picture presented here is thus approximate rather than exact, but it does provide a framework to evaluate alcohol consumption on a global basis.

Table 3.1 shows the most salient characteristics of alcohol consumption in these different regions of the world, beginning with the predominant beverage type. The third column in Table 3.1 shows the figures for recorded alcohol consumption per resident aged 15 and older in the 15 regional groupings. Clearly, recorded alcohol consumption is highest in the economically developed regions of the world. In contrast, recorded consumption is generally lower in Latin America, Africa, and parts of Asia, and particularly low in historically Moslem states and the Indian subcontinent.

Adding in estimates of unrecorded consumption changes the picture somewhat. The fourth column in Table 3.1 shows the estimated level of total alcohol consumption per resident aged 15 and older in the 15 regions. Western

Europe, Russia, and other non-Moslem parts of the former Soviet Union now show the highest *per capita* consumption levels, but Latin American levels are not far behind. In proportional terms, it is in Africa and the Indian subcontinent that unrecorded consumption makes the greatest contribution. In terms of estimated total consumption per resident aged 15 and over, there is a more than 13-fold difference between the region with the highest estimated consumption (Europe C) and the region with the lowest (Middle East D). Interestingly, these two regions are contiguous.

There are substantial differences among regions in the proportion of drinkers in the adult population. In most societies, men are much more likely than women to be drinkers. The fifth and sixth columns in Table 3.1 show the estimated proportions of drinkers among males and females for each region. As noted above, most adults in Western and Eastern Europe and in the region including Japan and Australasia are drinkers. In the Americas, a majority of adults are drinkers, but around one-third abstain. In the rest of the world, only a minority of adults are drinkers. Women are particularly unlikely to be drinkers in the Indian subcontinent and Indonesia, and in the Middle East. Differences between men and women in the proportion of drinkers are particularly marked in China and South-East Asia.

The seventh column in Table 3.1 shows the total consumption per drinker for each of the 15 regions; the abstainers are excluded from the population base on which alcohol consumption is calculated. On this basis, the range of variation between world regions is much diminished, with the groupings that include Russia, South Africa, and Western Europe now much more similar to the groupings that include China, Bolivia, and Pakistan. This means that, in a global perspective, a country's abstention rate has a very important influence on per adult consumption levels.

3.3 Trends and dramatic shifts in *per capita* alcohol consumption

3.3.1 Trends in *per capita* alcohol consumption

Looking at trends in recommended *per capita* alcohol consumption world-wide, there seems to have been a decline in drinking in many of the high alcohol consumption countries from the early 1970s to the mid-1990s (Figure 3.1). This is particularly the case in the traditional wine-producing countries in Europe, such as France, Italy, and Portugal, where the decrease is mostly due to reductions in wine consumption (Gual and Colom 1997). Similar trends are also seen in the wine-producing countries in South America such as Argentina and Chile. In

Table 3.1 Characteristics of alcohol consumption in different regions of the world (population-weighted averages)

(1) WHO region (see definitions below)	(2) Predominant beverage type	(3) Recorded consumption[a]	(4) Total consumption[b]	(5) % drinkers among males[c]	(6) % drinkers among females[d]	(7) Consumption per drinker[e]	(8) Average drinking pattern[f]	(9) % alcohol dependent[g]
Africa D (e.g., Nigeria, Algeria)	Mainly fermented beverages	2.3	4.9	47.0	27.0	13.3	2.5	0.7
Africa E (e.g., Ethiopia, South Africa)	Mainly other fermented beverages and beer	3.8	7.1	55.0	30.0	16.6	3.1	1.6
Americas A (Canada, Cuba, US)	>50% beer, about 25% spirits	8.3	9.3	73.0	58.0	14.3	2.0	5.1
Americas B (e.g., Brazil, Mexico)	Beer, followed by spirits	6.3	9.0	75.0	53.0	14.1	3.1	3.5
Americas D (e.g., Bolivia, Peru)	Spirits, followed by beer	3.3	5.1	74.0	60.0	7.6	3.1	3.2
Eastern Mediterranean B (e.g., Iran Saudi Arabia)	Spirits and beer	0.9	1.3	18.0	4.0	11.0	2.0	0.0
E. Mediterranean D (e.g., Afghanistan, Pakistan)	Spirits and beer	0.3	0.5	17.0	1.0	6.0	2.4	0.0
Europe A (e.g., Germany, France, UK)	Wine and beer	11.6	12.9	90.0	81.0	15.1	1.3	3.4
Europe B 1 (e.g., Bulgaria, Poland, Turkey)	Spirits	5.6	9.3	77.0	57.0	14.3	2.9	0.8
Europe B 2 (e.g., Armenia, Azerbaijan, Tajikistan)	Spirits and wine	2.1	4.3	54.0	33.0	9.9	3.0	0.2

Table 3.1 (continued)

(1) WHO region (see definitions below)	(2) Predominant beverage type	(3) Recorded consumption[a]	(4) Total consumption[b]	(5) % drinkers among males[c]	(6) % drinkers among females[d]	(7) Consumption per drinker[e]	(8) Average drinking pattern[f]	(9) % alcohol dependent[g]
Europe C (e.g., Russian Federation, Ukraine)	Spirits	8.6	13.9	89.0	81.0	16.5	3.6	4.8
South-East Asia B (e.g., Indonesia, Thailand)	Spirits	2.3	3.1	35.0	9.0	13.7	2.5	0.4
South-East Asia D (e.g., Bangladesh, India)	Spirits	0.4	2.0	26.0	4.0	12.9	3.0	0.8
Western Pacific A (e.g., Australia, Japan)	Beer and spirits	6.8	8.5	87.0	77.0	10.4	1.2	2.1
Western Pacific B (e.g., China, Philippines, Viet Nam)	Spirits	3.7	5.0	84.0	30.0	8.8	2.2	0.9

[a] Recorded alcohol consumption (in litres of absolute alcohol) per resident aged 15 and older.
[b] Estimated alcohol consumption per resident aged 15 and older.
[c] Estimated proportion of male drinkers aged 15 and older.
[d] Estimated proportion of female drinkers aged 15 and older.
[e] Estimated total alcohol consumption (in litres of absolute alcohol) per adult drinker.
[f] Estimated hazardous drinking score (1 = low level of risk, 4 = high level of risk associated with a country's predominant pattern of drinking).
[g] Estimated rate of alcohol dependence, among those aged 15+.

Source: Based on estimates (Rehm et al., in press) from the WHO Comparative risk analysis within the global burden of disease 2000 study. Recorded consumption is derived from official or industry figures; unrecorded consumption is estimated from a variety of sources. The percentages of drinkers (drinking at all in the last 12 months) among males and females are derived from population surveys, where possible. Where figures for a country were otherwise unavailable, they were extrapolated from nearby countries on the basis of similarity of alcohol culture. Hazardous drinking pattern is an estimate derived from survey data and expert judgements at the country level. Estimates of the total population alcohol dependent are derived from population surveys, especially the World Mental Health Survey (WHO 2002).

The 15 regional groupings below (which comprise the 191 WHO Member States) have been defined by WHO on the basis of geographical location as well as high, medium, or low levels of adult and of infant mortality. WHO's Europe B has been subdivided to separate out the relatively low consumption southern republics of the former Soviet Union.

Africa D	Algeria, Angola, Benin, Burkina Faso, Cameroon, Cape Verde, Chad, Comoros, Equatorial Guinea, Gabon, Gambia, Ghana, Guinea, Guinea-Bissau, Liberia, Madagascar, Mali, Mauritania, Mauritius, Niger, Nigeria, Sao Tome and Principe, Senegal, Seychelles, Sierra Leone, Togo
Africa E	Botswana, Burundi, Central African Republic, Congo, Côte d'Ivoire, Democratic Republic of the Congo, Eritrea, Ethiopia, Kenya, Lesotho, Malawi, Mozambique, Namibia, Rwanda, South Africa, Swaziland, Uganda, United Republic of Tanzania, Zambia, Zimbabwe
America A	Canada, Cuba, United States of America
America B	Antigua and Barbuda, Argentina, Bahamas, Barbados, Belize, Brazil, Chile, Colombia, Costa Rica, Dominica, Dominican Republic, El Salvador, Grenada, Guyana, Honduras, Jamaica, Mexico, Panama, Paraguay, Saint Kitts and Nevis, Saint Lucia, Saint Vincent and the Grenadines, Suriname, Trinidad and Tobago, Uruguay, Venezuela
America D	Bolivia, Ecuador, Guatemala, Haiti, Nicaragua, Peru
Eastern Mediterranean B	Bahrain, Cyprus, Iran (Islamic Republic of), Jordan, Kuwait, Lebanon, Libyan Arab Jamahiriya, Oman, Qatar, Saudi Arabia, Syrian Arab Republic, Tunisia, United Arab Emirates
Easter Mediterranean D	Afghanistan, Djibouti, Egypt, Iraq, Morocco, Pakistan, Somalia, Sudan, Yemen
Europe A	Andorra, Austria, Belgium, Croatia, Czech Republic, Denmark, Finland, France, Germany, Greece, Iceland, Ireland, Israel, Italy, Luxembourg, Malta, Monaco, Netherlands, Norway, Portugal, San Marino, Slovenia, Spain, Sweden, Switzerland, United Kingdom
Europe B 1	Albania, Bosnia and Herzegovina, Bulgaria, Georgia, Poland, Romania, Slovakia, The Former Yugoslav Republic Of Macedonia, Turkey, Yugoslavia
Europe B 2	Armenia, Azerbaijan, Kyrgyzstan, Tajikistan, Turkmenistan, Uzbekistan
Europe C	Belarus, Estonia, Hungary, Kazakhstan, Latvia, Lithuania, Republic of Moldova, Russian Federation, Ukraine
South-east Asia B	Indonesia, Sri Lanka, Thailand
South-east Asia D	Bangladesh, Bhutan, Democratic People's Republic of Korea, India, Maldives, Myanmar, Nepal
Western Pacific A	Australia, Brunei Darussalam, Japan, New Zealand, Singapore
Western Pacific B	Cambodia, China, Cook Islands, Fiji, Kiribati, Lao People's Democratic Republic, Malaysia, Marshall Islands, Micronesia (Federated States of), Mongolia, Nauru, Niue, Palau, Papua New Guinea, Philippines, Republic of Korea, Samoa, Solomon Islands, Tonga, Tuvalu, Vanuatu, Viet Nam

other developed countries with relatively high *per capita* alcohol consumption, a smaller but still significant decrease has been observed over the same period, for instance in Canada and in the US. Some developed countries have countered this trend, particularly countries with a traditionally low or medium consumption level, such as Japan, Finland, and Denmark (WHO 1999).

In contrast to the general trends in developed countries, increases in recorded *per capita* consumption have been noted for many developing countries (WHO 1999). However, to some extent these increases in recorded consumption are likely to be at the expense of unrecorded consumption. This implies a need to be especially cautious when making statements about global trends. Overall, there does appear to have been a convergence in consumption among the developed countries as well as between developed and developing countries over the past thirty years. This conclusion is supported by more systematic data compiled from the WHO Global Alcohol Database (WHO 1999), which is summarized for different world regions in Figures 3.1, 3.2, 3.3, and 3.4.

Adult *per capita* consumption in Europe A and B (Figure 3.1) seems to be driven by long-term trends (Mäkelä *et al.* 1981; Simpura 1998). There are indications that the current downward trend is levelling off. For Europe C, the curve shows more variation. As discussed in the next section, the sharp decline at the end of the 1980s is due to the anti-alcohol campaign of the Gorbachev

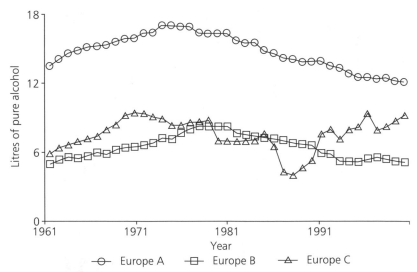

Fig. 3.1 Adult *per capita* consumption in selected WHO regions: Europe A (e.g., Germany, France, UK), Europe B (e.g., Bulgaria, Poland, Armenia), Europe C (e.g., Russian Federation, Ukraine). See Table 3.1 for full list of countries included in each WHO region.

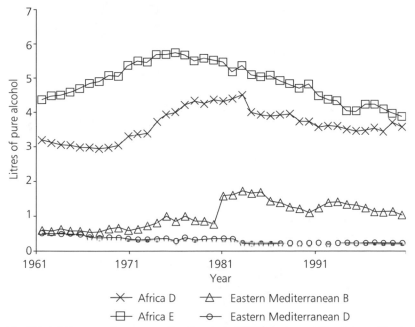

Fig. 3.2 Adult *per capita* consumption in selected WHO regions: Africa D (e.g., Nigeria, Algeria), Africa E (e.g., Ethiopia, South Africa), Eastern Mediterranean B (e.g., Iran, Saudia Arabia), Eastern Mediterranean D (e.g., Afghanistan, Pakistan) . See Table 3.1 for full list of countries included in each WHO region.

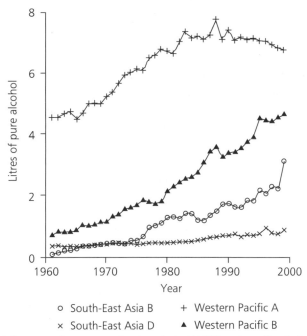

Fig. 3.3 Adult *per capita* consumption in selected WHO regions: South-East Asia B (e.g., Indonesia, Thailand), South-East Asia D (e.g., Bangladesh, India), Western Pacific A (e.g., Australia, Japan), and Western Pacific B (e.g., China, Philippines, Vietnam). See Table 3.1 for full list of countries included in each WHO region.

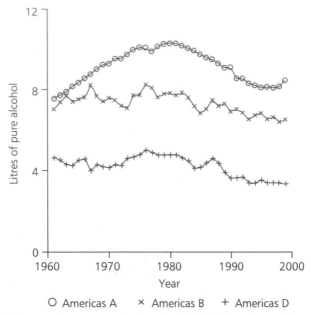

Fig. 3.4 Adult *per capita* consumption in selected WHO American regions: Americas A (e.g., Canada, Cuba, USA), Americas B (e.g., Brazil, Mexico), and Americas D (e.g., Bolivia, Peru). See Table 3.1 for full list of countries included in each WHO region.

period (1985–1988) in the former Soviet Union (White 1996). No trends are apparent for Eastern Mediterranean B and D, or for Africa D (Figure 3.2).

For the Western Pacific region shown in Figure 3.3, there was an upward trend that seems to have stopped at the end of the 1980s. For Western Pacific B and South-East Asia B, consumption has clearly increased.

For the Americas, Figure 3.4 shows a long wave for America A of increasing and then decreasing consumption, almost parallel to the Europe A consumption. For Americas B and D, slightly downward trends are apparent.

3.3.2 Remarkable changes in consumption

Some remarkable and sudden shifts in alcohol consumption have taken place in recent decades, changes that are of particular concern from a public health perspective. As already noted (Figure 3.2), a number of developing countries have witnessed marked increases in recorded *per capita* consumption. Moreover, in several **countries in transition** (Europe C, Figure 3.1), sudden changes over shorter periods of time have been observed. In Poland, the recorded *per capita* consumption decreased markedly from 1980 to 1981 (a drop of 24%, from 8.4 litres of pure alcohol to 6.4 litres per adult inhabitant), concurrent with the anti-alcohol campaign launched by the 'Solidarity' trade movement and co-opted in the government's declaration of martial law and its institution of alcohol rationing (Moskalewicz 2000). In the former Soviet Union, a similar decrease was observed in the mid-1980s during the aforementioned anti-alcohol campaign of the Gorbachev era (White 1996; Reitan 2000). The campaign was initiated in 1985 and gradually lost its momentum from 1987 onwards. The recorded *per capita* consumption of pure ethanol dropped from 8.4 litres in 1984 to 3.3 litres in 1987 (Ivanets and Lukomskaya 1990). Even when illicit consumption is taken into account, there seems to have been a large net reduction of some 25% during the anti-alcohol campaign (Shkolnikov and Nemtsov 1997). At the end of the campaign, alcohol consumption returned to former levels.

3.4 The impact of total alcohol consumption

3.4.1 The distribution of alcohol consumption in the population

Studies from a number of countries demonstrate that alcohol consumption is unevenly distributed across the population (and even across the drinking population). Most of the alcohol in a society is consumed by a relatively small minority of drinkers. Lemmens (1991) estimated for the Netherlands in the mid-1980s that the top one-tenth of drinkers consumed more than one-third of the total alcohol, and that the top 30% of drinkers accounted for up to three-quarters of all consumption. Greenfield and Rogers (1999) found even more extreme results with US data. They found that the top 20% drink almost 90% of all alcohol and that young adults (ages 18–29), comprising roughly one-quarter of the adult population, account for almost half of all adult consumption. In China, it has been estimated that the top 12.5% of the drinkers (or 7.5% of the total population) consume 60% of the total amount of alcohol (Wei *et al.* 1999).

In a comparison of Norway, a relatively low alcohol consumption country, and France, a high consumption country, Skog (1991) found that in both countries the upper 10% of the drinkers consumed a disproportionately large percentage of the alcohol. Nevertheless, the concentration of consumption was more pronounced in Norway (50%) than in France (30%). According to Skog, this exemplifies a general pattern. Consumption is likely to be more strongly concentrated in a small segment of the population in low consumption countries, whereas the concentration is less pronounced where *per capita* consumption is higher.

3.4.2 The relationship between total alcohol consumption and prevalence of heavy drinkers

When alcohol consumption levels increase in any given society, there tends to be an increase in the prevalence of heavy drinkers, defined in terms of a high annual alcohol intake. In Finland, total alcohol consumption increased by 46% from 1968 to 1969. The increase in consumption was influenced most by the addition of new heavy drinking occasions (Mäkelä 1970), and the increase was greater in heavier consumption groups (Mäkelä 2002). Because heavy drinkers account for a significant proportion of total alcohol consumption, it would be difficult for the total consumption level to increase without an increase in their drinking. The connection between heavy drinkers and the level of total consumption in the population has also been explained by the social nature of most drinking. People tend to influence each other's drinking with their own drinking behaviour, which implies that heavier drinkers, along with other drinkers, tend to drink more when consumption increases (Skog 1985, 2001).

3.5 Drinking patterns

As noted in Chapter 2, the term 'drinking pattern' refers to regularities in the frequency, amount, and type of alcohol consumed over a period of time. Drinking patterns are important because they have a direct effect on the drinker's blood alcohol level and other aspects of a person's drinking that are likely to lead to harm.

3.5.1 Type of beverage

One important aspect of the drinking pattern is the type of alcoholic beverage consumed. There are many varieties of alcoholic beverages, with varying levels of alcohol content. In many places, one or two beverage types account for most of the alcohol consumption. Predominant beverage types tend to change relatively slowly in a culture, although there are historical exceptions. For example, in 1917, a major tax increase in Denmark suddenly altered the predominant alcoholic beverage from spirits to beer (Bruun *et al.* 1975). The excise duty rate for distilled spirits was increased 12-fold and that of beer two-fold. The consumption of distilled spirits decreased much more than that of beer, so the share of beer as a per cent of total alcohol consumption increased, but there was definitely no substitution from distilled spirits to beer.

Historically, spirits drinking was often regarded as more problematic than the drinking of fermented beverages like wine or beer. From a medical perspective, the choice of beverage makes little difference in terms of most long-term health consequences, such as liver cirrhosis (Smart 1996). It is the total amount of pure alcohol consumed, regardless of beverage type, that accounts for the toxic effects. But spirits drinking does entail some special risks. Overdoses from strong spirits are much more common than overdoses from fermented beverages. Some health consequences, such as throat cancers, also seem to be particularly associated with spirits drinking (Tuyns *et al.* 1979). And yet, the harmful effects of specific beverages are less important than the specific cultural associations of different alcoholic beverages, and the drinking patterns associated with them. In the US and UK, beer, rather than stronger beverages, is most often involved in hazardous drinking (Rogers and Greenfield 1999), in part because of its cultural meaning as a recreational beverage.

The second column of Table 3.1 lists the predominant beverage types of the 15 world regions. On a global basis, grape wine is a relatively unimportant part of alcohol consumption, although it dominates in specific areas like southern Europe. Rice-based fermented beverages, traditionally called rice wines, are important beverages in some Asian countries like Japan, as are medium-strength spirits (~25%) such as *soju*. *Arrack* and other spirits tend to predominate in the lowest consumption areas (where their concentration facilitates concealment), and spirits such as vodka predominate in the highest consumption area, Slavic Europe.

In Africa and Latin America, traditional fermented beverages such as opaque beer, *pulque* (made from the maguey plant), and *chicha* (made from maize) play an important role, with much of their production now industrialized. But nearly everywhere in the developing world, European-style lager beer is the prestige commodity among everyday alcoholic beverages (Jernigan 2000). This style of beer, typically promoted and produced by multinational firms or their partners, shows growth in consumption levels in most parts of the developing world.

3.5.2 The drinking context

The extent to which alcohol is consumed in public settings (i.e., pubs, bars, restaurants) rather than in private settings has implications for harmful consequences (particularly violence), as well as prevention strategies. However, the association with alcohol problems probably varies by culture and over time. For instance, Finnish drinkers consumed more alcohol per occasion at home than in public drinking places in the 1950s, but by the mid-1960s, differences by location in amount consumed had diminished among Helsinki drinkers (Partanen 1975). While quantitative data on drinking contexts are sparse (Single *et al.* 1997), estimates from data on recorded consumption

Table 3.2 Per cent of alcohol consumed in public drinking places in different countries

Country	Per cent of alcohol consumed[a]
Belgium	55%
Canada	21%
Denmark	21%
Finland	24%
Ireland[b]	76%
Netherlands	29%
New Zealand	44%
Norway	30%
Spain	65%
Sweden	23%
Switzerland	37%
United States	24%

[a] Sources for estimates are all found in Brewers Association of Canada (1997). Estimates are mostly based on beverage-specific data on recorded alcohol sales and proportion of each beverage being consumed in public drinking places.

[b] The estimate for Ireland is based on figures for beer and spirits consumption only, which implies that the proportion of alcohol being consumed in public drinking places is probably somewhat higher. Wine consumption constitutes, however, only 9.5% of the total Irish alcohol consumption.

(Brewers Association of Canada 1997) show that the proportion of alcohol consumed in public places varies considerably across countries (Table 3.2). Survey studies in several countries have found that drinking in public places is particularly associated with heavy drinking and intoxication (Cosper *et al.* 1987; Single *et al.* 1997).

3.5.3 **Distribution of drinking occasions and intake per occasion**

Total consumption can be regarded as a combination of two dimensions, drinking frequency and average quantity per occasion, each with its own distribution. Two equal distributions of total consumption may thus be composed of different combinations of drinking frequency and quantity. If regular drinking has different health effects than occasional heavy drinking, two apparently equal overall levels of drinking may lead to different outcomes.

Simply assessing total consumption may thus lead to erroneous conclusions. For example, in epidemiological studies on cardiovascular risk, consumption is sometimes presented as average number of drinks per day, which can be misinterpreted as daily drinking of the particular amounts. As Knupfer (1987) has noted, however, such 'daily light' drinkers are rare, and those who drink daily are mostly heavy drinkers. Similar findings were reported by San José *et al.* (2000) for the Netherlands. But while Lemmens (1991) found drinking frequency to be positively associated with quantity per occasion, other studies in different populations have found little or no relation between these complementary components of total consumption (Leifman 2001).

3.5.4 Intoxication

As discussed in Chapter 2, intoxication is a major mechanism for damage from alcohol. Intoxication results from drinking a relatively large amount of alcohol on one particular occasion, although the term covers more than simply the amount of alcohol consumed. To understand the implications of total consumption, it is important to differentiate between drinkers whose amount consumed varies considerably from one occasion to another and drinkers who consistently drink about the same amount on each occasion. Risks will be quite different for a person who drinks three bottles of beer every evening and a person who drinks one bottle every day but 15 bottles on a Saturday night, though their average consumption will be the same.

Cultures vary in the extent to which drinking to intoxication is a characteristic of the drinking pattern. They also differ in how intoxicated people get, and how people behave while intoxicated (Room and Mäkelä 2000). The eighth column in Table 3.1 shows the average drinking pattern score for each of the 15 regions, compiled as a population-weighted average of the scores of the included nations. The score was derived from survey data, extrapolation, and expert judgement. Nations were assigned a score from 1 to 4, indicating the level of hazard associated with the predominant pattern of drinking (Rehm *et al.* 2001). Note that the score is independent of both the proportion of abstainers and the volume of alcohol consumption. In principle, it is intended to indicate the differential risk of problems associated with the dominant patterns of drinking in the country or region. It can be viewed as an indication of the extent to which intoxication is a characteristic mediator between alcohol consumption and social and casualty harms in that nation.

The two regions with the lowest average score for hazardous drinking pattern are Europe A and Western Pacific A. Europe A, especially, includes countries assigned a higher drinking pattern score than the average. For instance, the score assigned to Sweden, Norway, and Finland is three, but the score for the region as a whole is brought down by more populous countries with lower hazardous drinking pattern scores.

The region including Russia and Ukraine (Europe C) has the highest drinking pattern score, but the scores are also high in Africa, Latin America, Eastern Europe, and India. The level of hazard thus has relatively little relationship to the per adult level of consumption. A hazardous pattern can be associated with either high or low consumption levels in the population at large.

3.5.5 Intoxication among young persons

Intoxication is a particularly marked characteristic of drinking by teenagers and young adults in many cultures. As they are relative neophytes to drinking, their episodes of intoxication may be particularly prone to harmful consequences. A recent multinational study of drinking habits and drug use among school children provides a basis for comparisons among European countries as well as the US (Hibell *et al.* 2000). The second column in Table 3.3 shows the number of drinking events in the last year reported by 15-year-olds in each country in 1995, and the fifth column shows the same data for 1999. The average number of drinking occasions increased between 1995 and 1999 in 20 of 24 countries. The respondents were also asked about the number of occasions when they were 'drunk' in the last year. The results are shown for 1995 in the third column, and for 1999 in the sixth column. Again, the average number of occasions increased in 20 of 24 countries.

The fourth and seventh columns in Table 3.3 show, for 1995 and 1999 respectively, the ratio of intoxication frequency to drinking frequency. This ratio thus represents the proportion of drinking occasions that become occasions of drunkenness. There is no general trend from 1995 to 1999. With a few notable exceptions, the ratio in a particular country seems quite stable, suggesting that the number of intoxication occasions in a particular country increases or decreases in relation to the number of drinking occasions. Nevertheless, there are large differences between countries, and they tend to fall in a quite distinct north–south gradient across Europe. In the southern European countries, approximately one out of ten drinking occasions lead to a state of subjective intoxication, whereas intoxication is reported to be the result in a majority of drinking occasions in the most northern European countries. Results for eastern and central European countries, the United Kingdom, and the US fall somewhere in between.

A similar picture emerges when the same methods are applied to data assembled from a variety of separate but comparable surveys of adult populations in 13 countries (Table 3.4). The ratios in the last two columns of the table tend to be higher in northern than in southern Europe. However, because these data have not been collected as part of a coordinated study, the comparisons are likely to be less precise than those of the Hibell *et al.* (2000) study.

Table 3.3 Drinking frequency and alcohol intoxication among 15–16 year olds in 31 countries[a,b]

(1) Country	(2) Drinking occasions (D) 1995	(3) Intoxication occasions (I) 1995	(4) Ratio I/D 1995	(5) Drinking occasions (D) 1999	(6) Intoxication occasions (I) 1999	(7) Ratio I/D 1999
Bulgaria				8.4	2.9	0.35
Croatia	6.6	1.9	0.29	8.6	2.5	0.29
Cyprus	14.3	1.3	0.09	10.3	0.6	0.06
Czech Republic	14.4	4.2	0.29	17.6	5.3	0.30
Denmark	22.1	10.2	0.46	25.8	12.7	0.49
Estonia	7.7	2.6	0.34	10.5	4.0	0.38
Faroe Islands	10.9	6.5	0.60	11.3	6.1	0.54
Finland	9.4	8.2	0.88	10.9	9.1	0.83
France				10.2	1.6	0.15
Greece	14.7	1.6	0.11	17.6	2.2	0.12
Greenland				9.0	6.6	0.73
Hungary	8.2	2.4	0.29	7.4	2.7	0.36
Iceland	8.3	6.7	0.82	7.2	6.3	0.88
Ireland	17.1	7.3	0.43	20.1	9.3	0.46
Italy	11.4	2.0	0.17	8.7	1.3	0.15
Latvia	8.4	2.4	0.29	9.5	3.7	0.39
Lithuania	6.5	3.3	0.50	10.8	3.6	0.33
Malta	15.7	1.9	0.12	17.8	2.0	0.11
Netherlands				17.0	3.5	0.20
Norway	6.7	4.0	0.60	9.1	5.6	0.61
Poland	8.4	2.9	0.34	11.9	4.0	0.34
Portugal	7.9	0.8	0.10	8.3	1.9	0.22
Romania				8.5	1.6	0.19
Russia				13.0	3.7	0.29
Slovak Republic	8.5	2.3	0.27	11.2	3.1	0.28
Slovenia	7.4	2.8	0.38	10.8	4.5	0.41
Sweden	9.1	5.7	0.63	9.6	6.0	0.62
Turkey	4.9	1.2	0.24			
Ukraine	7.4	0.8	0.11	7.9	5.2	0.66
United Kingdom	17.7	8.8	0.49	19.5	9.4	0.48
USA	7.1	3.2	0.45	7.7	3.4	0.44

[a] Average number of drinking occasions (past year), average number of occasions involving intoxication (past year), and ratio of intoxication (I) frequency to drinking (D) frequency by country for the years 1995 and 1999.

[b] Data from the two ESPAD studies. Figures on average drinking frequency and average frequency of being drunk were calculated on the basis of published distributions of drinking frequency and frequency of having been drunk (Hibell et al. 1997, 2000).

Table 3.4 Drinking and intoxication among adults in 11 countries[a]

(1) Country	(2) Drinking occasions in 12 months	(3) Intoxication occasions in 12 months	(4) Occasions of drinking 6+/ 5+ drinks in 12 months	(5) Ratio: intoxication occasions/ drinking occasions	(6) Ratio: 6+/5+ occasions/ drinking occasions
Denmark[b]	139	7	11	0.05	0.08
Finland[b]	77	9	7	0.12	0.09
Finland[e]	53		13		0.25
France[e]	91		7		0.07
Germany[e]	76		9		0.11
Italy[e]	150		18		0.12
Norway[b]	47	7	6	0.14	0.13
Russia[c]		20		0.25	
Sweden[e]	31		8		0.27
United Kingdom[e]	92		32		0.33
USA[d]	103	3	12	0.03	0.12

[a] Average annual number of drinking occasions, occasions of subjective intoxication, occasions of drinking 5+ or 6+ drinks per occasion (about 60 gm pure ethanol), and the proportions of drinking occasions involving intoxication and involving 5+/6+ drinks, for a selection of countries.
[b] Data from Mäkelä *et al*. (1999).
[c] Data from Simpura *et al*. (1997): figures for males in Moscow.
[d] Dawson (2000): figures for non-Hispanic white drinkers who are neither abusers nor dependent.
[e] Data from Leifman (2002). Note: Data from the UK may be problematic (i.e., surprisingly high levels).

3.5.6 **Alcohol dependence**

As discussed in Chapter 2, alcohol dependence may be viewed as a mediator between alcohol consumption and alcohol-related problems. That is, someone who has become alcohol dependent is more likely to continue to drink in ways that result in health or social harm. On the basis of advances in psychiatric epidemiology, it is now possible to estimate alcohol dependence rates from surveys conducted in the WHO global regions (last column of Table 3.1) (Rehm and Eschmann 2002).

In general, there is a strong relationship between the estimated per adult total consumption in a global region and the estimated rate of alcohol dependence. Patterns of drinking reflected in high hazardous drinking scores may also lead to dependence. It is also likely that cultural differences in attributions and in the experience and recognition of affective states are related to dependence rates, as suggested by a WHO study of the cross-cultural comparability of the criteria for alcohol dependence (Room *et al.* 1996).

3.6 Distribution of drinking across demographic sub-groups and over the life-span

3.6.1 Gender

A large research literature, based primarily on survey studies of drinking habits, has consistently shown that there are significant differences in drinking patterns between men and women, between younger and older people, and often between ethnic or religious groups. As Table 3.1 suggests, there are striking gender differences in whether a person drinks, with men more likely to be drinkers and women abstainers. Among drinkers, men drink on average significantly more than women do. There is variation among countries in the proportion of total alcohol consumed by men, but the range of variation in Europe and North America is not great: from less than 70% (in Denmark, Switzerland, and the US) to over 80% (in France and Russia) (Simpura *et al.* 1997, p. 102). In some developing countries, men's share of the overall consumption is much greater. For instance, survey data from China indicate that around 95% of alcohol is consumed by men (Wei *et al.* 1999), and a similar figure has been reported from the Seychelles (Perdrix *et al.* 1999).

Moreover, men drink 'heavily' (i.e., to intoxication, or large quantities per occasion) much more often than women. This is consistently reported from a number of different countries, such as the US (Dawson 2000; Weisner *et al.* 2000), Russia (Bobak *et al.* 1999), the Nordic countries (Mäkelä *et al.* 1999), Brazil (Moreira *et al.* 1996), China (Wei *et al.* 1999), India (Mohan and Sharma 1995), Japan (Tsunoda 1988), Mexico (Natera Rey 1995), South Africa (van der Burgh and Rocha Silva 1988), the Netherlands (Neve *et al.* 1996), and Germany (Bloomfield 1998). Hence, there are more heavy drinkers and more heavy drinking occasions among men, and consequently harmful drinking is more likely to characterize men than women. Although the evidence is still sparse, it seems that this phenomenon may be even more distinctive in developing countries (Room *et al.* 2002).

3.6.2 Age groups and life cycle

Drinking habits in various age groups are difficult to compare across countries because different measures of drinking and age groupings have been used in population surveys. Moreover, most surveys that compare drinking in various age groups have been conducted in the established market economies of

Europe and North America, so the findings may not necessarily apply to other regions of the world. Nevertheless, a common picture emerges from these studies: abstinence and infrequent drinking are more prevalent in older age groups, and intoxication and heavy drinking episodes are more frequent among adolescents and young adults. This has been reported from the Nordic countries (Mäkelä et al. 1999), Canada (Demers 1997), the US (Dawson 1998), and the Netherlands (San José et al. 2000). On the other hand, studies from Germany (Bloomfield 1998), the US (Weisner et al. 2000), the Nordic countries (Mäkelä et al. 1999), and the Seychelles (Perdrix et al. 1999) have found that the average consumption or the proportions of high-volume consumers do not vary much across age groups.

Of particular concern in many countries is hazardous drinking among youth. In most of the countries where alcohol consumption is widespread (e.g., most European and American countries, New Zealand and Australia), a large proportion of adolescents drink alcohol, at least from time to time (WHO 1999; Hibell et al. 2000; Jernigan 2001). Data from the 1999 European School Survey Project on Alcohol and Drugs (ESPAD; Hibell et al. 2000) showed that in all 29 participating countries more than half of the 15- and 16-year-old students reported drinking in the previous year. Among the drinkers in most countries, the majority reported less than 10 drinking occasions in the preceding year. Yet in some countries (Denmark, Greece, Ireland, and United Kingdom) more than half of the 15- and 16-year-olds had 10 or more such occasions in the past year. In most of the countries, the majority of the students had their first drink before the age of 14. Iceland and Norway were notable exceptions, with drinking onset before age 14 reported by less than one-third of the students (Hibell et al. 2000). As noted above, it is evident that in most of the countries the frequency of drinking, as well as the frequency of drinking to intoxication, increased among youth between 1995 and 1999 (Table 3.3).

A number of studies from Western industrialized countries have shown that young people consume alcohol in public drinking places more often than middle-aged and older people (Cosper et al. 1987; Single 1993; Demers 1997), and a large proportion of young people's consumption tends to take place in bars and pubs (Engels et al. 1999).

The age gradient in drinking level and abstinence described in recent cross-sectional studies may be interpreted as an age effect (i.e., people tend to drink less heavily or become abstinent as they get older), a cohort effect (i.e., those who grew up in the second half of the 20th century were exposed to heavier drinking cultures than older cohorts), or a combination of both. Longitudinal studies have shown that middle-aged and elderly people are more likely than younger people to reduce their drinking or become abstinent, and much less likely than younger people to increase their drinking or take up heavy drinking (Fillmore *et al.* 1991; Hajema *et al.* 1997; Mulder *et al.* 1998). In a study of drinking careers in a Native American (Navajo) population, Kunitz *et al.* (1994) found that young people who would have been classified as alcoholic tended to moderate or quit drinking as they became older. But there appear to be cultural differences in the extent and timing of reducing heavy drinking with increasing age. A cross-ethnic study by Caetano (1997) showed that the stability and incidence of problem drinking was higher among Hispanics and Blacks than among Whites in the US general population.

3.6.3 Indigenous minority groups

Of particular concern in a number of developed countries is the pattern of consumption among indigenous minority groups. Some studies of Aborigines in Australia and Maoris in New Zealand show two or three times the average alcohol consumption of the general population. Studies of indigenous populations in North America have shown that these groups also have a significantly higher alcohol intake than the general population (see Brady 2000 for a review), although there is considerable variation between groups (Heath 1983). In the 1980s, the *per capita* consumption in Greenland (with a mainly Inuit population) was almost twice as high as in the rest of Denmark (National Institute for Alcohol and Drug Research 2001). However, no differences in amount of consumption have been found, for instance, between the Saami population and the general population in Norway (Larsen and Saglie 1996). Apart from consumption level, drinking patterns reported from various indigenous populations also tend to be more hazardous, with any drinking at all often implying drinking to intoxication (Dawson 1998; Brady 2000). On the other hand, rates of abstention are often higher in indigenous minority groups than in the surrounding population (e.g., Hunter *et al.* 1992).

3.7 Summary and implications

Sales data from established market economies show a slight overall decrease in alcohol consumption in recent years, as well as converging trends in traditional high consumption and low consumption countries. Of particular concern, however, is the increasing consumption in some of the emerging economies of the developing world, given that the drinking appears to be concentrated in a smaller fraction of the population in these countries.

While levels of alcohol consumption vary greatly from one part of the world to another, it appears that much of this variation is attributable to differences in the proportions of adults who abstain from drinking altogether. On a base limited to drinkers, the consumption level of the highest consuming region is less than three times that of the lowest consuming region. This suggests that registered *per capita* consumption will increase steeply if the proportion of abstainers declines, particularly in places where abstention is very common, as is true in much of the developing world.

It is not only the level of total alcohol consumption that is relevant to the health and social problems from drinking; the drinking pattern is also of considerable importance. Thus, the same amount of consumption may be associated with quite different problem levels in different societies. The large variation in total consumption and drinking patterns across population subgroups also implies that alcohol-related problems will be very unevenly distributed within a given country.

In terms of the mediators between alcohol consumption and social and health problems discussed in Chapter 2, there are large variations in the extent to which drinking is concentrated into occasions of intoxication. The hazardous drinking pattern score for global regions (Table 3.1) gives an indication of the relative prominence of intoxication occasions in different regions of the world. We have also presented estimates for the rates of alcohol dependence, a second mediator between levels of consumption and the occurrence of social and health problems. The global regions appear to cluster into two groups when the proportion of drinkers who report being alcohol dependent is compared to the consumption level per drinker. Some parts of the world—the Americas, Eastern Europe, and the Indian subcontinent—report higher rates of dependence than the consumption per drinker would suggest. Within each group of regions, however, there seems to be an association between the overall consumption per drinker and a drinker's probability of being dependent.

The differences in amounts and patterns of drinking between different countries and global regions imply differences in the composition and mixture of social and health problems from drinking, the issue addressed in the next chapter. The differences also imply that it may be necessary for the mixture of prevention and intervention strategies to vary from one society to another.

References

Bloomfield K. (1998) West German drinking patterns in 1984 and 1990. *European Addiction Research* 4, 163–71.

Bobak M., McKee M., Rose R., *et al.* (1999) Alcohol consumption in a national sample of the Russian population. *Addiction* 94, 857–66.

Brady M. (2000) Alcohol policy issues for indigenous people in the United States, Canada, Australia and New Zealand. *Contemporary Drug Problems* 27, 435–509.

Brewers Association of Canada (1997) *Alcoholic beverage taxation and control policies. International survey,* 9th edn. Ottawa: Brewers Association of Canada.

Bruun K., Edwards G., Lumio M., *et al.* (1975) *Alcohol control policies in public health perspective.* Helsinki: The Finnish Foundation for Alcohol Studies.

Caetano R. (1997) Prevalence, incidence and stability of drinking problems among Whites, Blacks and Hispanics: 1984–1992. *Journal of Studies on Alcohol* **58**, 565–72.

Cosper R.L., Okraku I.O., and Neumann B. (1987) Tavern going in Canada: A national survey of regulars at public drinking establishments. *Journal of Studies on Alcohol* **48**, 252–9.

Dawson D.A. (1998) Beyond black, white and Hispanic: Race, ethnic origin and drinking patterns in the United States. *Journal of Substance Abuse* **10**, 321–39.

Dawson D.A. (2000) Drinking patterns among individuals with and without DSM-IV alcohol use disorders. *Journal of Studies on Alcohol* **61**, 111–20.

Deelertyenyong M., Udomprasertgui V., Onthuam Y., *et al.* (1992) Incidence rate of alcoholic drink consumption in seven occupations of Surin province. In: Wongphanich M. *et al.* (eds.) *Research perspectives in occupational health and ergonomics in Asia,* pp. 583–94. Bangkok: Occupational Health Department, Mahidol University.

Demers A. (1997) When at risk? Drinking contexts and heavy drinking in the Montreal adult population. *Contemporary Drug Problems* **24**, 449–71.

Dunn J. and Laranjeira R. (1996) Memorandum to World Health Organization, Geneva.

Engels R.C.M.E., Knibbe R.A., and Drop M.J. (1999) Visiting public drinking places: An explorative study into the functions of pub-going for late adolescents. *Substance Use and Misuse* **34**, 1261–80.

Fillmore K.M., Hartka E., Johnstone B.M., *et al.* (1991) Meta-analysis of life course variation in drinking: The collaborative alcohol-related longitudinal project. *British Journal of Addiction* **86**, 1221–68.

Greenfield T.K. and Rogers J.D. (1999) Who drinks most of the alcohol in the US? The policy implications. *Journal of Studies on Alcohol* **60**, 78–89.

Gual A. and Colom J. (1997) Why has alcohol consumption declined in countries of southern Europe? *Addiction* **92** (Suppl. 1), 21–31S.

Hajema K.-J., Knibbe R.A., and Drop M.A. (1997) Changes in alcohol consumption in a general population in the Netherlands: A 9 year follow-up study. *Addiction* **92**, 49–60.

Heath D.B. (1983) Alcohol use among North American Indians. In: Smart R.G., Glasser F., and Israel Y. (eds.) *Research advances in alcohol and drug problems,* Vol. 7, pp. 343–96. New York, New York: Plenum Press.

Hettige S.T. (1991) *Alcoholism, poverty and health in rural Sri Lanka: Some empirical evidence.* Paper presented at the International Congress on Alcoholism and the Addictions, Stockholm, Sweden.

Hibell B., Andersson B., Bjarnason T., *et al.* (1997) *The 1995 European school survey project on alcohol and other drugs (ESPAD) report: Alcohol and other drug use among students in 26 countries.* Stockholm: Swedish Council for Information on Alcohol and Other Drugs (CAN).

Hibell B., Andersson B., Ahlström S., *et al.* (2000) *The 1999 ESPAD report: Alcohol and other drug use among students in 30 European countries.* Stockholm: Swedish Council for Information on Alcohol and Other Drugs (CAN).

Hunter E.M., Hall W.D., and Spargo R.M. (1992) Patterns of alcohol consumption in the Kimberley Aboriginal population. *Medical Journal of Australia* **156**, 764–8.

Ivanets N.N. and Lukomskaya M.I. (1990) USSR's new alcohol policy. *World Health Forum* 11, 246–52.

Jernigan D.H. (2000) Applying commodity chain analysis to changing modes of alcohol supply in a developing country. *Addiction* 95 (Suppl. 4), 465–75S.

Jernigan D.H. (2001) *Global status report: Alcohol and young people.* WHO/MSD/MSB/01.1. Geneva: Mental Health and Substance Abuse Department, World Health Organization.

Knupfer G. (1987) Drinking for health: The daily light drinker fiction. *British Journal of Addiction* 82, 547–55.

Kunitz S.J., Levy J.E., Andrews T., *et al.* (1994) *Drinking careers: A twenty-five year study of three Navajo populations.* New Haven, CT: Yale University Press.

Larsen S. and Saglie J. (1996) Alcohol use in Saami and non-Saami areas in northern Norway. *European Addiction Research* 2, 78–82.

Leifman H. (2001) Estimations of unrecorded alcohol consumption levels and trends in 14 European countries. *Nordic Studies on Alcohol and Drugs* 18 (English Suppl.), 54–70.

Leifman H. (2002) A comparative analysis of drinking patterns in 6 EU countries in the year 2000. *Contemporary Drug Problems* 29, 501–48.

Lemmens P.H. (1991) *Measurement and distribution of alcohol consumption* (dissertation). Maastricht: University of Limburg.

Mäkelä K. (1970) Dryckegångernas frekvens enligt de konsumerade drykerna och mängden före och efter lagreformen (The frequency of drinking occasions according to type of beverage and amount consumed before and after the new alcohol law). *Alkoholpolitik* 33, 144–53.

Mäkelä K., Room R., Single E.R., *et al.* (1981) *Alcohol, society, and the state: I. A comparative study of alcohol control.* Toronto: Addiction Research Foundation.

Mäkelä P. (2002) Whose drinking does a liberalization of alcohol policy increase? Change in alcohol consumption by the initial level in the Finnish panel survey in 1968 and 1969. *Addiction* 97, 701–6.

Mäkelä P., Fonager K., Hibell B., *et al.* (1999) *Drinking habits in the Nordic countries.* SIFA Rapport 2/99. Oslo: National Institute for Alcohol and Drug Research.

Mohan D. and Sharma H.K. (1995) India. In: Heath D.W. (ed.) *International handbook of alcohol and culture*, pp. 128–41. Westport, CT: Greenwood Press.

Moreira L.B., Fuchs F.D., Moraes R.S., *et al.* (1996) Alcoholic beverage consumption and associated factors in Porto Alegre, a southern Brazilian city: A population-based survey. *Journal of Studies on Alcohol* 57, 253–9.

Moskalewicz J. (2000) Alcohol in the countries in transition: The Polish experience and the wider context. *Contemporary Drug Problems* 27, 561–92.

Mulder M., Ranchor A.V., Sanderman R., *et al.* (1998) Stability of lifestyle behaviour. *International Journal of Epidemiology* 27, 199–207.

Murray C.J.L. and Lopez A.D. (eds.) (1996) *The global burden of disease: A comprehensive assessment of mortality and disability from diseases, injuries and risk factors in 1990 and projected to 2020.* Cambridge, MA: Harvard School of Public Health on behalf of the World Health Organization and the World Bank (Global Burden of Disease and Injury Series, Vol. I).

Natera Rey G. (1995) Mexico. In: Heath D.W. (ed.) *International handbook of alcohol and culture*, pp. 179–89. Westport, CT: Greenwood Press.

National Institute for Alcohol and Drug Research (2001) *Alcohol and drugs in Norway.* Oslo: National Institute for Alcohol and Drug Research.

Neve R.J.M., Drop M.J., Lemmens P.H., *et al.* (1996) Gender differences in drinking behaviour in the Netherlands: Convergence or stability? *Addiction* 91, 357–73.

Partanen J. (1975) On the role of situational factors in alcohol research: Drinking in restaurants vs. drinking at home. *Drinking and Drug Practices Surveyor* 10, 14–16.

Perdrix J., Bovet P., Larue D., *et al.* (1999) Patterns of alcohol consumption in the Seychelles Islands (Indian Ocean). *Alcohol and Alcoholism* 34, 773–85.

Rehm J.T. and Eschmann S. (2002) International comparison of health determinants: Global monitoring of average volume of alcohol consumption. *Soziale- und Präventivmedizin* 47, 1–11.

Rehm J., Monteiro M., Room R., *et al.* (2001) Steps towards constructing a global comparative risk analysis for alcohol consumption: Determining indicators and empirical weights for patterns of drinking, deciding about the theoretical minimum, and dealing with differential consequences. *European Addiction Research* 7, 138–47.

Rehm J., Room R., Monteiro M., *et al.* (2003) Alcohol as a risk factor for burden of disease. In: World Health Organization (ed.) *Comparative quantification of health risks: Global and regional burden of disease due to selected major risk factors.* Geneva: World Health Organization.

Reitan T.C. (2000) Does alcohol matter? Public health in Russia and the Baltic countries before, during, and after the transition. *Contemporary Drug Problems* 27, 511–60.

Rogers J.D. and Greenfield T.K. (1999) Beer drinking accounts for most of the hazardous alcohol consumption reported in the United States. *Journal of Studies on Alcohol* 60, 732–9.

Room R. and Mäkelä K. (2000) Typologies of the cultural position of drinking. *Journal of Studies on Alcohol* 61, 475–83.

Room R., Janca A., Bennett L.A., *et al.* (1996) WHO cross-cultural applicability research on diagnosis and assessment of substance use disorders: An overview of methods and selected results. *Addiction* 91, 199–220.

Room R., Jernigan D., Carlini-Marlatt B., *et al.* (2002) *Alcohol and the developing world: A public health perspective.* Helsinki: Finnish Foundation for Alcohol Studies.

San José B., van Oers J.A.M., van de Mheen H., *et al.* (2000) Drinking patterns and health outcomes: Occasional versus regular drinking. *Addiction* 95, 865–72.

Shkolnikov V.M. and Nemtsov A. (1997) The anti-alcohol campaign and variations in Russian mortality. In: Bobadilla J.L., Costello C.A., and Mitchell F. (eds.) *Premature death in the New Independent States*, pp. 239–61. Washington, DC: National Academy Press.

Simpura J. (1998) Mediterranean mysteries: Mechanisms of declining alcohol consumption. *Addiction* 93, 1301–4.

Simpura J., Levin B., and Mustonen H. (1997) Russian drinking in the 1990s: Patterns and trends in international comparison. In: Simpura J. and Levin B. (eds.) *Demystifying Russian drinking: Comparative studies from the 1990s*, pp. 79–107. Helsinki: STAKES.

Simpura J., Tigerstedt C., Hanhinen S., *et al.* (1999) Alcohol misuse as a health and social issue in the Baltic Sea region: A summary of findings from the Baltica Study. *Alcohol and Alcoholism* 34, 805–23.

Single E. (1993) Public drinking. In: Galanter M. (ed.) *Recent developments in alcoholism*, Vol. 11, *Ten years of progress*, pp. 143–52. New York: Plenum Press.

Single E., Beaubrun M., Mauffret M., *et al.* (1997) Public drinking, problems and prevention measures in twelve countries: Results of the WHO project on public drinking. *Contemporary Drug Problems* 24, 425–48.

Skog O.-J. (1985) The collectivity of drinking cultures. A theory of the distribution of alcohol consumption. *British Journal of Addiction* 80, 83–99.

Skog O.-J. (1991) Drinking and the distribution of alcohol consumption. In: Pittman D.J. and White H. (eds.) *Society, culture, and drinking patterns reexamined*, pp.135–56. New Brunswick: Alcohol Research Documentation.

Skog O.-J. (2001) Commentary on Gmel and Rehm's interpretation of the theory of collectivity in drinking culture. *Drug and Alcohol Review* 20, 325–31.

Smart R.G. (1996) Behavioral and social consequences related to the consumption of different beverage types. *Journal of Studies on Alcohol* 57, 77–84.

Tsunoda T. (1988) Survey of drinking patterns and alcohol-related problems in Japan. In: NIAAA Research Monograph No. 19: *Cultural influences and drinking patterns—A focus on Hispanic and Japanese populations*, pp. 63–78. Rockville, MD: US Department of Health and Human Services, Public Health Service, Alcohol, Drug Abuse, and Mental Health Administration, National Institute on Alcohol Abuse and Alcoholism.

Tuyns A.J., Pequignot G., and Abbatucci J.S. (1979) Oesophageal cancer and alcohol consumption; importance of type of beverage. *International Journal of Cancer* 23, 443–7.

Van der Burgh C. and Rocha Silva L. (1988) Drinking in the Republic of South Africa, 1962–1982. *Contemporary Drug Problems* 15, 447–70.

Wei H., Derson Y., Shuiyuan X., *et al.* (1999) Alcohol consumption and alcohol-related problems: Chinese experience from six area samples, 1994. *Addiction* 94, 1467–76.

Weisner C., Conell C., Hunkeler E.M., *et al.* (2000) Drinking patterns and problems of the 'stably insured': A study of the membership of a health maintenance organization. *Journal of Studies on Alcohol* 61, 121–9.

White S. (1996) *Russia goes dry: Alcohol, state and society.* Cambridge: Cambridge University Press.

Willis J. (2001) *Alcohol in East Africa, 1850–1999.* Durham: Durham University, History Department. Website: http://www.dur.ac.uk/History/web/cover.htm

WHO. See World Health Organization.

World Health Organization (1999) *Global status report on alcohol.* WHO/HSC/SAB/99.11. Geneva: WHO Substance Abuse Department.

World Health Organization (2000a) *International guide for monitoring alcohol consumption and related harm.* Geneva, Switzerland: WHO Department of Mental Health and Substance Dependence, Noncommunicable Diseases and Mental Health Cluster.

World Health Organization (2000b) *The World Health Report 2000—Health systems: Improving performance.* Geneva, Switzerland: WHO.

World Health Organization (2002) *The World Mental Health (WMH2000) initiative.* Geneva: Assessment, Classification, and Epidemiology Group, WHO. Website: http://www.hcp.med.harvard.edu/icpe/WMH2000.html

Chapter 4

The global burden of alcohol consumption

4 1 Introduction

This chapter describes the enormous range of alcohol-related consequences within two broad categories: alcohol's contribution to the burden of illness carried by individuals and societies, and alcohol's harmful effect on the social fabric of families, communities, and nations. It also discusses the beneficial effects of alcohol, and considers their implications for estimating the burden of illness.

Establishing that alcohol consumption is a direct cause of various social and health problems is a task with great significance for public health. If a social or health problem is at least in part attributable to drinking, the evidence generally helps to suggest specific measures to prevent or control the problem. Quantifying the strength of the relationship is an additional tool in making decisions about policy priorities, also taking into account the prevalence of the particular problem. For instance, the invention of reliable instruments to measure **blood alcohol concentration (BAC)** opened the way for the scientific study of drinking–driving behaviour. The result was a recognition that drinking was implicated in a much larger share of traffic fatalities than had been previously thought. This eventually led to substantial policy changes concerning drinking–driving. On the other hand, routine measurement of BAC can also result in overestimation of alcohol's role, as when alcohol's presence in the situation is equated with causality.

We begin with a discussion of methodological issues in establishing causal relations between drinking and its consequences. We then consider the evidence on health consequences in three areas:

1. Alcohol's role in the global burden of disease and disability.

2. Alcohol and all-cause mortality.

3. Alcohol's relation to some specific causes of death and disease.

The relation of drinking to different types of social problems is then considered. A case study of the Russian experience in the anti-alcohol campaign of

1985–1987 is used to illustrate the potential changes in health and social problems that follow from reductions in alcohol consumption. Before turning to conclusions, the available evidence is considered on the relative magnitude of health and social problems from drinking.

4.2 Measurement and inferential issues

4.2.1 The nature of health and social problems

To varying degrees, different health and social problems have both an objective element and an element that is a matter of social definition. At one end of the continuum, the fact of death can be measured objectively and reliably. But when it is necessary to divide deaths into different categories (or 'causes of death', as they are conventionally called), social definition becomes important. In standard medical classifications, a death from a gunshot wound, for instance, can be variously coded as an open wound of the head or as a suicide by firearms. For both acute and chronic causes of death, national recording and coding practices often vary from one country to another (e.g., Ramstedt 2002). For health problems short of death, social definition plays an even larger role. The threshold at which a potential disability is socially noticeable varies between cultures (Room *et al.* 2001). Despite these difficulties, there has been substantial progress in international efforts to employ codes for causes of death and disease that are cross-culturally applicable (see WHO 1992). While this effort has contributed to the advance of epidemiology and other health sciences (WHO 2001), the apparent objectivity of the international classification system should not obscure the fact that an element of social definition is still present.

While internationally comparable statistics by causes of death have long been available, and there are now similar data on hospitalizations by cause (at least for established market economies), there are no cross-nationally comparable data on disabilities (Goerdt *et al.* 1996; Rehm and Gmel 2000a), since the revised system for classifying and recording disability has only recently been adopted by the World Health Organization, that is, the *International classification of function, disability and health* (ICF; cf. WHO 2001). The paucity of data on morbidity and disability is especially problematic for estimates of alcohol's role, as there are indications that alcohol is more related to disability than to mortality (Murray and Lopez 1996; see below).

For social problems, as the term itself implies, the element of social definition becomes more prominent. Child marriage and polygamy are accepted customs in some societies, but would be defined as social problems and indeed crimes in others. Even within a given society, the existence of a social problem is itself often a matter of judgement and dispute—the partners in a couple may disagree about whether there is a marital problem at all. And often the way social matters are thought about in a given society changes over time. In English-speaking societies around 1900, for instance, divorce was commonly viewed as a social problem, and the then-difficult process of getting a divorce created legally defined categories of divorce, such as divorce due to the partner's inebriety. The shift in many jurisdictions in recent decades to 'no-fault divorce' abolished these categories (Room 1996).

Scientific progress depends on objective definitions and measures. For this reason, the role of alcohol as a causal factor in disease is presently more clearly understood scientifically than the role of alcohol in the causation of social harm. Nevertheless, reliable measurement and cross-national comparisons are not only possible for many social problems, but are also useful for public policy purposes.

4.2.2 Alcohol as a cause

In classifications of disease and crime, some categories are alcohol specific. For instance, the category of 'alcohol poisoning' in the *International classification of diseases* (ICD) specifies a causal role of alcohol in the death or injury; this causal attribution is usually accepted without question. The 'attributable fraction', defined as the proportion of cases in the category assumed to be caused by drinking, is thus set at 1.0 or 100% for these conditions. But the causal attribution built into these categories is substantially influenced by social factors. The doctor or health worker making the attribution to alcohol may be over-sensitive to a potential alcohol attribution. More commonly, however, alcohol's involvement in a death may be missed by those certifying the death, or may deliberately not be mentioned in order to protect the reputation of the deceased. Thus a landmark study of death recording in 12 cities in 10 countries found that, after supplementing data from the death certificate with data from hospital records and interviews with attending physicians and family members, the net number of deaths assigned to the ICD category 'liver cirrhosis with mention of alcoholism' rose by 135%, with the majority of the new cases recoded from categories of cirrhosis without mention of alcoholism (Puffer and Griffith 1967, p. 167).

For other categories of death, disease, disability, and crime, alcohol's involvement may be a matter of increased probability rather than certainty. Thus, some of those who die in traffic accidents where a driver had been drinking would have died even if there had been no drinking (Reed 1981) because the other driver may have been at fault. To measure the role of alcohol in this wider range of categories, then, it is necessary to draw on epidemiological and other studies to estimate relative risk (i.e., how much particular levels and patterns of drinking increase the risk) for each of the disease categories where alcohol is potentially involved. For some causes of death—notably for casualties—the relative risk varies between cultures and countries. After combining information on the relative risk with prevalence data on the relevant levels and patterns of drinking, the attributable fraction (i.e., the proportion of the disease attributable to drinking) can then be calculated for a particular society or group of similar societies.

It should be noted that alcohol's causal role in social and health problems is usually contributory, being only one of several factors responsible for the problem. For example, hepatitis and malnutrition may be involved in a cirrhosis death, as well as heavy drinking. Ice on the road and poor street lighting may play a causal role in a traffic crash, along with drinking by a driver. The kind of causation of interest to epidemiologists is based on the following question: Would the event or condition have occurred in the absence of the drinking?

Determination of causality may vary between classes of consequences and, implicitly, according to the causal logic of the underlying sciences (Rehm and Fischer 1997; Pernanen 2001). For health outcomes, the usual epidemiological definitions have been used, which stress not only consistent relations but also biological pathways (Rothman and Greenland 1998). Thus, the consistent relationship between alcohol and lung cancer found in many epidemiological studies (English *et al.* 1995) is not included here as an alcohol-attributable disease because no biological pathway has yet been identified, and because the higher incidence of lung cancer in drinkers is believed to be caused by smoking (Bandera *et al.* 2001).

This example is interesting from another perspective. One might argue that smoking, or the persistence of smoking, is part of a causal chain linked to alcohol (Rothman and Greenland 1998). If such a causal relationship could be established, then some cases of lung cancer would be attributable to drinking. Despite the consistent relationship between alcohol and smoking, lung cancer has not been included in this overview because the evidence of alcohol *causing* smoking was not judged to be sufficient. Current knowledge seems to indicate that both behaviours stem from common third causes (Little 2000). In this decision, as in other decisions underlying this chapter, care was taken not to overstate the impact of alcohol.

While the causal status of the relationship between alcohol and health outcomes often depends on the plausibility of potential biological pathways, the causal status of the relationships between alcohol and social harm cannot usually be determined this way. An exception is aggressive behaviour. A causal link between alcohol intoxication and aggression has been supported by epidemiological and experimental research, as well as by research indicating specific biological mechanisms linking alcohol to aggressive behaviour. For example, several epidemiological studies have found that the relationship between usual drinking pattern and aggression disappears when drinking at the time of the violence is taken into account (Collins and Schlenger 1988; Wiley and Weisner 1995). This indicates that the positive association between heavy drinking and aggression is related to the effects of alcohol, and is not just an artefact of heavier drinkers being more aggressive people generally. Experimental studies of the effects of alcohol on aggressive behaviour in controlled conditions also suggest a causal relationship between alcohol and aggression (Bushman and Cooper 1990; Bushman 1997), although this relationship is clearly moderated by a number of variables, including sex and personality of the drinker as well as situational and cultural factors (Lipsey *et al.* 1997; Graham *et al.* 1998). There is also a growing body of evidence supporting several potential biological pathways for alcohol to increase aggressive behaviour. One pathway links the effects of alcohol on risk-taking and aggression to the anxiolytic effects of alcohol, which are mediated through the GABA brain receptors (Pihl *et al.* 1993). In support of this mechanism, animal research has found that benzodiazepine agonists potentiate the effects of alcohol on aggression while benzodiazepine antagonists reduce this effect (Miczek *et al.* 1993, 1997). Alcohol has a number of other effects on the brain, including the impairment of cognitive functioning (Peterson *et al.* 1990), which can reduce problem-solving ability (Sayette *et al.* 1993) and thereby contribute to aggression.

For other social problems, the issue of alcohol attribution, and how much of a given problem should be attributed to alcohol, has no easy solution. As already noted, there are some social problems that are by definition wholly attributable to alcohol; for instance, arrests for public drunkenness or for drinking in public, where these are against the law. For some social problems, an alternative is to define an attributable fraction by aggregate-level studies, examining how much the rate of the social problem changes in a population when drinking patterns or the level of alcohol consumption change. For many social problems, there may be record keeping attribution by a police officer, social worker, or other professional dealing with the problem. Other possible sources of attribution, much used in population surveys, are the drinker's own attribution of causality to alcohol, and the attributions of the drinker's family members, friends, bystanders, or victims. There is often considerable variation in attribution between observers of the same phenomenon, and this methodology has been criticized because respondents' attributions may not be sufficient evidence of causality (see Gmel *et al.* 2000). But such attributions sometimes constitute the essence of the social problem and thus become part of the data. For example, if someone considers that his or her spouse's drinking causes problems, then that belief, in itself, tends to mean that there is a relationship problem connected to the drinking.

In addition to the consistency of empirical evidence from all these sources, theoretical underpinnings and methodology play an important role in making inferences about alcohol's contribution to social harm.

4.2.3 The role of average volume and drinking patterns

So far we have only spoken about relationships between alcohol and problems in general terms. Clearly, different dimensions of alcohol consumption have to be distinguished to arrive at a better understanding of such relationships. In this chapter, as in the previous one, we distinguish between two dimensions: average alcohol consumption and drinking patterns. Drinking patterns include but are not limited to heavy drinking occasions. For each category of alcohol-related consequences, the potential influence of these two broad dimensions of alcohol consumption will be examined.

For instance, one study showed that **all-cause mortality** in light-to-moderate male drinkers (<2 drinks a day) was about twice as high if they had occasional heavy drinking episodes (Rehm *et al.* 2001a). Heavy drinking occasions not only play a role in mortality, but also are very important contributions to acute consequences, particularly accidents and injuries. Thus, any discussion of the relationship between alcohol consumption and consequences needs to take into account both the nature of the problem (health vs. social), and the dimension of drinking involved (average volume vs. pattern of drinking).

4.2.4 Evidence on alcohol's role: individual- and population-level research

Death, disability, and social problems affect individuals, and there is thus an inherent interest in the following question: At the individual level, what is alcohol's causal role in harm or benefits? An equally important question, especially from a public health perspective, is the following: At the population level, what happens if there is an increase or decrease in alcohol consumption, or a change in the drinking pattern? The answers to these two questions often point in the same direction, but not always (Skog 1996). A change that is beneficial for some individuals may be harmful for the population as a whole, and vice versa. Complicating this issue is the fact that each level of analysis has its own difficulties in measurement and in causal attribution. Establishing causality from aggregate changes is quite complex because it is difficult to control for other factors as confounders (Morgenstern 1998).

To better understand these phenomena, epidemiologists have developed a variety of research methods that can be roughly divided into medical epidemiology and population-level analyses. With many of the health and social problems related to drinking, the causal role of alcohol cannot be discerned from the individual case. Since the role of alcohol in these circumstances is neither necessary nor sufficient, the establishment of cause depends in part on the degree of statistical association in a large sample of cases. Thus the material of an aetiological study in medical epidemiology commonly involves summarizing and comparing the individual outcomes across a large sample of cases.

Nevertheless, in most of these studies the sample does not represent the experience of a whole population. This experience is represented by another type of evidence, population-level analyses, particularly **time–series analyses** looking at the co-variation from one point in time to another between an alcohol variable and a potential outcome variable. In recent years, the number of time–series analyses has grown considerably in the alcohol field. But like other aggregate-level research methods, time–series studies have problems controlling for confounding variables and **disaggregating** the exposure variable into sex- or age-specific measures. Another limitation is ambiguity in the interpretation of the theoretical meaning of the exposure (especially in the interpretation of the contribution of heavy drinkers).

On the other hand, medical epidemiological studies at the individual level suffer from their own characteristic faults (Edwards *et al.* 1994, pp. 44–50). The measurement of alcohol consumption typically depends on self-report, with all the problems of underestimation that this entails. Most such studies have paid little attention to drinking pattern. It is uncommon for studies to measure consumption at more than one point in the lifetime, although amounts consumed and patterns of drinking often vary over time. For health conditions or social problems with a chronic aspect, the cumulative impact of drinking over time has not been studied extensively. And even when such studies are carried out, they are conducted in a limited range of countries, with highly selected cohorts (e.g., doctors or nurses) that may not be representative of the general population.

If the results from individual-level and population-level studies point in the same direction, our confidence in the findings is increased substantially. Such is the case, for instance, with studies of the relation of drinking to homicide. But if the results do not point in the same direction, judgements must be made about the relative weight of evidence from the different studies. Despite the complexity involved in establishing causal relations between alcohol and problems, and the difficulties of estimating the strength and prevalence of these relations, the science of alcohol epidemiology has advanced to the point that alcohol's specific role in a variety of health and social problems is now much more clearly understood, as the remainder of this chapter will show.

4.3 Alcohol consumption and health consequences

To estimate the burden of disease attributable to alcohol-related health consequences, it is necessary to take into account both its deleterious and beneficial effects. Deleterious effects stem from alcohol's contribution to many chronic disease conditions (see English *et al.* 1995; Gutjahr *et al.* 2001; or Rehm *et al.* 2003), as well as accidents, injuries, and acute toxic effects. Box 4.1 describes the major conditions associated with alcohol-related morbidity and mortality. In addition, some specific drinking patterns have been found to have beneficial effects on coronary heart disease and ischaemic stroke (see contributions in Chadwick and Goode 1998; Puddey *et al.* 1999). The relationship between alcohol consumption and diabetes is not clear, but there is suggestive evidence for a beneficial effect of light-to-moderate drinking (see Ashley *et al.* 2000).

Box 4.1 Major alcohol-related health conditions contributing to morbidity and mortality[a]

1. **Cancers:** head and neck cancers as well as cancers of the gastrointestinal tract, liver cancer, and female breast cancer.

2. **Neuropsychiatric conditions:** alcohol-dependence syndrome, alcohol abuse, depression, anxiety disorder, organic brain disease.

3. **Cardiovascular conditions:** ischaemic heart disease, cerebrovascular disease.

4. **Gastrointestinal conditions:** alcoholic liver cirrhosis, cholelithiasis, pancreatitis.

5. **Maternal and perinatal conditions:** low birth weight, intrauterine growth retardation.

6. **Acute toxic effects:** alcohol poisoning.

7. **Accidents:** road and other transport injuries, fall, drowning and burning injuries, occupational and machine injuries.

8. **Self-inflicted injuries:** suicide.

9. **Violent deaths:** assault injuries.

[a] Based on overview studies (see Gutjahr *et al.* 2001 for details).

4.3.1 **Alcohol and all-cause mortality**

All-cause mortality is one potential summary measure for combining different alcohol effects. Using this measure, some of the complex relations between alcohol consumption and mortality rate can be illustrated. Figure 4.1 shows the effects of alcohol on male adults under 45 in the US (Rehm *et al.* 2001b). The relationship between average volume of alcohol consumed and all-cause mortality is almost linear in this age group. This reflects the fact that most beneficial effects of alcohol on mortality concern older age groups only.

Figures 4.2 and 4.3 show the relationship between average volume consumed and all-cause mortality for older age groups of men and women, respectively (Rehm *et al.* 2001a, b). For both genders, relationships are J-shaped, with the females experiencing deleterious effects at lower levels of alcohol consumption. These curves can be interpreted as reflecting the beneficial effects of moderate alcohol consumption on coronary heart disease (see Box 4.2) and ischaemic stroke, together with the detrimental effects of alcohol on many other chronic diseases.

Up to this point, only average volume has been considered. Based on recent research on drinking patterns and all-cause mortality, there should be no beneficial effects for patterns with heavy drinking occasions and more pronounced beneficial effects for patterns without such occasions (Rehm *et al.* 2001a). Thus sex, age, and different dimensions of alcohol consumption influence the effect of alcohol on all-cause mortality. In addition, the underlying mix of causes of death for all-cause mortality influences the exact shape of the risk curve (Rehm 2000; Rehm *et al.* 2001a).

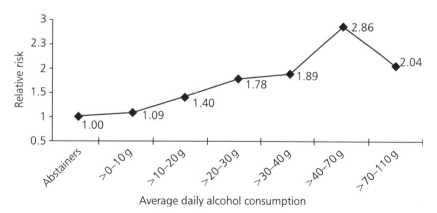

Fig. 4.1 Average daily alcohol consumption (in grams) and risk of all-cause mortality (males below age 45) (Rehm *et al.* 2001a, b).

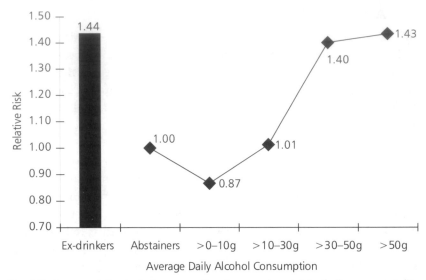

Fig. 4.2 Average daily alcohol consumption (in grams) and risk of all-cause mortality (females age 45 and over) (Rehm *et al.* 2001a, b).

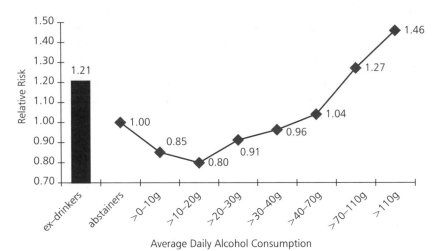

Fig. 4.3 Average daily alcohol consumption (in grams) and risk of all-cause mortality (males age 45 and over) (Rehm *et al.* 2001a, b).

In the following paragraphs (and in Boxes 4.2 to 4.5), we consider the evidence for some of the most important disease conditions related to alcohol: coronary heart disease, breast cancer, motor vehicle accidents, and suicide. Each box summarizes the research evidence derived from individual-level studies and studies based on population (aggregate-level) time–series analyses. Except for traffic accidents, the focus of this research is primarily on mortality. Evidence from **meta-analytic reviews** and key studies is summarized in terms of the effects of total volume of alcohol consumed, moderate drinking, drinking pattern, plausible biological mechanisms, and interactions with factors that mediate or moderate the relationship between alcohol and the condition. Boxes 4.6 through 4.9 summarize the evidence for physical, psychological, and social effects of alcohol on violence, marital problems, child abuse, and work-related problems.

4.3.2 Coronary heart disease (CHD)

Box 4.2 summarizes the evidence for coronary heart disease. In individual-level studies, which have been carried out mainly in developed societies, the

---

Box 4.2 **Effects of alcohol on coronary heart disease (ICD-9 410–414)**

Individual-level studies

1. **Volume of alcohol.** All meta-analytic reviews found significant beneficial effects (Maclure 1993; English *et al.* 1995; Single *et al.* 1999; Corrao *et al.* 2000). There is some indication of detrimental effects of heavy drinking (Rehm *et al.* 1997; Corrao *et al.* 2000).

2. **Moderate drinking.** Significant beneficial effect in meta-analytic studies.

3. **Patterns of drinking.** Binge drinking was detrimentally related to CHD (Bondy 1996; Puddey *et al.* 1999).

4. **Mechanisms.** Plausible hypotheses (blood lipids, blood coagulation) not yet fully clarified but increasing biological evidence (Alcohol Health and Research World 1997; Single *et al.* 2000).

5. **Interactions.** No consistent interaction found; some beverages found to be more protective but this may only indicate that beverage preference is a marker for other factors (see also Rimm *et al.* 1996).

Aggregate-level studies

Skog (1983) found a weak negative association between *per capita* alcohol consumption and ischaemic heart disease mortality for those 60 years and older (Norway), suggesting a cardioprotective effect.

Hemström (2001) found mainly random co-variation between *per capita* consumption of alcohol and CHD in 15 countries. A slight indication of a cardioprotective effect of alcohol among 30- to 44-year-old women in high consumption countries was observed (significant for Italy). Mean alcohol effect estimates were close to zero (absent alcohol effect) among men and otherwise weakly positive among women.

relationship between alcohol consumption and CHD is negative overall, indicating a cardioprotective effect. As noted above, this effect explains the lower death rate of light drinkers relative to abstainers. It has been found consistently in many studies, even after adjusting for potential confounders (e.g., diet, see Rehm *et al.* 1997; social isolation, Murray *et al.* 1999), and after correcting for the **sick-quitter effect** (Shaper *et al.* 1988; Shaper 1990a, b). The evidence for biological mechanisms is strong but not fully conclusive (Zakhari 1997). At least half of the effect seems to be short-term (mainly in terms of preventing blood clots), so there may be little benefit from sporadic drinking, the most common drinking pattern in developing countries.

With respect to heavy drinking, the results are less clear, with some studies indicating detrimental effects, especially for females (Rehm *et al.* 1997; Corrao *et al.* 2000). Heavy binge drinking, as is common in Russia, is associated with increased deaths from CHD. Thus when total consumption dropped by an estimated 25% in Russia between 1985 and 1988, deaths from circulatory disease, including CHD, dropped by 9% among males and 6% among females (Shkolnikov and Nemtsov 1997; Leon *et al.* 1998).

Aggregate level studies reveal no significant effect beyond that expected from random variation (Hemström 2001). This result is consistent with the postulate that changes in the level of drinking in a population are spread through the whole population (Skog 1996), so that those whose hearts benefit from a rise in consumption are matched by those whose hearts are harmed by the rise. A recent multi-level analysis produced results consistent with individual-level studies, i.e., beneficial effects for countries where drinking patterns are mainly regular (often with meals), and detrimental effects for countries with more irregular patterns and heavy drinking occasions (Rehm *et al.* 2003).

Overall, there is general support for the cardioprotective effect of regular, light, and moderate alcohol consumption at the level of the individual drinker. This effect applies mainly to the age group of 40 years and older, where the overwhelming majority of CHD occurs (e.g., Murray and Lopez 1996; for the relationship to alcohol by age, see Rehm and Sempos 1995a, b). However, the public health implications of this conclusion are limited. The aggregate-level studies suggest that there may be no net protective effect at the population level from an increase in the level of consumption, and little protective or even a detrimental effect in societies where drinking patterns are sporadic.

In considering the public health implications of the individual-level cardio-protective findings, attention must be paid to strategies that increase the number of light regular drinkers without significantly increasing the number of heavy drinkers. If a segment of the population could successfully be encouraged to have one drink every day or every second day, they would obtain most of the heart benefits (Criqui 1994, 1996) without experiencing alcohol-related problems. But there is very little evidence for effective strategies to accomplish this goal (as discussed later in this book): if there is an increase in consumption in the light-drinking segment of the population, there tends to be an increase in the heavier-drinking segment as well. As noted above, this tendency is consistent with the finding of no significant effect in the aggregate-level CHD studies.

4.3.3 **Breast cancer**

As shown in Box 4.3, alcohol seems to have a small dose-dependent effect on breast cancer (Singletary and Gapstur 2001). There is a likely interaction with hormones, especially oestrogen. With respect to drinking patterns, binge drinking may be related to higher risks, but the evidence is only suggestive. Some studies show differences among alcoholic beverages in the relationship to breast cancer, but beverage preference may be a marker for other factors. We conclude that there is a modest relationship of volume of drinking to breast cancer.

Box 4.3 **Effects of alcohol on breast cancer and/or breast carcinoma (ICD-9 174; 233.0)**

Individual-level studies

1. **Volume of alcohol.** All meta-analytic reviews after English *et al.* (1995) found significant detrimental effects (Smith-Warner *et al.* 1998; Corrao *et al.* 1999; Single *et al.* 1999; Gutjahr *et al.* 2001).

2. **Moderate drinking.** Significant detrimental effect in meta-analytic studies, even if tested not as a linear trend but categorically (Corrao *et al.* 1999).

3. **Patterns of drinking.** Trend for binge drinking (Kinney *et al.* 2000); hypotheses by Kohlmeier and Mendez (1997).

4. **Mechanisms.** Plausible hypotheses; not yet fully clarified (Single *et al.* 2000).

5. **Interactions.** Oestrogen, oestradiol (pre- vs. post-menopausal women) in many studies (Ginsburg *et al.* 1996; Ginsburg 1999).

Aggregate-level studies

No studies available.

4.3.4 **Traffic injuries and deaths**

Motor vehicle crashes are clearly linked to alcohol (Box 4.4). A dose–response relationship has been demonstrated with respect to level of consumption prior to driving, with a threshold for negative consequences estimated at 40 mg% (0.04%) (Eckardt *et al.* 1998). Biological evidence supports this relationship. There is some indication of positive effects below this threshold for experienced drinkers, but the evidence is not extensive. There is a relationship between accidents and average volume, but it is not clear whether this relationship is independent of drinking patterns. At the population level, changes in the legal BAC

Box 4.4 **Effects of alcohol on injuries and deaths from motor vehicle crashes (ICD 9 E810–E819)**

Individual-level studies

1. **Volume of alcohol.** Volume of drinking is related to risk of traffic crashes (Midanik *et al.* 1996). It is not clear if this effect is independent of patterns of drinking (see Rehm and Gmel 2000b); e.g., if the relationship is only a reflection of the correlation between heavy drinking occasions and volume and between such occasions and crashes.

2. **Moderate drinking.** Threshold for negative effect of alcohol on subjective and psychomotor performance measures when alcohol blood alcohol concentrations are 40 mg%[a] or higher (around 0.4 gm pure alcohol/kg). Subjective feelings of being 'intoxicated' occur as low as 0.25 gm pure alcohol/kg or BACs from 10 mg% to 30 mg% (Eckardt *et al.* 1998). There are indications of a J-shaped dose–response curve on subjective measures and psychomotor performance measures. The positive effects occur at very low levels of consumption, however.

3. **Patterns of drinking.** As psychomotor performance is linked to acute intake of alcohol, there is a strong effect of patterns (Gruenewald *et al.* 1996; Eckardt *et al.* 1998; Rossow *et al.* 2001).

4. **Mechanisms.** At the neurochemical level, consumption of ethanol affects the function of GABA, glutamatergic, serotonergic, dopaminergic, cholinergic, and opioid neuronal systems. Ethanol can affect these systems directly, and the interactions among these systems become important in the expression of ethanol's actions (Eckardt *et al.* 1998).

Effects of alcohol on injuries and deaths from motor vehicle crashes (ICD 9 E810–E819) *(continued)*

5. **Interactions.** There is some evidence that there is adaptation or learning, and that the adverse effect on performance is less in experienced drinkers (Cherpitel 1996; Rossow *et al.* 2001). There is some indication of differences between beverages, but beverages may just be proxies for other variables (e.g., Gruenewald and Ponicki 1995).

Aggregate-level studies

Fatal accident rates increase with increased *per capita* consumption in many European countries (Skog 2001). Numerous studies show that interventions like reducing legal BAC limits are associated with reductions in traffic crashes (Mann *et al.* 2001).

[a] This corresponds to 0.04 gm/100 ml (0.04%) or 0.4 gm/1000 ml.

level have an effect on rates of motor vehicle crashes, especially single-vehicle night-time crashes associated with drinking–driving (Mann *et al.* 2001). This strongly supports the findings from individual-level case-control studies of the important role of alcohol in motor vehicle accidents.

4.3.5 Suicide

The relationship between alcohol and suicide or parasuicide (attempted suicide) is well established for heavy drinkers (Rossow 2000), both from individual- and aggregate-level studies (Box 4.5). The strength of the overall relationship seems to vary between cultures. Individual- and aggregate-level studies both suggest that more 'explosive' drinking patterns (e.g., irregular, heavy drinking occasions) are linked to a higher incidence of suicide.

4.3.6 Alcohol in the global burden of disease

According to the Global Burden of Disease study sponsored by the World Health Organization and the World Bank (Murray and Lopez 1996; Murray and Lopez 1997b; WHO 2002), in 2000 alcohol-related death and disability accounted for 4.0% of the total cost to life and longevity. Ranking as the fifth most detrimental risk factor of 26 examined, alcohol accounts for about the same amount of global burden of disease as tobacco (4.1%) (Ezzati *et al.* 2002). In developed countries, alcohol was the third most detrimental risk factor, accounting for 9.2% of all burden of disease, with only tobacco (12.2%) and

Box 4.5 Effects of alcohol on suicide (ICD-9 E950–E959)

Individual-level studies

1. **Volume of alcohol.** Some studies indicate a linear relationship between consumption level and risk of suicidal behaviour (e.g., Andréasson *et al.* 1988; Dawson 1997). A large number of studies have demonstrated a significantly increased risk of suicide and parasuicide among alcohol abusers/heavy drinkers (Rossow 2000; Rossow *et al.* 2001).

2. **Moderate drinking.** No protective effect of moderate drinking, but rather a slightly increased risk (e.g., Andréasson *et al.* 1988; Dawson 1997).

3. **Patterns of drinking.** Some studies have demonstrated increased risk of suicide with increasing frequency of intoxication (Rossow and Wichstrøm 1994; Dawson 1997), and an apparently stronger association with intoxication frequency than with consumption level (Dawson 1997).

4. **Theoretical underpinnings.** Plausible hypotheses: social disintegration, social losses, and mental illness suggested as intermediate factors (Skog 1991; Murphy 2000).

5. **Interactions.** Psychiatric co-morbidity increases the risk of suicidal behaviour among alcohol abusers (Murphy 2000). The relationship also seems to vary based on cultural norms (see aggregate-level studies).

Aggregate-level studies

Suicide rates are found to increase with increased *per capita* consumption in a number of studies (Rossow 2000; Ramstedt 2001), yet the strength of the association varies considerably, tending to be higher in countries with an 'explosive' drinking pattern than in other countries, and remaining insignificant in some countries (Norström 1988; Gmel *et al.* 1998; Ramstedt 2001). The impact of drinking pattern is supported by cross-cultural comparisons of the aggregate-level associations, i.e., a stronger association in drinking cultures where intoxication is a more prominent characteristic (Norström 1988; Norström 1995; Ramstedt 2001).

high blood pressure (10.9%) causing more harm. In emerging economies like China, alcohol in the year 2000 was the most detrimental risk factor, with 6.2% of the burden of disease attributable to drinking, followed by blood pressure (5.0%) and tobacco (4.0%) (see Ezzati *et al.* 2002 for details). It should be noted that the figures for alcohol reported here take into account the beneficial effects on CHD. Burden of disease in all these estimates is quantified in terms of Disability Adjusted Life Years (DALYs), a composite health summary measure used to estimate the burden of disease in a given country (Murray *et al.* 2000), that combines years of life lost to premature death with years of life lost due to disability. In this calculation, disability is indirectly calculated from morbidity, where the time lived with disease is multiplied by a disease-specific weight. For example, major depression has a weight of 0.6, which means that an episode of depression in a single individual lasting two years would be counted as 1.2 DALYs (2 × 0.6). Disease-specific weights were derived from expert evaluations (for details see Murray and Lopez 1997a) using standard methodologies (Drummond *et al.* 1997).

Global alcohol-attributable DALYs are summarized in Table 4.1. Overall, injuries account for the largest portion of alcohol-attributable disease burden as measured in DALYs, at 40%, with unintentional injuries far outweighing intentional injuries. The second largest category in alcohol-attributable disease burden is neuropsychiatric disease, comprising 38% of the burden. Neuropsychiatric diseases and disorders such as depression are often disabling, but not lethal, and this is reflected in the markedly higher proportion of overall disease burden caused by this category, compared to alcohol-attributable mortality (38% of alcohol-attributable DALYs; 6% of alcohol-attributable deaths) (see Rehm *et al.* 2003). The next categories are about equal in size and each accounts for 6–8% of the global disease burden. These categories cover 'other non-communicable diseases' (diabetes and liver cirrhosis), malignant neoplasms, and cardiovascular disease. The DALYs in Table 4.1 again are net figures, where the alcohol-related beneficial effects on disease have already been subtracted. Overall, the detrimental effects of alcohol on disease burden by far outweigh the beneficial effects.

Males have a far higher alcohol-related disease burden than females, with a ratio of about 5 to 1. This ratio is much larger in developing regions, as the vast majority of drinking is confined to males in most of these countries. As shown in Table 4.2, there are also tremendous differences between regions. The alcohol-attributable disease burden ranges from close to zero among females in the predominantly Moslem Eastern Mediterranean regions to more than 20% for males in the eastern part of Europe, with Russia as the largest country in this region (Rehm *et al.* 2003).

Table 4.1 Global burden of disease (DALYs in 1000s) in 2000 attributable to alcohol by major disease categories (adapted from Rehm *et al.* 2003)

Disease conditions	Males		Females		Both genders	
	DALYs	**%**	**DALYs**	**%**	**DALYs**	**%**
Conditions arising during the perinatal period	68	0.14	55	0.62	123	0.21
Malignant neoplasm	3180	6.44	1021	11.44	4201	7.20
Neuropsychiatric conditions	18 090	36.62	3814	42.73	21 904	37.56
Cardiovascular diseases	4411	8.93	−428	−4.79	3983	6.83
Other non-communicable diseases (diabetes, liver cirrhosis)	3695	7.48	860	9.63	4555	7.81
Unintentional injuries	14 008	28.36	2487	27.86	16 495	28.28
Intentional injuries	5945	12.04	1117	12.51	7062	12.11
Alcohol-related disease burden all causes (DALYs)	49 397	100.00	8926	100.00	58 323	100.00

Table 4.2 Alcohol-attributable disease burden in DALYs (in 1000s) in 2000 by WHO region (from Rehm *et al.* 2003)

Region[a]	Total alcohol-attributable DALYs		Per cent of all disease burden	
	Male	**Female**	**Male**	**Female**
Africa D	1441	393	2.0	0.6
Africa E	3621	785	3.5	0.8
The Americas A	2925	702	11.9	3.2
The Americas B	7854	1443	17.3	4.1
The Americas D	789	170	8.6	2.2
Eastern Mediterranean B	162	22	1.3	0.2
Eastern Mediterranean D	328	36	0.6	0.1
Europe A	3103	416	11.1	1.6
Europe B	2183	446	10.2	2.5
Europe C	7543	1570	21.5	6.5
South-East Asia B	1793	284	5.3	1.0
South-East Asia D	4927	675	2.8	0.4
Western Pacific A	708	43	8.1	0.6
Western Pacific B	12 020	1941	9.1	1.8
World	49 397	8926	6.5	1.3
World (TOTAL)	58 323		4.0	

[a] See Table 3.1 for a list of countries included in each WHO region.

4.3.7 Alcohol and health consequences

The results presented thus far point to the following conclusions:

1. Volume of drinking is linked to most disease outcomes through specific dose–response relationships. These relationships can be linear (as in the case of breast cancer or suicide), accelerating (as in the case of liver cirrhosis or motor vehicle accidents), or J-shaped (as in the case of heart disease or all-cause mortality).

2. Patterns of drinking also play an important role in both the disease burden and the health benefits of drinking; thus patterns of drinking have been linked to CHD, motor vehicle accidents, and suicide, and are suspected to be linked to breast cancer.

3. Moderate drinking has negative as well as positive health outcomes. It has been linked to an increased risk of cancer and other disease conditions.

4. Many disease conditions have interactions with other factors, which make it difficult to estimate the contribution of alcohol to causation of disease.

5. For some disease conditions, individual- and aggregate-level study results do not converge. This is the case for CHD, where individual-level studies suggest a biologically plausible beneficial effect, and the limited evidence from aggregate studies does not show this effect.

4.4 Alcohol consumption and social harm

Although public discussion has often concentrated on alcohol-related problems connected with disease and other medical conditions, alcohol is also linked to consequences in the social realm, which have been called 'the forgotten dimension' (Klingemann and Gmel 2001). Box 4.6 describes the areas included within this dimension.

The conceptual diversity of these social consequences makes it difficult to evaluate this field systematically. As suggested above, there is no common metric that would allow comparisons between social and medical outcomes, or even within social outcomes alone. Social cost studies have been suggested as such a metric, but these have often excluded social problems (e.g., family problems), for lack of data (Single *et al.* 1998). The overall figures from the cost studies also depend heavily on indirect costs such as productivity losses, which are difficult to estimate (Gutjahr and Gmel 2001a, b).

A second possibility is to work from employment records, social welfare data, and law-court reports. Here, an attribution of the problem to drinking is often made by a third party, such as a social worker, police officer, or employer.

Box 4.6 **Categories of alcohol-related social harm**

Harm category

Violence.[a]

Vandalism.

Public disorder.

Family problems: divorce/marital problems; child abuse.

Other interpersonal problems.

Financial problems.

Work-related problems other than work accidents.[b]

Educational difficulties.

Social costs.

[a] Injuries from violence are also part of accidents and injuries in the morbidity and mortality section.

[b] Work-related accidents are part of accidents and injuries in the morbidity and mortality section.

But alcohol attributions in such records are usually not kept or not available. The main social records system that still routinely provides some data on social problems related to alcohol is police arrests and other criminal justice actions (Aarens *et al.* 1977). In the police records system, the crime may be alcohol specific, or there may be an attribution of it to drinking by the arresting officer, although this is often under-attributed. Victimization surveys supply an alternative method of estimating alcohol-related crimes, but these methods too raise the question of the validity of respondents' attributions.

Boxes 4.7 through 4.10 give some insight into the evidence for selected social consequences. Except for violence, the epidemiological evidence on the extent of alcohol's role in social problems is quite weak.

4.4.1 **Violence**

Individual- as well as aggregate-level studies (Box 4.7) indicate a causal relationship between alcohol consumption and violence (Room and Rossow 2001). The strength of the relationship seems to be culturally dependent. Patterns of drinking, especially drinking to intoxication, seem to play an important role in causing violence. As discussed above, biological and psychological studies support the epidemiological findings.

Box 4.7 **Effects of alcohol on violence**

Individual-level studies

1. **Volume of alcohol.** A number of studies indicate a linear relationship between consumption level and risk of involvement in violent incidents (Dawson 1997; Rossow 2000; Wells *et al.* 2000). A large number of studies have demonstrated a significantly increased risk of involvement in violence among alcohol abusers/heavy drinkers (Pernanen 1991; Rossow *et al.* 2001). Several studies have also shown that heavy drinkers are more likely to be the victims of violence (Room and Rossow 2001; Rossow *et al.* 2001).

2. **Moderate drinking.** Survey studies indicate no protective effect of moderate drinking, but rather a slightly increased risk (Dawson 1997; Rossow 2000; Wells *et al.* 2000). However, experimental research suggests that alcohol does not have a reliable effect on aggression at very low blood alcohol concentrations (BACs) (Graham *et al.* 1998).

3. **Patterns of drinking.** Studies have demonstrated increased risk of violent events with increasing frequency of intoxication (Dawson 1997; Rossow *et al.* 1999; Wells *et al.* 2000), and an apparently stronger association with intoxication frequency than with consumption level (Dawson 1997; Wells *et al.* 2000).

4. **Theoretical underpinnings.** Several underlying mechanisms are probable (see Pernanen 1991; Gustafson 1993; Galanter 1997; Graham *et al.* 1998, 2000).

5. **Interactions.** A number of individual and environmental characteristics moderate the relationship between alcohol and violence (Gustafson 1993; Pernanen 1996; Graham *et al.* 1996, 1998).

Aggregate-level studies

Rates of reported (non-fatal) violence have been found to increase with increased *per capita* consumption in a few studies (Skog and Bjørk 1988; Lenke 1990; Norström 1993, 1998), and homicide rates have also been found to increase with increased *per capita* consumption. Again, the strength of the association varies, and tends to be higher in countries with 'explosive' drinking patterns than in other countries (Lenke 1990; Norström 1998; Parker and Cartmill 1998; Rossow 2001).

The impact of drinking pattern is supported by cross-cultural comparisons of the aggregate-level magnitude of the association, i.e., a stronger association in drinking cultures where intoxication is a more prominent characteristic (Lenke 1990; Rossow 2001).

4.4.2 Divorce and marital problems

The epidemiological evidence for any causal relationship between alcohol consumption and marital problems such as divorce is weak (Box 4.8). In some countries, a partner's heavy drinking is a legal justification for divorce and subjective attributions are common (Rehm *et al.* 1999). The proposition that alcohol consumption is a cause for divorce lacks confirming or refuting evidence from well-controlled epidemiological studies.

Box 4.8 Effects of alcohol on divorce and marital problems

Individual-level studies

1. **Volume of alcohol.** A large number of cross-sectional studies have demonstrated a significant positive association between heavy drinking and divorce, but only a few well-designed studies have demonstrated a significantly increased risk of separation or divorce among married alcohol abusers/heavy drinkers as compared to others (Leonard and Rothbard 1999). No studies of a dose–response relationship between volume of consumption and divorce risk was found. Fu and Goldman (2000) found no significant association between alcohol consumption and risk of divorce. A few longitudinal studies on alcohol consumption and marital aggression (see Quigley and Leonard 1999) have shown that husbands' heavy drinking is predictive of marital violence.

2. **Moderate drinking.** No systematic study on this relationship was found.

3. **Patterns of drinking.** The impact of alcohol consumption on marital relation and divorce has been related to aspects of heavy drinking/alcohol abuse, but not to drinking patterns beyond that.

4. **Theoretical underpinnings.** No systematic theory.

5. **Interactions.** Effects probably mediated by marital satisfaction (marital functioning, marital aggression, etc.) (Leonard 1990).

Aggregate-level studies

Divorce rates are found to increase with increased *per capita* consumption in one US study (Cacses *et al.* 1999), and rates of domestic violence (mostly partner violence) are also found to increase with increased *per capita* consumption (Norström 1993).

4.4.3 Child abuse

The systematic empirical evidence for any causal relationship between alcohol consumption and child abuse is weak (Box 4.9) (Rossow 2000). Only the effect of heavy drinking or abuse/dependence seems to be substantiated.

4.4.4 Work-related problems (other than work accidents)

Clearly, there is an association between alcohol consumption and different outcome variables at the workplace (Box 4.10). However, the direction and nature of causality often are not clear. Most findings suggest rather complex interactions with both individual characteristics and environmental factors, including work characteristics (Rehm and Rossow 2001).

Box 4.9 Effects of alcohol on child abuse

Individual-level studies

1. **Volume of alcohol.** A large number of studies have reported a variety of childhood adversities to be more prevalent among children of heavy drinkers than others, although many of these studies have been criticized for inadequate methodology (Barber and Gilbertson 1999; Rossow 2000). A few recent reports from well-designed studies have shown a higher risk of indicators of child abuse in families with heavy drinking caretakers (see Rossow 2000 for a review). There is little research to suggest any specific relationship between drinking level and risk of child abuse.

2. **Moderate drinking.** No systematic study on this relationship was found.

3. **Patterns of drinking.** The impact of alcohol consumption on child abuse has been related to aspects of heavy drinking/alcohol abuse, but not to drinking patterns beyond that.

4. **Theoretical underpinnings.** No systematic theory.

5. **Interactions.** May probably interact with family resources and functioning (Windle 1996).

Aggregate-level studies

Norström (1993) analysed the association between *per capita* consumption and physical abuse of children in a time–series analysis of Swedish data, and found a weak and positive but not statistically significant association.

Box 4.10 Effects of alcohol on work-related problems other than work accidents

Individual-level studies

1. Volume of alcohol:[a]

    (a) Absenteeism (including tardiness and leaving work early) due to illness, or disciplinary suspension, resulting in loss of productivity.

    (b) Turnover due to premature death, disciplinary problems or low productivity from the use of alcohol.

    (c) Inappropriate behaviour (such as behaviour resulting in disciplinary procedures).

    (d) Theft and other crime.

    (e) Poor co-worker relations and low company morale.

2. **Moderate drinking.** There is some indication that some negative effects are related to moderate drinking as well (Mangione *et al.* 1999).

3. **Patterns of drinking.** Intoxication and heavy drinking occasions are related to work problems even after control of volume (Rehm and Rossow 2001). Alcohol abuse and dependence has been linked to many work problems (Rehm and Rossow 2001).

4. **Theoretical underpinnings.** Diverse, often weak, theoretical underpinnings. Often 'eclectic' theories like Ames and Janes (1992).

5. **Interactions.** Many factors have been found to interact with alcohol in producing work problems. These can be broadly classified under the following headings:

    * individual factors

    * environmental factors

    * work-related factors (Rehm and Rossow 2001)

Aggregate-level studies

No studies found.

[a] The following effects have not always been clearly linked to volume, but to alcohol in general (see Single *et al.* 1998; Rehm and Rossow 2001).

4.4.5 **Alcohol and social problems: the overall findings**

The situation with respect to social consequences of alcohol can be summarized as follows. Clearly, alcohol is related to many social outcomes. This is evidenced by the correlation between different alcohol variables (especially alcohol abuse and dependence) and different social outcomes. However, causal relationships to alcohol are not established for many of these outcomes. In many instances, weak research designs have been used, and longitudinal and experimental studies are scarce. The situation is complicated by the fact that alcohol seems to be part of a complex causal web (Murray and Lopez 1999; Rehm 2000), where its effects depend on or are modified by a multitude of other factors on different levels.

4.5 **Problem rates in relation to changes in alcohol consumption: the Russian experience**

After 1960, mortality rates in Russia and other parts of Eastern Europe began to increase, while in Western Europe they were gradually declining. Then, in the period from 1985 to 1988, mortality in Russia and other parts of the Soviet Union took a sudden sharp turn for the better. The trend then reversed again, and in the period from 1990 to 1994 mortality dramatically increased, to an extent never seen before in peacetime in industrialized societies. Since 1995, the rates have improved somewhat; by 1998 they had returned to approximately the rate of 1984 (Shkolnikov *et al.* 2001).

The improving trend in mortality in the 1980s corresponds to the period of the anti-alcohol campaign of the Gorbachev era (see Chapter 3, Section 3.3.2). The subsequent declining trend corresponds to the dissolution of the Soviet Union, and the state's subsequent loss of control of the alcohol market. Shkolnikov *et al.* (2001) attribute the rebound in the late 1990s to a reduction in drinking. But many other changes also took place in the period after 1989, besides changes in the availability of alcohol, and it is likely that alcohol bears only part of the responsibility for the dramatic mortality crisis of the early 1990s.

To understand the role of alcohol in health, it is important to understand what happened in the period between 1984 and 1988. This was a period of *glasnost* (political openness) and *perestroika* (restructuring). One can argue that there was a new spirit of hope in the Soviet Union. But it was not a time of great social changes; the political and economic system was still intact and functioning much as it had earlier in the decade. The most obvious change in 1985, from a health perspective, was the advent of the anti-alcohol campaign. The events of this period offer an unusually well developed picture of what can happen to a population's health when there is a substantial change in the amount of alcohol in the society.

As shown in Table 4.3, the changes in this period were quite dramatic. Between 1984 and 1987, age-standardized death rates fell among males by 12% and among females by 7% (Leon *et al.* 1998). There was a quite specific pattern in terms of which causes of death were affected. Cancer deaths did not follow the general trend; they actually rose slightly. Deaths among males from alcohol-specific causes were most affected (Leon *et al.* 1998); they fell by 56%. Deaths from accidents and violence fell by 36%. Deaths from pneumonia (40%), other respiratory diseases (20%), and infectious diseases (25%) also fell. And deaths from circulatory diseases, which accounted for over half of all deaths, fell among males by 9%. The trends were similar among females, but the changes were less dramatic.

Estimates of the actual alcohol consumption (Shkolnikov and Nemtsov 1997) show a decline in total consumption, combining legal and illegal sources, from 14.2 litres *per capita* in 1984 to 10.7 litres *per capita* in 1987— much less than the decline in officially recorded sales, but still a decline of about 25% (see also Chapter 3, Figure 3.1).

The experience of the Soviet Union in the latter half of the 1980s suggests that a substantial cut in the alcohol supply can produce dramatic beneficial effects on the population's health. For each litre of ethanol by which *per capita* consumption dropped in Russia, the age-standardized mortality dropped by

Table 4.3 Age-standardized mortality rates per million for Russia by gender, comparing 1987 to 1984 and 1994 to 1987 (standardized to European population)[a]

Cause of death	1984 (rate/million)		Ratio, 1987/1984 rates		Ratio, 1994/1987 rates	
	Male	Female	Male	Female	Male	Female
All causes	21 293	11 606	0.88	0.93	1.37	1.2
Accidents and violence	2519	597	0.64	0.76	2.26	1.91
Alcohol-specific causes	455	123	0.44	0.48	4.29	3.9
Pneumonia	279	118	0.6	0.68	2.29	1.26
Other respiratory diseases	1531	523	0.8	0.78	1.16	0.94
Infectious and parasitic diseases	308	88	0.75	0.77	1.6	1.15
Circulatory diseases	11 798	8037	0.91	0.94	1.29	1.17
All neoplasms	5252	1488	1.04	1.03	1.04	1.05

[a] Recalculated from Leon *et al.* (1998).

2.7%. Given appropriate circumstances, alcohol can have a much greater net impact on a population's health than findings from previous studies have suggested. The figure is considerably higher than the estimated Western European experience showing a 1.3% net decrease in mortality from a one-litre drop in *per capita* consumption (Norström 1996; Her and Rehm 1998). This discrepancy illustrates that the effects of a given volume of alcohol on health and disease can vary from one society to another. Among the factors that can have a major effect on this relationship are the dominant patterns of drinking in a society. In Russia and in a number of other newly independent states, there is a longstanding tradition of repeated heavy binge drinking, particularly among males. This pattern of drinking seems to be strongly implicated in the finding that a litre of ethanol has about twice as much effect on mortality in Russia as it does in Western Europe.

The second major lesson from this experience pertains to the relation between drinking and heart disease. The lesson is that drinking pattern matters. Deaths from heart disease actually declined in Russia during the anti-alcohol campaign of the 1980s, before rising again dramatically in the early 1990s. And yet the medical epidemiological literature was so committed to the idea that alcohol had predominantly protective effects for the heart that at first this finding was interpreted as showing that alcohol could not have played a role in the changes in Soviet mortality in the late 1980s and early 1990s. It has taken some time to come to the realization that, in cultural contexts like the former Soviet Union, alcohol is detrimental rather than beneficial for the mature heart. The exact mechanisms by which intoxication can cause heart disease are still a matter of some discussion (Kupari and Koskonen 1998; McKee and Britton 1998), but by now there is a developing consensus that the data from the former Soviet Union, as well as elsewhere (Kauhanen *et al.* 1997), show that alcohol can be very bad for the heart, given a cultural pattern of repeated binge drinking.

4.6 **Comparing health and social harm from drinking**

Although at present there is no adequate comparative measure of the relative magnitude of social and health problems attributable to drinking, some comparisons can be made that are relevant to the issue, primarily in terms of estimates of the relative burden of alcohol problems in social and health services. Such estimates do not take account of private costs and problems, such as disruption of family life or work roles, except as they come to the attention of public agencies.

Cost-of-illness studies of the economic costs attributable to alcohol include estimates of the 'direct costs' of health and social services used by those with alcohol-related problems. Typically, the ongoing cost to the society for handling these cases is larger in the social welfare and criminal justice sectors than in the health sector. For instance, a study of Scotland health and social services (CATALYST 2001, p. 3) estimated alcohol-attributable health care costs of 95.6 million pounds, social work service costs of 85.9 million pounds, and criminal justice and fire service costs of 267.9 million pounds.

In a mixed urban, suburban, and rural county in northern California, those reporting 'problem drinking' (defined in terms of having heavy drinking occasions, serious social consequences of drinking, or dependence symptoms among persons obtaining services from one or another system), were distributed as follows: 41.0% were seen by the criminal justice system, 8.0% by the social welfare system, 42.1% by the general health system (primary health clinics and emergency rooms), 3.1% by the public mental health system, and 5.9% by public alcohol or drug treatment agencies (Weisner 2001). It seems that in California, the resources devoted to dealing with alcohol-related social problems are at least as extensive as those devoted to alcohol-related health problems.

A third way of estimating the relative burden of health and social harm is from survey research, where the attribution is by the drinker or those around the drinker. A telephone survey, for instance, found that 7.2% of Canadians reported that they had been pushed, hit, or assaulted by someone who had been drinking, 6.2% had had friendships break up as a result of someone else's drinking, and 7.7% had had family problems or marriage difficulties due to someone else's drinking, all within the previous 12 months. In the same study, 2.3% reported that their own drinking had had a harmful effect on their home life or marriage in the past year, 3.7% said that it had harmed their friendships or social life, while 5.5% reported that it had harmed their physical health (derived from Eliany *et al.* 1992, pp. 258 and 274). While questions have been raised about the accuracy of these kinds of survey data, particularly in terms of what respondents mean by 'health' problems (Greenfield 1995; Bondy and Lange 2000), a consistent finding from survey studies is that social problems due to someone's drinking extend more broadly in the population than health problems due to drinking.

4.7 Conclusions

Alcohol accounts for a significant disease burden world-wide and is related to many negative social consequences. Although direct causality is not established unequivocally for some of these consequences, the conclusions for alcohol policy are the same, whether alcohol is the sole causal factor for a consequence, a causal factor among many others, or a factor mediating the influence of another causal factor. In all cases alcohol contributes to social burden, and public policy must strive to reduce this burden, as well as the alcohol-related burden of disease. While there may be some offsetting psychological benefits from drinking (Peele and Brodsky 2000), from the point of view of minimizing the social harm from drinking, the general conclusion is that the lower the consumption, the better.

Considerations are more complicated for the health side. There is the beneficial effect on CHD at the individual level, with plausible biological pathways and some experimental evidence. This becomes an issue in public health policymaking, although the implications at the population level are debatable. The CHD protective effect also has to be balanced in policymaking against the detrimental consequences, even at low levels of drinking (e.g., the effects of alcohol on breast cancer and the risk of developing alcohol abuse or dependence).

Overall, the conclusion must be that alcohol consumption levels affect the health of a population as a whole. In addition to this, the predominant pattern of drinking in a population can have a major influence on the extent of damage from alcohol consumption. Patterns that seem to add to the damage are drinking to intoxication, and recurrent binge drinking.

References

Aarens M., Cameron T., Roizen J., *et al.* (1977) *Alcohol, casualties and crime.* Report C18. Berkeley, CA: Social Research Group.

Alcohol Health and Research World (1997) Alcohol's effect on organ function. *Alcohol Health and Research World* 21, 1–96.

Ames G.M. and Janes C. (1992) Cultural approach to conceptualizing alcohol and the workplace. *Alcohol Health and Research World* 16, 112–19.

Andréasson S., Allebeck P., and Romelsjö A. (1988) Alcohol and mortality among young men: longitudinal study of Swedish conscripts. *British Medical Journal* 296, 1021–5.

Ashley M.J., Rehm J., Bondy S., *et al.* (2000). Beyond ischemic heart disease: are there other health benefits from drinking alcohol? *Contemporary Drug Problems* 27, 735–77.

Bandera E.V., Freudenheim J.L., and Vena J.E. (2001) Alcohol and lung cancer: a review of the epidemiologic evidence. *Cancer Epidemiology, Biomarkers and Prevention* 10, 813–21.

Barber J.G. and Gilbertson R. (1999) Drinker's children. *Substance Use and Misuse* 34, 383–402.

Bondy S.J. (1996) Drinking patterns and their consequences: report from an international meeting—Overview of studies on drinking patterns and consequences. *Addiction* 91, 1663–74.

Bondy S.J. and Lange P. (2000) Measuring alcohol-related harm: test-retest reliability of a popular measure. *Substance Use and Misuse* 35, 1263–75.

Bushman B.J. (1997) Effects of alcohol on human aggression: validity of proposed mechanisms. In: Galanter M. (ed.) *Recent developments in alcoholism*, Vol. 13, *Alcohol and violence*, pp. 227–44. New York: Plenum Press.

Bushman B.J. and Cooper H.M. (1990) Effects of alcohol on human aggression: An integrative research review. *Psychological Bulletin* 107, 341–54.

Cacses F.M., Harford T.C., Williams G.D., *et al.* (1999) Alcohol consumption and divorce rates in the United States. *Journal of Studies on Alcohol* 60, 647–52.

CATALYST Health Economics Consultants Ltd. (2001) *Alcohol misuse in Scotland: Trends and costs: Final report.* Northword, Middlesex: Catalyst Health Economics Consultants. Web address: www.scotland.gov.uk/health/alcoholproblems

Chadwick D.J. and Goode J.A. (eds.) (1998) *Alcohol and cardiovascular disease.* Novartis Foundation Symposium No. 216, London, 7–9 October 1997. Chichester, UK: John Wiley and Sons, Ltd.

Cherpitel C.J. (1996) Drinking patterns and problems and drinking in the event: An analysis of injury by cause among casualty patients. *Alcoholism: Clinical and Experimental Research* 20, 1130–7.

Collins J.J. and Schlenger W.E. (1988) Acute and chronic effects of alcohol use on violence. *Journal of Studies on Alcohol* 49, 516–21.

Corrao G., Bagnardi V., Zambon A., *et al.* (1999) Exploring the dose–response relationship between alcohol consumption and the risk of several alcohol-related conditions: a meta-analysis. *Addiction* 94, 1551–73.

Corrao G., Rubbiati L., Bagnardi V., *et al.* (2000) Alcohol and coronary heart disease: a meta-analysis. *Addiction* 95, 1505–23.

Criqui M.H. (1994) Alcohol and the heart: Implications of present epidemiologic knowledge. *Contemporary Drug Problems* 21, 125–42.

Criqui M.H. (1996) Alcohol and coronary heart disease: Consistent relationship and public health implications. *Clinica Chimica Acta* 246, 51–7.

Dawson D.A. (1997) Alcohol, drugs, fighting and suicide attempt/ideation. *Addiction Research* 5, 451–72.

Drummond M.F., O'Brien B., Stoddart G.L., *et al.* (1997) *Methods for the economic evaluation of health care programmes*, 2nd edn. Oxford, New York, Toronto: Oxford University Press.

Eckardt M.J., File S.E., Gessa G.L., *et al.* (1998) Effects of moderate alcohol consumption on the central nervous system. *Alcoholism: Clinical and Experimental Research* 22, 998–1040.

Edwards G., Anderson P., Babor T.F., *et al.* (1994) *Alcohol policy and the public good.* Oxford: Oxford University Press.

Eliany M., Giesbrecht N., Nelson M., *et al.* (1992) *Alcohol and other drug use by Canadians: A national alcohol and other drugs survey (1989) Technical report.* Ottawa: Health and Welfare Canada.

English D., Holman D., Milne E., *et al.* (1995) *The quantification of drug caused morbidity and mortality in Australia, 1992.* Canberra: Commonwealth Department of Human Services.

Ezzati M., *et al.* and the Comparative Risk Assessment Collaborating Group (2002) Selected major risk factors and global and regional burden of disease. *Lancet* 360, 1347–60.

Fu H. and Goldman N. (2000) Association between health-related behaviours and the risk of divorce in the USA. *Journal of Biosocial Science* 32, 63–88.

Galanter M. (ed.) (1997) *Recent developments in alcoholism*, Vol. 13, *Alcohol and violence.* New York: Plenum Press.

Ginsburg E.S. (1999) Estrogen, alcohol and breast cancer risk. *Journal of Steroid Biochemistry and Molecular Biology* **69**, 299–306.

Ginsburg E.S., Mello N.K., and Mendelson J.H. (1996) Effects of alcohol ingestion on estrogens in postmenopausal women. *Journal of the American Medical Association* **276**, 1747–51.

Gmel G., Rehm J., and Ghazinouri A. (1998) Alcohol and suicide in Switzerland—an aggregate-level analysis. *Drug and Alcohol Review* **17**, 27–37.

Gmel G., Rehm J., Room R., *et al.* (2000) Dimensions of alcohol-related social harm in survey research. *Journal of Substance Abuse* **12**, 113–38.

Goerdt A., Koplan J.P., Robine J.M., *et al.* (1996) Non-fatal health outcomes: concepts, instruments and indicators. In: Murray C.J.L. and Lopez A.D. (eds.) *The global burden of disease: A comprehensive assessment of mortality and disability from diseases, injuries and risk factors in 1990 and projected to 2020*, pp. 201–46. Boston: Harvard School of Public Health.

Graham K., Schmidt G., and Gillis K. (1996) Circumstances when drinking leads to aggression: An overview of research findings. *Contemporary Drug Problems* **23**, 493–557.

Graham K., Leonard K.E., Room R., *et al.* (1998) Current directions in research in understanding and preventing intoxicated aggression. *Addiction* **93**, 659–76.

Graham K., West P., and Wells S. (2000) Evaluating theories of alcohol-related aggression using observations of young adults in bars. *Addiction* **95**, 847–63.

Greenfield T. (1995) *What's in a problem? Type and seriousness of harmful effects of drinking on health, based on a pilot US national telephone survey*. Paper presented at the 21st annual Alcohol Epidemiology Symposium, Kettil Bruun Society, Porto, June 5–9.

Gruenewald P.J. and Ponicki W.R. (1995) Relationship of the retail availability of alcohol and alcohol sales to alcohol-related traffic crashes. *Accident Analysis and Prevention* **27**, 249–59.

Gruenewald P.J., Mitchell P.R., and Treno A.J. (1996) Drinking and driving: Drinking patterns and drinking problems. *Addiction* **91**, 1637–49.

Gustafson R. (1993) What do experimental paradigms tell us about alcohol-related aggressive responding? *Journal of Studies on Alcohol* **Suppl. 11**, 20–9S.

Gutjahr E. and Gmel G. (2001a) The social costs of alcohol consumption. In: Klingemann H. and Gmel G. (eds.) *Mapping the social consequences of alcohol consumption*, pp. 133–43. Dordrecht: Kluwer Academic Publishers.

Gutjahr E. and Gmel G. (2001b) *Die sozialen Kosten des Alkoholkonsums in der Schweiz. Epidemiologische Grundlagen 1995–1998* (The social costs of alcohol consumption in Switzerland: epidemiological foundations 1995–1998) Forschungsbericht Nr. 36 im Auftrag des Bundesamtes für Gesundheit, Vertrag Nr. 98.000794 (8120). Lausanne, Switzerland: SFA (Schweizerische Fachstelle für Alkohol- und andere Drogenprobleme).

Gutjahr E., Gmel G., and Rehm J. (2001) The relation between average alcohol consumption and disease: an overview. *European Addiction Research* **7**, 117–27.

Hemström Ö. (2001) *Per capita* alcohol consumption and ischaemic heart disease. *Addiction* **96** (Suppl. 1), 93–112S.

Her M. and Rehm J. (1998) Alcohol and all-cause mortality in Europe 1982–1990: a pooled cross-section time-series analysis. *Addiction* **93**, 1335–40.

Kauhanen J., Kaplan G.A., Goldberg D.E., *et al.* (1997) Beer bingeing and mortality: results from the Kuopio ischaemic heart disease risk factor study, a prospective population-based study. *British Medical Journal* 315, 846–51.

Kinney A.Y., Millikan R.C., Lin Y.H., *et al.* (2000) Alcohol consumption and breast cancer among black and white women in North Carolina (United States). *Cancer Causes Control* 11, 345–57.

Klingemann H. and Gmel G. (2001) Introduction: Social consequences of alcohol—the forgotten dimension? In: Klingemann H. and Gmel G. (eds.) *Mapping the social consequences of alcohol consumption*, pp. 1–9. Dordrecht: Kluwer Academic Publishers.

Kohlmeier L. and Mendez M. (1997) Controversies surrounding diet and breast cancer. *Proceedings of the Nutrition Society* 56, 369–82.

Kupari M. and Koskinen P. (1998) Alcohol, cardiac arrhythmias and sudden death. In: Chadwick D.J. and Goode J.A. (eds.) *Alcohol and cardiovascular disease*, pp. 68–79. Novartis Foundation Symposium No. 216, London, 7–9 October 1997. Chichester, UK: John Wiley and Sons, Ltd.

Lenke L. (1990) *Alcohol and criminal violence: Time series analysis in a comparative perspective.* Stockholm: Almquist and Wiksell International.

Leon D.A., Chenet L., Shkolnikov V.M., *et al.* (1998) Huge variation in Russian mortality rates 1984–94: artifact, alcohol, or what? *Lancet* 350, 383–8.

Leonard K.E. (1990) Marital functioning among episodic and steady alcoholics. In: Collins R.L., Leonard K.E., and Searless J.S. (eds.) *Alcohol and the family: Research and clinical perspectives*, pp. 220–43. New York, NY: The Guilford Press.

Leonard K.E. and Rothbard J.C. (1999) Alcohol and the marriage effect. *Journal of Studies on Alcohol* Suppl. 13, 139–46S.

Lipsey M.W., Wilson D.B., Cohen M.A., *et al.* (1997) Is there a causal relationship between alcohol use and violence? In: Galanter M. (ed.) *Recent developments in alcoholism*, Vol. 13, *Alcohol and violence*, pp. 245–82. New York: Plenum Press.

Little H.J. (2000) Behavioral mechanisms underlying the link between smoking and drinking. *Alcohol Research and Health* 24, 215–24.

Maclure M. (1993) Demonstration of deductive meta-analysis: Ethanol intake and risk of myocardial infarction. *Epidemiologic Reviews* 15, 328–51.

Mann R.E., Macdonald S., Stoduto G., *et al.* (2001) The effects of introducing or lowering legal per se blood alcohol limits for driving: an international review. *Accident Analysis and Prevention* 33, 569–83.

Mangione T.W., Howland J., Amick B., *et al.* (1999) Employee drinking practices and work performance. *Journal of Studies on Alcohol* 60, 261–70.

McKee M. and Britton A. (1998) The positive relationship between alcohol and heart disease in Eastern Europe: potential physiological mechanisms. *Journal of the Royal Society of Medicine*, 91, 402–7.

Miczek K.A., Weerts E.M., and DeBold J.F. (1993) Alcohol, benzodiazepine-GABA receptor complex and aggression: Ethological analysis of individual differences in rodents and primates. *Journal of Studies on Alcohol* Suppl. 11, 170–9S.

Miczek K.A., DeBold J.F., van Erp A.M.M., *et al.* (1997) Alcohol, $GABA_A$: benzodiazepine receptor complex, and aggression. In: Galanter M. (ed.) *Recent developments in alcoholism*, Vol. 13, *Alcohol and violence*, pp. 139–71. New York: Plenum Press.

Midanik L.T., Tam T.W., Greenfield T., *et al.* (1996) Risk functions for alcohol-related problems in a 1988 US national sample. *Addiction* 91, 1427–37.

Morgenstern H. (1998) Ecologic studies. In: Rothman K.J. and Greenland S. (eds.) *Modern epidemiology*, pp. 459–80. Philadelphia, PA: Lippincott-Raven Publishers.

Murphy G.E. (2000) Psychiatric aspects of suicidal behaviour: Substance abuse. In: Hawton K. and van Heeringen K. (eds.) *The international handbook of suicide and attempted suicide*, pp. 135–46. Chichester, UK: John Wiley and Sons.

Murray C.J.L. and Lopez A. (1996) Quantifying the burden of disease and injury attributable to ten major risk factors. In: Murray C.J.L. and Lopez A. (eds.) *The global burden of disease: A comprehensive assessment of mortality and disability from diseases, injuries and risk factors in 1990 and projected to 2020*, pp. 295–324. Boston: Harvard School of Public Health on behalf of the World Health Organization and the World Bank.

Murray C.J.L. and Lopez A. (1997a) Mortality by cause for eight regions of the world: Global burden of disease study. *Lancet* 349, 1269–76.

Murray C.J.L. and Lopez A. (1997b) Global mortality, disability, and the contribution of risk factors: Global burden of disease study. *Lancet* 349, 1436–42.

Murray C.J.L. and Lopez A. (1999) On the comparable quantification of health risks: lessons from the Global burden of disease study. *Epidemiology* 10, 594–605.

Murray C.J.L., Salomon J.A., and Mathers C. (2000) A critical examination of summary measures of population health. *Bulletin of the World Health Organization* 78, 981–94.

Murray R.P., Rehm J., Shaten J., *et al.* (1999) Does social integration confound the relation between alcohol consumption and mortality in the Multiple Risk Factor Intervention Trial (MRFIT)? *Journal of Studies on Alcohol* 60, 740–5.

Norström T. (1988) Alcohol and suicide in Scandinavia. *British Journal of Addiction* 83, 553–9.

Norström T. (1993) Family violence and total consumption of alcohol. *Nordisk Alkoholtidskrift* 10, 311–18.

Norström T. (1995) Alcohol and suicide: a comparative analysis of France and Sweden. *Addiction* 90, 1463–9.

Norström T. (1996) *Per capita* consumption and total mortality: an analysis of historical data. *Addiction* 91, 339–44.

Norström T. (1998) Effects on criminal violence of different beverage types and private and public drinking. *Addiction* 93, 689–99.

Parker R.N. and Cartmill R.S. (1998) Alcohol and homicide in the United States 1934–1995—or one reason why US rates of violence may be going down. *Journal of Criminal Law and Criminology* 88, 1369–98.

Peele S. and Brodsky A. (2000) Exploring psychological benefits associated with moderate alcohol use: Necessary corrective to assessments of drinking outcomes? *Drug and Alcohol Dependence* 60, 221–47.

Pernanen K. (1991) *Alcohol in human violence.* New York, NY: Guilford Press.

Pernanen K. (1996) *Sammenhengen Alkohol-Vold* (The relationship between alcohol and violence). Oslo: National Institute for Alcohol and Drug Research.

Pernanen K. (2001) What is meant by 'alcohol-related' consequences? In: Klingemann H. and Gmel G. (eds.) *Mapping the social consequences of alcohol consumption*, pp. 21–31. Dordrecht, Kluwer Academic Publishers.

Peterson J.B., Rothfleisch J., Zelazo P., *et al.* (1990) Acute alcohol intoxication and neuropsychological functioning. *Journal of Studies on Alcohol* 51, 114–22.

Pihl R.O., Peterson J.B., and Lau M.A. (1993) A biosocial model of the alcohol-aggression relationship. *Journal of Studies on Alcohol* Suppl. 11, 128–39S.

Puddey I.B., Rakic V., Dimmitt S.B., *et al.* (1999) Influence of pattern of drinking on cardiovascular disease and cardiovascular risk factors: A review. *Addiction* **94**, 649–63.

Puffer R. and Griffith G.W. (1967) *Patterns of urban mortality*, Scientific Publication No. 151. Washington DC: Pan American Health Organization.

Quigley B.M. and Leonard K.E. (1999) Husband alcohol expectancies, drinking, and marital conflict styles as predictors of severe marital violence among newlywed couples. *Psychology of Addictive Behaviors* **13**, 49–59.

Ramstedt M. (2001) Alcohol and suicide in 14 European countries. *Addiction* **96** (Suppl. 1), 59–75S.

Ramstedt M. (2002) Alcohol-related mortality in 15 European countries in the postwar period. *European Journal of Population* **18**, 307–23.

Reed D.S. (1981) Reducing the costs of drinking and driving. In: Moore M.H. and Gerstein D.R. (eds.) *Alcohol and public policy: Beyond the shadow of prohibition*, pp. 336–87. Washington, DC: National Academy Press.

Rehm J. (2000) Alcohol consumption and mortality. What do we know and where should we go? *Addiction* **95**, 989–95.

Rehm J. and Fischer B. (1997) Measuring harm: implications for alcohol epidemiology. In: Plant M., Single E., and Stockwell T. (eds.) *Alcohol: Minimising the harm: What works?*, pp. 248–61. London: Free Association Books Ltd.

Rehm J. and Gmel G. (2000a) Gaps and needs in international alcohol epidemiology. *Journal of Substance Use* **5**, 6–13.

Rehm J. and Gmel G. (2000b) Aggregating dimensions of alcohol consumption to predict medical and social consequences. *Journal of Substance Abuse* **12**, 155–68.

Rehm J. and Rossow I. (2001) The impact of alcohol consumption on work and education. In: Klingemann H. and Gmel G. (eds.) *Mapping the social consequences of alcohol consumption*, pp. 67–77. Dordrecht: Kluwer Academic Publishers.

Rehm J. and Sempos C.T. (1995a) Alcohol consumption and mortality—questions about causality, confounding and methodology. *Addiction* **90**, 493–8.

Rehm J. and Sempos C.T. (1995b) Alcohol consumption and all-cause mortality. *Addiction* **90**, 471–80.

Rehm J., Bondy S., Sempos C.T., *et al.* (1997) Alcohol consumption and coronary heart disease morbidity and mortality. *American Journal of Epidemiology* **146**, 495–501.

Rehm J., Frick U., and Bondy S. (1999) A reliability and validity analysis of an alcohol-related harm scale for surveys. *Journal of Studies on Alcohol* **60**, 203–8.

Rehm J., Greenfield T.K., and Rogers J.D. (2001a) Average volume of alcohol consumption, patterns of drinking and all-cause mortality. Results from the US National Alcohol Survey. *American Journal of Epidemiology* **153**, 64–71.

Rehm J., Gutjahr E., and Gmel G. (2001b) Alcohol and all-cause mortality: a pooled analysis. *Contemporary Drug Problems* **28**, 337–61.

Rehm J., Room R., Monteiro M., *et al.* (2003) Alcohol as a risk factor for burden of disease. In: World Health Organization (ed.) *Comparative quantification of health risks: Global and regional burden of disease due to selected major risk factors.* Geneva: World Health Organization.

Rimm E.B., Klatsky A.L., Grobbe D., *et al.* (1996) Review of moderate alcohol consumption and reduced risk of coronary heart disease: Is the effect due to beer, wine, or spirits? *British Medical Journal* **312**, 731–6.

Room R. (1996) Alcohol consumption and social harm: conceptual issues and historical perspectives. *Contemporary Drug Problems* 23, 373–88.

Room R. and Rossow I. (2001) The share of violence attributable to drinking. *Journal of Substance Use* 6, 218–28.

Room R., Rehm J., Trotter R.T., II, *et al.* (2001) Cross-cultural views on stigma, valuation, parity, and societal values towards disability. In: Üstün T.B., Chatterji S., Bickenbach J.E., *et al.* (eds.) *Disability and culture: Universalism and diversity*, pp. 247–91. Seattle: Hoigrefe and Huber.

Rossow I. (2000) Suicide, violence and child abuse: review of the impact of alcohol consumption on social problems. *Contemporary Drug Problems* 27, 397–434.

Rossow I. (2001) Drinking and violence: a cross-cultural comparison of the relationship between alcohol consumption and homicide in 14 European countries. *Addiction* 96 (Suppl. 1), 77–92S.

Rossow I. and Wichstrom L. (1994) Parasuicide and use of intoxicants among Norwegian adolescents. *Suicide and Life-Threatening Behavior* 24, 174–83.

Rossow I., Pape H., and Wichstrøm L. (1999) Young, wet and wild? Associations between alcohol intoxication and violent behaviour in adolescence. *Addiction* 94, 1017–31.

Rossow I., Pernanen K., and Rehm J. (2001) Alcohol, suicide and violence. In: Klingemann H. and Gmel G. (eds.) *Mapping the social consequences of alcohol consumption*, pp. 93–112. Dordrecht: Kluwer Academic Publishers.

Rothman K.J. and Greenland S. (1998) *Modern epidemiology*, 2nd edn. Philadelphia, PA: Lippincott-Raven Publishers.

Sayette M.A., Wilson T., and Elias M.J. (1993) Alcohol and aggression: A social information processing analysis. *Journal of Studies on Alcohol* 54, 399–407.

Shaper A.G. (1990a) Alcohol and mortality: a review of prospective studies. *British Journal of Addiction* 85, 837–47.

Shaper A.G. (1990b) A response to commentaries: the effects of self-selection. *British Journal of Addiction* 85, 859–61.

Shaper A.G., Wannamethee S.G., and Walker M. (1988) Alcohol and mortality in British men: explaining the U-shaped curve. *Lancet II* 8623, 1267–73.

Shkolnikov V.M. and Nemtsov A. (1997) The anti-alcohol campaign and variations in Russian mortality. In: Bobadilla J.L., Costello C.A., and Mitchell F. (eds.) *Premature death in the New Independent States*, pp. 239–61. Washington, DC: National Academy Press.

Shkolnikov V., McKee M., and Leon D.A. (2001) Changes in life expectancy in Russia in the mid-1990s. *Lancet* 357, 917–21.

Single E., Robson L., Xie X., *et al.* (1998) The economic costs of alcohol, tobacco and illicit drugs in Canada, 1992. *Addiction* 93, 991–1006.

Single E., Robson L., Rehm J., *et al.* (1999) Morbidity and mortality attributable to alcohol, tobacco, and illicit drug use in Canada. *American Journal of Public Health* 89, 385–90.

Single E., Rehm J., Robson L., *et al.* (2000) The relative risks and etiologic fractions of different causes of death and disease attributable to alcohol, tobacco and illicit drug use in Canada. *Canadian Medical Association Journal* 162, 1669–75.

Singletary K.W. and Gapstur S.M. (2001) Alcohol and breast cancer: Review of epidemiologic and experimental evidence and potential mechanisms. *Journal of the American Medical Association* 286, 2143–51.

Skog O.-J. (1983) Methodological problems in the analysis of temporal covariation between alcohol consumption and ischemic heart disease. *British Journal of Addiction* 78, 157–72.

Skog O.-J. (1991) Alcohol and suicide: Durkheim revisited. *Acta Sociologica* 34, 193–206.

Skog O.-J. (1996) Public health consequences of the J-curve hypothesis of alcohol problems. *Addiction* 91, 325–37.

Skog O.-J. (2001) Alcohol consumption and mortality rates from traffic accidents, accidental falls, and other accidents in 14 European countries. *Addiction* 96 (Suppl. 1), 49–58S.

Skog O.-J. and Bjørk E. (1988) *Alkohol og Voldskriminalitet. En Analyse av Utviklingen i Norge 1931–1982* (Alcohol and violent crimes. An analysis of the 1931–1982 trends in Norway). Oslo: SIFO.

Smith-Warner S.A., Spiegelman D., Yaun S.-S., *et al.* (1998) Alcohol and breast cancer in women: a pooled analysis of cohort studies. *Journal of the American Medical Association* 279, 535–40.

Weisner C. (2001) The provision of services for alcohol problems: a community perspective for understanding access. *Journal of Behavioral Health Services and Research* 28, 130–42.

Wells S., Graham K., and West P. (2000) Alcohol-related aggression in the general population. *Journal of Studies on Alcohol* 61, 626–32.

Wiley J.A. and Weisner C. (1995) Drinking in violent and nonviolent events leading to arrest: Evidence from a survey of arrestees. *Journal of Criminal Justice* 23, 461–76.

Windle M. (1996) Effect of parental drinking on adolescents. *Alcohol Health and Research World* 20, 181–4.

WHO. See World Health Organization.

World Health Organization (1992) *International statistical classification of diseases and related health problems—10ᵗʰ revision (ICD-10). Tabular list.* Geneva, Switzerland: World Health Organization.

World Health Organization (1999) *Global status report on alcohol.* Geneva, Switzerland: World Health Organization.

World Health Organization (2001) *The international classification of functioning, disability and health.* Geneva: World Health Organization.

World Health Organization (2002) *The world health report 2002 – Reducing risks, promoting healthy life.* Geneva, Switzerland: World Health Organization.

Zakhari S. (1997) Alcohol and the cardiovascular system: molecular mechanisms for beneficial and harmful action. *Alcohol Health and Research World* 21, 21–9.

Section III

The toolkit: strategies and interventions

Chapter 5

Section overview: strategies and interventions to reduce alcohol-related harm

5.1 Introduction

As indicated in Chapter 1, alcohol policy is broadly defined as any purposeful effort or authoritative decision on the part of governments or non-government groups to minimize or prevent alcohol-related consequences. Policies may involve the implementation of a specific strategy with regard to alcohol problems (e.g., increase alcohol taxes), or the allocation of resources that reflect priorities with regard to prevention or treatment efforts. Although the focus of the chapters in this section is on policies that reduce alcohol-related harm, policies that result in increasing harm are also examined in this book (see Chapter 14), thus providing insight into the public health risks associated with ill-advised policy decisions. This chapter considers research conducted not only to evaluate the effects of specific alcohol policies, but also studies of prevention strategies (e.g., alcohol education in schools) and other interventions (e.g., screening and brief counselling for high-risk drinkers) that have been evaluated prior to being implemented as formal alcohol policies.

Drawing on an extensive literature involving both original research and integrative literature reviews, the chapters in this section provide ample evidence of a wide variety of effective strategies that can be translated into alcohol policies. However, in some cases policies persist despite evidence that the strategy is flawed, and the outcome with regard to reducing alcohol-related problems is thus inconsequential. To understand why policies succeed or fail to accomplish their aims, the field of alcohol policy analysis has begun to consider the mechanisms that relate policies to outcomes, as demonstrated by the research reviewed in this section.

5.2 Rules of evidence

A variety of methodological approaches have been used to assess the impact of alcohol policies as well as policy-relevant prevention and treatment strategies.

These include experimental studies, survey research, analysis of archival and official statistics, time–series analyses, qualitative research, and **natural experiments**. In many studies **quasi-experimental** research designs have been used. This type of research typically involves before and after measurement of a group, community, or other jurisdiction that is exposed to an intervention, and similar measurement is conducted in comparable groups or communities where no intervention took place. Natural experiments have played a large role in this literature. For example, when sobriety checks (see Chapter 9) are implemented in one jurisdiction and not in an adjacent one, the relative impact of the policy can be examined over time through comparative analysis of archival data such as accident rates or drinking–driving arrests.

The appropriateness of any given research methodology for alcohol policy evaluation depends on the phenomena under study, the current state of knowledge, the availability of valid measurement procedures, and the ways in which the information will be put to use (McKinley 1992). Generally, the most conclusive evidence in the behavioural and medical sciences derives from **randomized clinical trials** where an untreated control group is compared to an intervention group. A close example from the prevention field is the evaluation of a school-based preventive intervention that randomly assigns some students to a no-intervention control group and other students to a program that teaches alcohol resistance skills. Yet even such a well-accepted design has pitfalls when applied to alcohol prevention research, because the individual is often not the proper unit of analysis. For instance, the teaching of the resistance skills in a school-based intervention will usually be done by a teacher in a classroom full of students, and the social interaction taking place at the level of the class should be taken into account as part of the design and the analysis. Though they are still rare, there are now some evaluation studies that take the community as the unit to be randomized (e.g., Wagenaar *et al.* 2000). One study even tested the effects of an alcohol control measure by random assignment of different regions of a country to the intervention and the control condition (Norström and Skog 2001).

Randomized-control studies are rare in the prevention field because of political, ethical, and cost considerations. Most of the evidence on this topic comes from quasi-experimental studies where the possibility of bias and **confounding** always exists. For this reason, it is particularly important to undertake several studies, each with a different design, and to examine whether there is convergence in the findings.

The most direct evidence on the effects of an intervention comes from studying what happens when the intervention is applied or removed, in comparison with another time or place when there is no change in the intervention. When a study of such an intervention is planned in advance, consideration can be given to what kinds of data will be most appropriate to collect. Where possible, data would likely include population surveys before and after the change (if possible with a longitudinal panel component), the compilation of event data on cases coming to the attention of health, police, and other social response agencies, and observational and qualitative interview material concerning social processes in the period of change. However, a useful evaluation can often be done even in the absence of such planning, when the political process throws up what, from the researcher's perspective, is a natural experiment. In this case, the researcher is dependent on matching post-intervention data with data that was collected for other purposes prior to the change.

Studies of what happens when there is a change—an intervention implemented or discontinued—provide the most valuable evidence on the effects of alcohol policy. Yet one can also learn from cross-sectional studies comparing sites where different policies are in effect. Given the potential sources of confounding, however such studies provide only weak evidence of effectiveness.

The various modes of data collection have different advantages and drawbacks. Social surveys, for example, generally measure attitudes and behaviours through the direct questioning of individual drinkers. Studies based on survey data tend to be descriptive, correlational, and subject to the limitations of self-report methods. Data collected by social and health agencies (e.g., police statistics, hospital discharge data, mortality records) have a different set of strengths and weaknesses. By definition, they give a good picture of the agency response in an area, but the available data are influenced by cultural perceptions, agency priorities, and recording practices.

Quantitative research methods, such as social surveys, can be complemented by qualitative studies, such as ethnographic interviewing, participant observation, case studies, and focus group activities. As long as standard scientific principles of confirmation, refutation, causal inference, and generalizability are applied, research, using a number of methods and strategies, is able to produce a firm evidence base on which effective alcohol policy can be developed.

The value of combining different types of evidence is that each method has its own advantages. In general, as one moves from individual-level to population-level interventions, the utility of experimental methods becomes problematic. One reason is that it is often not feasible to manipulate people or policies at the level of the general population or even the community. For this reason different research approaches, measurement procedures, and data collection techniques can all contribute to an understanding of alcohol policy.

Evaluation research is necessary in order to measure whether the policy has any impact, and to provide a 'reality-check' to high expectations often attached to promising new initiatives in this area. Evaluation also needs to be ongoing.

Evidence from one time period may not necessarily be applicable to situations emerging in another era. And evidence from developed countries may not always be applicable to developing countries. Furthermore, communities often want locally based evidence, or at least evidence that is close to home to justify their interventions, rather than relying on dated findings from far afield. While there may be general agreement about the scientific support for a specific strategy, there may be doubt among policy-makers that these findings will apply to their jurisdiction.

Evaluation research provides a useful but often under-utilized resource to decision-makers. Should resources be devoted to those policies that have at best a modest effect, or should they be directed to policies that have a chance for a broader and more substantial impact? Decisions about which strategies to implement, phase out, or modify should be informed by findings from systematic evaluation.

With these methodological considerations in mind, the policies, strategies, and interventions discussed in this section of the book were systematically evaluated on the basis of the following rules of evidence. First, the world literature on each area was reviewed and critically appraised by the authors with other experts serving as external reviewers. Special attention was given to research developments during the last decade, in part because of the dramatic increase in research during this period, and in part because the prior literature had been reviewed critically and systematically in *Alcohol policy and the public good* (Edwards *et al.* 1994). Reviews of the literature were either commissioned as background papers (Babor 2000), or conducted by the authors themselves. The emphasis was always on studies with better research designs (e.g., experimental or quasi-experimental designs with control groups or comparison conditions). The variety of approaches, wide scope of the searches, and expert involvement have led to detailed evaluations and careful weighting of the existing evidence. Still, potential biases may be present due to missed studies and selectivity of inclusion. Given the origins of the scientific literature in the alcohol field, most of the research reviewed in this section of the book originated in English-speaking countries. To compensate for the relative lack of research in other parts of the world, the authors were asked to give careful consideration to the cross-national generalizability of findings from particular studies. Finally, a series of meetings were held to review and critique the contents, findings, and conclusions of each chapter.

5.3 Section overview

The policies, strategies, and interventions discussed in the next seven chapters cover the most currently favoured policy options where there is a related research base available for review. Chapter 6 focuses on policies aimed at changing the economic environment through price and taxation. Chapter 7 examines policies aimed at changing the physical availability of alcohol. Chapters 8 and 9 address a broad range of strategies aimed at preventing or minimizing important alcohol-related harms and consequences. Chapter 10, on regulating alcohol promotion, and Chapter 11, on addressing education and persuasion, both cover strategies that generally try to change behavior by influencing public perceptions about alcohol. Finally, Chapter 12 discusses the effectiveness of treatment and other therapeutic interventions in preventing alcohol problems from a public health perspective.

References

Babor T.F. (ed.) (2000) Alcohol and public policy: Research contributions. *Contemporary Drug Problems* 27, 393–668.

Edwards G., Anderson P., Babor T.F., *et al.* (1994) *Alcohol policy and the public good.* New York: Oxford University Press, Inc.

McKinlay J.B. (1992) Health promotion through healthy public policy: The contribution of complementary research methods. *Canadian Journal of Public Health* 83 (Suppl.), 11–19S.

Norström T. and Skog O.-J. (2001) *Effekter av lördagsöppna Systembolagsbutiker: uppföljning av de först tio månaderna* (Effects of Saturday opening of the alcohol monopoly shops: follow-up of the first 10 months). Stockholm: Social and Health Ministry. http://social.regeringen.se/pressinfo/pdf/folkhalsa/rapport_lordagsoppet.pdf

Wagenaar A.C., Murray D.M., Gehan J.P., *et al.* (2000) Communities mobilizing for change on alcohol: Outcomes from a randomized community trial. *Journal of Studies on Alcohol* 61, 85–94.

Chapter 6

Pricing and taxation

6.1 Introduction

Among the various strategies that states and nations use to control alcohol-related problems, the regulation of **alcohol taxes** and prices has been by far the most popular. This is not simply because governments need financial resources and by tradition acquire them by taxation; regulations on taxes and prices are relatively easy to establish in law and to enforce in practice. For more than a century, taxation of alcoholic beverages by many governments has also been used to reduce rates of harm from drinking. Economic studies conducted in many developed and some developing regions of the world have demonstrated that increased alcoholic beverage taxes and prices are related to reductions in alcohol use and related problems.

This chapter considers the aims, mechanisms, and effects of alcohol taxation and pricing, two important economic strategies that have strong implications for the prevention of alcohol-related problems. Economic research and other studies are reviewed to evaluate how alcohol prices affect alcohol consumption and what aspects of the marketplace moderate the effects of price increases.

6.2 Aims and mechanisms of formal controls over beverage prices

In the absence of any formal controls over production, distribution, and sales, the price of an alcoholic beverage would be set by market conditions purely on the basis of its supply and demand. However, most countries increase alcoholic beverage retail prices over their production and distribution costs and control profit through special alcohol taxes or other price controls. Quite often there is no explicitly stated public health rationale for taxes on alcoholic beverages, such as special excise duties, value added taxes, or sales taxes higher than the normal rate. But in many countries, alcohol and other dependence-producing substances have been treated differently from other consumer products.

In some countries, during certain time periods, taxation of alcoholic beverages has been a very important source of state revenue. Between 1911 and

1917, for example, over one-third of the total revenues from taxes levied by the US government came from alcoholic beverages (Landis 1945). Similar figures can be found for the Netherlands, the United Kingdom, and the Nordic countries (Denmark, Finland, Iceland, Norway, and Sweden). The relative importance of alcohol taxation as a source of state revenues declined in most established market economies during the 20th century, particularly after the advent of modern income taxation and general value added or sales taxes. In many market economies, the share of alcohol taxes in state budgets has also declined because of decreases in alcohol tax rates. For instance, Ireland experienced a clear decrease in alcohol tax revenues relative to total state revenues between 1970, when its share was 16.5% (Davies and Walsh 1983), and 1996, when it was estimated at 5.0% (Hurst *et al.* 1997). Despite these trends, alcohol tax revenues are still of considerable fiscal significance in many developed countries (Hurst *et al.* 1997).

In some developing countries, alcohol taxation remains an important source of government revenue. In India, alcohol taxes are one of the main sources of state revenue, accounting for as much as 23% of the total collected in some states (see Room *et al.* 2002). In Cameroon, 43% of government revenue in 1990 came from taxes on beer and soft drinks. In other developing countries, the proportion of government revenue is in the same range as the developed economies: 2% in Nigeria, 2.3% in South Africa, 4% in Sri Lanka, and 10% in Kenya (Room *et al.* 2002). The equivalent figure for the 12 countries of the European Community (EC) in 1991 was 2.4%. A crucial issue in developing countries is the effect of tax increases on other aspects of the market. For example, after increasing taxes on lager beer, Zimbabwe had to lower its tax because consumers switched to untaxed cottage-produced opaque beer (Jernigan 1997).

6.3 **Supply and demand**

Basic economic theory posits that alcohol prices represent an equilibrium between the demand for alcoholic beverages and their supply or their availability through retailers (Pindyck and Rubinfeld 1989). Reduced supply with a constant demand, or increased demand with a constant supply, will result in higher prices. In a similar manner, increased supply with a constant demand, or decreased demand with a constant supply, will result in lower prices. It is also the case that deliberate changes in prices will affect supply and demand relationships. Alcoholic beverage prices that are increased through external means, such as heavier excise duties, will reduce alcohol consumption, as consumers can only afford a smaller amount of drinking with higher prices.

In order to generate more revenue, a state may impose or increase alcohol excise duties, or increase the price of alcoholic beverages in some other way, to obtain more financial gain from each unit sold. Increased excise duty rates usually lead to increases in alcoholic beverage prices, and the increase in beverage prices usually leads to a reduction in alcohol consumption. If alcohol consumption remains unchanged despite increased tax rates and alcohol prices, the state receives all the new consumer expenditures on alcoholic beverages in the form of new tax revenues. In this example, the demand for alcoholic beverages is not at all responsive to any price change from the increased taxes. In reality, however, this is very seldom the case. How responsive the demand for alcoholic beverages is to increases or decreases in price will determine how the change in price will affect alcohol consumption.

Economists use the term **price elasticity of demand** when measuring the sensitivity of consumption to changes in price. The price elasticity of demand is defined as the percentage change in consumption resulting from a 1% change in price. For example, a price elasticity for alcohol of −0.5 implies that a 1% increase in price would reduce alcohol consumption by 0.5%. Three types of elasticity are distinguished. If the price elasticity of demand has a value between 0.0 and −1.0, the demand for a commodity is said to be 'inelastic' with respect to its own price, as a change in its price results in a relatively smaller change in its consumption. If the own-price elasticity has a value of −1.0, the demand is said to be **unit price elastic**, as the change in its price results in an equal relative change in its consumption. Finally, with values below −1.0, the demand is said to be **price elastic**, as the change in its price leads to a proportionally greater change in its consumption. Obviously, commodities with very inelastic demand are the best alternatives for the purposes of revenue generation. As will be discussed later in this chapter, the demand for alcoholic beverages is often inelastic. Note, however, that a rise in price will produce some reduction in consumption even if the commodity is **price inelastic**, so long as the value is not zero or higher.

The responsiveness of alcohol consumption to its price affects not only the efficiency with which special alcohol taxes generate revenue, but also the potential health benefits to be reaped from higher alcohol prices. Highly elastic demand for alcohol would indicate more than proportionate decreases in alcohol use relative to increases in its price, suggesting that substantial health benefits may accrue with higher alcohol prices, assuming a monotonic positive relationship between overall alcohol consumption and related problems. As the elasticity value increases towards zero, these benefits decrease, and if it reaches zero, health benefits from alcohol prices are eliminated. Thus, though revenue generation and reduced alcohol problems are somewhat different benefits of increases in alcohol prices, they can be optimized with respect to one another by how alcohol taxes are set and changed.

6.4 **The distribution of alcohol beverage prices**

As products on the market, alcoholic beverages are heterogeneous commodities, sharing only the inclusion of ethyl alcohol. In economic terms, they are composed of many different products and brands with a broad spectrum of qualities and use values. As such, alcoholic beverages can satisfy consumer needs in many different ways. They can be used as thirst quenchers, as appetizers, as drinks with meals, and as digestives. Alcoholic beverages can also be used as medicine, as a way to organize recreation and enjoyment, and as a means of getting intoxicated (Mäkela 1983).

Complex markets can take on rather different profiles with respect to prices, as reflected in the range of prices relative to an average price, and the correlated or uncorrelated movement of prices in related market components (Deaton 1988). Thus, tax increases may or may not be realized in uniform price increases across related alcohol products and brands. Indeed, in a complex market, tax increases may be partially neutralized by market-oriented decisions by producers, distributors, or sellers about pricing (Gruenewald and Treno 2000).

The breadth of alcoholic beverage qualities observed in the alcohol market is reflected in numerous products and brand divisions. Typically, the market for alcoholic beverages is divided into three product categories: distilled beverages, wine, and beer. To be sure, there are alcoholic beverages not fitting into these categories, such as cider and the often home-made fermented beverages that account for a significant amount of the alcohol consumed in Africa (WHO 1999).

Even within the usual trichotomy of distilled beverages, wine, and beer, alcoholic beverages can be further divided into numerous brands of widely differing quality, from very cheap to very expensive. One study found that prices for the top ten market leaders for distilled spirits, wine, and beer differed by a factor of 60 (Treno *et al.* 1993). Looking across an entire alcohol market, even greater price ranges can be observed (e.g., Ponicki *et al.* 1997). With prices per unit of ethanol also differing widely between on-premise (e.g., bars) and off-premise (e.g., grocery stores) establishments, quite often by factors of two to four, consumers are free to purchase alcohol at a very wide range of qualities, and to substitute purchases between one form of alcohol and another (Gruenewald and Treno 2000). The manner in which changes in special alcohol taxes affect the average level and distribution of alcoholic beverage prices is still relatively unknown (Kenkel and Manning 1996).

A number of other market factors affect alcoholic beverage prices. Differential taxation by product type is common, with distilled spirits usually taxed more heavily per unit of alcohol than wine or beer (see Hurst *et al.* 1997; Karlsson and Österberg 2001). Production, storage, and distribution costs vary between products and brands. The economic geography of alcohol distribution systems affects the average prices of alcoholic beverages sold in different places. It is more expensive to transport a bottle of beer 1000 kilometres from the brewery than to transport it next door, and it is more expensive to transport one litre of alcohol in the form of beer than in the form of distilled spirits. Alcohol prices may even differ by time of day, being less expensive during afternoon 'happy hours' and other sales promotions than during regular hours.

6.5 **Taxing alcoholic beverages**

Alcoholic beverages are viewed as especially suitable commodities for taxation because of their detrimental social and public health consequences. In some countries, particularly where the control of alcohol consumption is attuned to public health concerns, monopoly rights have been granted to state-owned companies, in part to provide better state control over production, import, wholesale, and retail sale of alcoholic beverages, and to improve state revenues from the sale of alcoholic beverages. This policy approach has been particularly favoured in the Nordic countries and in North America, but similar monopolies have been established in Costa Rica, Paraguay, Uruguay, the former Soviet Union, and the other eastern European countries (Kortteinen 1989). In a monopoly arrangement, prices may be adjusted by directly setting or fixing prices and establishing minimum price requirements. In the former case, monopolies may radically alter pricing patterns to meet certain objectives. For instance, in Finland, the State Alcohol Monopoly had the right to set alcoholic beverage prices. This privilege was used quite generally in favouring lighter beverages (wine and beer) at the expense of distilled spirits. Furthermore, if the monopoly felt that some specific beverage had become too popular among youth or alcoholics, the price of the beverage was raised in order to decrease its consumption (Holder *et al.* 1998). This is also an example of how monopolies may act to affect the lowest prices paid for alcohol so as to most efficiently curtail alcohol use (Gruenewald and Treno 2000).

Where the alcohol distribution system is under private rather than state control, taxes, tariffs, and licensing fees generate revenue for the state without restricting pricing actions at the wholesale and retail levels, although they reduce the efficiency of alcohol markets. Except to the extent that the state requires otherwise, wholesalers and retailers remain free to set prices to compete with each other, including considerable price differentiation between quality classes. In some places, price fixing and minimum pricing requirements are also allowed or imposed, which further restrict pricing choices in the alcohol market. In Canada, for instance, minimum price levels set by the provinces of Quebec and Ontario for beer have been justified as contributing to public health and order (McCarthy 1992).

6.6 Changes in alcoholic beverage prices

In many countries, real prices for alcohol have been in almost continuous decline since 1950 (Cook 1981). Using data from the US as an example, the average price in 1982 dollars of a six-pack of beer (containing a little over 2 litres) in 37 states is presented in Figure 6.1. The figure demonstrates the decline in real prices of beer that took place between 1982 and 1990, a reduction of 7% over eight years. In comparable series for wine and distilled spirits, reductions in real prices were 21% over eight years for wine and 32% over 14 years for distilled spirits. To provide further indication of the complex changes that take place in beverage prices over time, Figure 6.1 also presents the same relationships for two selected states. It can be noted that, despite the overall decline in average beverage prices nationally, different states move differently over time, sometimes influenced by changes in the state tax rate.

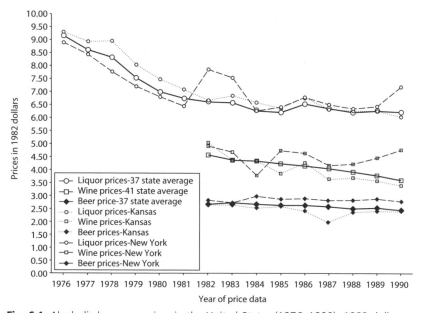

Fig. 6.1 Alcoholic beverage prices in the United States (1976–1990), 1982 dollars.

Even greater decreases in real prices of alcoholic beverages have occurred in other parts of the world in the period after World War II (see Leppänen *et al.* 2001; Österberg and Karlsson 2002). A major cause of this decline is that excise taxes are commonly set at a fixed amount of the local currency, so that inflation automatically reduces their value, unless there is new legislation to set a new tax level. A solution to the tendency of inflation to reduce the tax rate in real terms is to provide that the tax is tied to a cost-of-living index, rising and falling with it, rather than being set at a fixed value.

6.7 **Investigating and interpreting elasticity values**

The effect of price changes on alcohol consumption has been more extensively investigated than any other potential alcohol control measure. **Econometric methods** have been the most common tool used to study these effects. Combining the studies referenced in different reviews, econometric data dealing with all alcoholic beverages or certain categories of alcoholic beverages are currently available at least from the following countries: Australia, Belgium, Canada, Denmark, Germany, Finland, France, Ireland, Italy, Kenya, The Netherlands, New Zealand, Norway, Poland, Portugal, Spain, Sweden, the United Kingdom, and the United States (see Huitfeldt and Jorner 1972; Lau 1975; Ornstein 1980; Ornstein and Levy 1983; Godfrey 1986; Clements and Selvanathan 1991; Olsson 1991; Edwards *et al.* 1994; Yen 1994; Österberg 1995, 2000). This list indicates that information about the effects of changing alcohol prices on alcohol consumption chiefly derives from the developed countries.

In econometric studies, the responsiveness or sensitivity of the quantity purchased to the determinants of demand is measured by an estimate of elasticity. The price elasticities for alcoholic beverages estimated in different studies have shown that when other factors remain unchanged, an increase in price has generally led to a decrease in alcohol consumption, and that a decrease in price has usually led to an increase in alcohol consumption. In other words, alcoholic beverages appear to behave in the market like most other consumer goods and in the way presupposed by the theory of consumer demand.

While demonstrating that the use of alcohol is constrained by economic circumstances, studies dealing with different countries and time periods have also found different values for price elasticity with respect to both total alcohol consumption and the consumption of different categories of alcoholic beverages. These variations are partly due to the methods applied, the accuracy of the basic data, and the statistical uncertainties related to elasticity estimates. However, different elasticity values are also related to social, cultural, and economic circumstances prevailing in different countries in different time periods (Bruun *et al.* 1975).

Nevertheless, in the last two decades far more data on alcohol taxes, prices, and sales have become available, along with information about social and economic considerations and cross-border purchases. Combined with the use of more sophisticated analytical procedures (e.g., Gruenewald *et al.* 1993), there is now a much better scientific understanding of the complex relationship between alcohol prices and alcohol consumption.

6.8 Alcohol prices and the consumption of alcoholic beverages

There appear to be substantial differences between countries, and within countries over time, in the way alcohol consumers have reacted to changes in the price of alcoholic beverages. This is reflected in the diversity of price elasticity values cited across studies from any given nation. For instance, in the United States, estimated values of price elasticity for beer range from approximately zero to −1.4; similarly, estimates for wine range from −0.4 to −1.8, and estimates for distilled spirits from −0.1 to −2.0 (Österberg 1995).

A recent study by Grossmann *et al.* (1998) found that increases in the **full price** of alcohol resulting from either monetary prices or higher minimum legal drinking age significantly reduced drinking among young adults. Moreover, they found evidence that past and future consumption of alcohol have a positive effect on current consumption. Thus, Grossman and his colleagues estimate an average price elasticity of −0.3 from models that ignore addictive aspects of consumption, and of −0.7 for long-run price elasticity of demand. From a public policy perspective, it is the long-term effects, taking into account alcohol's dependence-producing properties, that are more important.

Godfrey's reviews of demand models from 1989 and 1990 discuss three alcohol studies in the United Kingdom, as well as her own estimates and the elasticity values used by the British treasury in their alcohol tax revenue calculations (Godfrey 1989, 1990). She found that the demand for beer, wine, and spirits has generally been price inelastic, while the demand for wines and distilled spirits has been more responsive to prices than the demand for beer (Godfrey 1989). Later studies appear to be in agreement with this interpretation (see Österberg 1995; Chaloupka *et al.* 2002). Consequently, studies from the United States and the United Kingdom give the impression that beer may be less price elastic than wine or distilled spirits, and may be quite price inelastic, at least in developed countries preferring beer.

In other countries of the world, own-price elasticity values for different beverages vary from place to place. As stated above, one reason for the low degree of elasticity for beer in Britain and the United States may be that these are beer-preferring countries, and beer sales have the largest market share in both nations. In wine-preferring countries such as France, Italy, and Spain, wine is a beverage taken with meals. One would therefore expect that in these countries wine sales would be inelastic with respect to changes in its price, as wine belongs to the basic dietary commodities like bread or pasta (Österberg 1995; see also Leppänen *et al.* 2001).

A second explanation for the variations in elasticity values from place to place is that other alcohol control measures, such as the overall physical availability of alcohol or conditions of use, affect the price elasticity values. This argument suggests that the removal of other alcohol control measures would give alcohol prices more power over consumption. In Sweden, for instance, the lifting of the **Bratt rationing system** led to a rise in the value of the price elasticity for distilled spirits (Huitfeldt and Jorner 1972).

In Finland, Ahtola and his colleagues (1986) found that price elasticity decreased for alcoholic beverages for the period 1955–1980. Their interpretation of this trend was that alcoholic beverages had come to be seen more and more as everyday commodities, as alcohol consumption had increased more than three-fold during this period. But these data could also indicate that price elasticity has a tendency to decrease as incomes and the standard of living increase, which leads to higher alcohol consumption. In addition, these trends may also reflect a shift to more expensive beverages inside certain beverage categories, just as when the price of alcoholic beverages increases, and consumers may both give up some of their drinking and move down the beverage price scale, decreasing the money put into alcoholic beverages but still getting the same amount of liquid and of ethyl alcohol as before (Gruenewald and Treno 2000).

The effect of changing prices on alcohol consumption has been studied primarily by means of data from Western industrialized nations. According to one study of an African nation, beer in Kenya was more price elastic than in North America and Europe (Partanen 1991). It is also possible that when developing countries become more industrialized, price elasticities of alcoholic beverages move towards those found in developed countries, rather than in the opposite direction. And, as noted in Chapter 3, there are substantial differences between recorded and unrecorded alcohol consumption in many parts of the world, particularly in the developing regions (cf. Table 3.1). To the extent that existing capabilities for home production and smuggling can respond rapidly to price changes, elasticity values may be affected.

6.9 **Price elasticities across drinking groups**

In econometric studies based on time–series data, the price elasticity values in many ways reflect the average reactions of consumers to changes in prices. It is particularly the treatment of alcohol consumers as a single homogeneous group that has raised concerns about the policy implications of price elasticity estimates. One example of these concerns is the disagreement in the literature on whether heavy drinkers are responsive to changes in alcohol prices. Econometric research in the United States, for example, has been extended to the study of the relationships between beverage taxes and self-reported use of alcohol among specific demographic groups, particularly young drinkers. These studies typically relate some measure of beverage prices or taxes to self-reports of alcohol use obtained from large national surveys. Grossman and colleagues were the first to estimate the effects of price on youth alcohol use (Grossman *et al.* 1987; Coate and Grossman 1988). Their studies conclude that youth beer consumption is inversely related to both the monetary price and the minimum legal drinking age. In addition, they conclude that frequent or heavy drinkers are more sensitive to price than infrequent or light drinkers (Grossman *et al.* 1987). Similar research indicates that higher beer excise taxes significantly reduce both the frequency of youth drinking and the probability of heavy drinking (Laixuthai and Chaloupka 1993), and that beer prices have a significant effect on underage drinking and binge drinking among female college students (Chaloupka and Wechsler 1996). An important issue for policy is the extent to which adult heavy and problematic drinkers are responsive to changes in alcohol prices. Manning *et al.* (1995) have argued that they are not, but with an analysis using cross-sectional data, which is weak in terms of causal significance. Studies of the effects of tax changes on problem outcomes, reviewed in the next section, provide much stronger evidence that changes in taxes do influence rates of problematic drinking.

As noted in earlier sections of this book (see Chapters 4 and 5), in recent years a variety of different methodological approaches have been applied to the study of drinking behaviour and alcohol-related problems, including experimental methods that provide insights into the causal mechanisms involved in changes in drinking. The new field of behavioural economics (Chaloupka *et al.* 1999), for example, has shown that while the relationship between price and drinking is complex, the cost of alcohol is an important determinant of alcohol consumption under carefully controlled laboratory conditions. This research (e.g., Babor 1985; Vuchinich and Simpson 1999) also demonstrates that alcoholics and heavy drinkers tend to be as responsive to short-term changes in the price of alcohol as moderate drinkers, a finding that supports the relationships observed at the population level.

6.10 **Alcohol prices and problems related to alcohol use**

While measures of alcohol sales are not routinely available for sub-groups of the population, measures of alcohol-related problems are often more specific. These include measures of morbidity and mortality focusing on alcohol-related liver disease, traffic accidents, violence, and suicide. Thus, one way to get indirect evidence of the effects of price policy on heavy consumers is to examine harmful outcomes related to heavy use, such as cirrhosis mortality (Cook and Tauchen 1982). One benefit of this kind of study design is that it takes care of the problems caused by possible substitution of recorded alcohol consumption by unrecorded alcohol consumption like home-made or privately imported alcoholic beverages (see Nordlund and Österberg 2000).

In the United States, Cook (1981) used changes in the state liquor excise duties legislated between 1960 and 1975 to study the effects of price changes on cirrhosis mortality. This quasi-experimental study indicated that the states that raised their liquor tax had a greater reduction or smaller increase in cirrhosis mortality than other states in the corresponding year. Cook and Tauchen (1982) studied the relationship between tax changes, consumption of distilled spirits, cirrhosis mortality, and car accidents using a sophisticated panel design tracking changes in these variables across many states over time. They observed a price elasticity for liquor of -1.8, and concluded that liquor consumption, including that of heavy drinkers as indicated by cirrhosis mortality, was quite responsive to price. Furthermore, a liquor tax increase tended to reduce the rate of fatal car accidents (see also Chaloupka *et al.* 1992). Sloan *et al.* (1994) considered the effects of changing prices of alcoholic beverages on deaths from motor vehicle traffic accidents, homicides, and suicides, all of which are considered to be primarily related to alcohol use. They found that higher alcoholic beverage prices did not lead to significant reductions in these kinds of mortality statistics.

In an attempt to get more directly at the relationship between beverage taxes and problem outcomes, particularly among youth, Saffer and Grossman (1987a, b) examined the impact of beer excise duties on youth motor vehicle fatality rates. Both studies concluded that increases in beer taxes significantly reduced youth motor vehicle fatalities. Chaloupka *et al.* (1993) further concluded that higher beer excise duties are among the most effective means to reduce drinking–driving in all segments of the population. Other studies using individual data also concluded that increases in beer taxes are effective in reducing drinking–driving as well as involvement in non-fatal traffic accidents. For example, Kenkel (1993) estimated that a 10% increase in the price of alcoholic beverages in the United States would reduce the probability of drinking–driving by about 7% for males and 8% for females, with even larger reductions among those 21 years and under.

Several studies have examined the impact of the price of alcoholic beverages on homicides and other crimes, including rape, robbery, assaults, motor vehicle thefts, domestic violence, and child abuse (Cook and Moore 1993; Sloan *et al.* 1994; Chaloupka *et al.* 1998; Markowitz and Grossman 1998, 2000). These studies suggest that raising the price of alcohol is likely to result in a reduction in violence. What is most striking about these studies is their convergence upon a single theme: raising alcohol taxes will lead to a reduction in a host of undesirable outcomes related to alcohol use.

6.11 **Summary**

This chapter has reviewed the role of alcohol prices as a means to curb total alcohol consumption and alcohol-related problems. The evidence suggests that alcohol prices do have an effect on the level of alcohol consumption and related problems. Consumers of alcoholic beverages respond to changes in alcohol prices, and heavy or problem drinkers appear to be no exception to this rule.

Despite these findings, the real price of alcoholic beverages has decreased in many countries during the last decades, at the same time as many other alcohol control measures have been liberalized or abandoned completely. A major reason for this price decline has been the failure of governments to increase tax levels in accordance with inflation. But in some cases alcohol taxes have been reduced to compete with cross-border smuggling and imports, or as required by trade dispute decisions (see Chapter 14).

Alcohol taxes are thus an attractive instrument of alcohol policy as they can be used to both generate direct revenue and to reduce alcohol-related harms. The most important downside to raising alcohol taxes is the possibility of potential alternatives or substitutions to taxed alcoholic beverages, particularly in terms of illegal smuggling or illegal in-country alcohol production. The net effects of taxation and price increases, however, are to reduce alcohol use and related problems.

References

Ahtola J., Ekholm A., and Somervuori A. (1986) Bayes estimates for the price and income elasticities of alcoholic beverages in Finland from 1955 to 1980. *Journal of Business and Economic Statistics* 4, 199–208.

Babor T.F. (1985) Alcohol, economics and the ecological fallacy: toward an integration of experimental and quasi-experimental research. In: Single E. and Storm T. (eds.) *Public drinking and public policy*, pp. 161–89. Toronto: Addiction Research Foundation.

Bruun K., Edwards G., Lumio M., *et al.* (1975) *Alcohol control policies in public health perspective.* Helsinki: Finnish Foundation for Alcohol Studies.

Chaloupka F.J. and Wechsler H. (1996) Binge drinking in college: The impact of price, availability, and alcohol control policies. *Contemporary Economic Policy* 14, 112–24.

Chaloupka F.J., Grossman M., Becker G.S., *et al.* (1992) *Alcohol addiction: An econometric analysis.* Presented at the Annual Meeting of the Allied Social Science Associations, Anaheim, CA, December.

Chaloupka F.J., Saffer H., and Grossman M. (1993) Alcohol-control policies and motor-vehicle fatalities. *Journal of Legal Studies* 22, 161–86.

Chaloupka F.J., Grossman M., and Saffer H. (1998) Effects of price on the consequences of alcohol use and abuse. In: Galanter M. (ed.) *Recent developments in alcoholism*, Vol. 14, *The consequences of alcoholism*, pp. 331–46. New York, NY: Plenum Press.

Chaloupka F.J., Grossman M., Bickel W.K., *et al.* (eds.) (1999) *The economic analysis of substance use and abuse: An integration of econometric and behavioral economic research.* Chicago, IL: University of Chicago Press.

Chaloupka F.J., Grossman M., and Saffer H. (2002) The effects of price on alcohol consumption and alcohol-related problems. *Alcohol Research and Health* 26, 22–34.

Clements K.W. and Selvanathan S. (1991) The economic determinants of alcohol consumption. *Australian Journal of Agricultural Economics* 35, 209–31.

Coate D. and Grossman M. (1988) Effects of alcoholic beverage prices and legal drinking ages on youth alcohol use. *Journal of Law and Economics* 31, 145–71.

Cook P.J. (1981) The effect of liquor taxes on drinking, cirrhosis and auto fatalities. In: Moore M. and Gerstein D. (eds.) *Alcohol and public policy: Beyond the shadow of prohibition*, pp. 255–85. Washington, DC: National Academy of Sciences.

Cook P.J. and Moore M.J. (1993) Taxation of alcoholic beverages. In: Hilton M.E. and Bloss G. (eds.) *Economics and the prevention of alcohol-related problems*, pp. 33–58. Research Monograph No. 25. NIH Pub. No. 93-3513. Rockville, MD: National Institute of Alcohol Abuse and Alcoholism (NIAAA).

Cook P.J. and Tauchen G. (1982) The effect of liquor taxes on heavy drinking. *Bell Journal of Economics* 13, 379–90.

Davies P. and Walsh D. (1983) *Alcohol problems and alcohol control in Europe.* New York: Gardner.

Deaton A. (1988) Quality, quantity and spatial variation of price. *American Economic Review* 78, 418–30.

Edwards G., Anderson P., Babor T.F., *et al.* (1994) *Alcohol policy and the public good.* Oxford: Oxford University Press.

Godfrey C. (1986) *Factors influencing the consumption of alcohol and tobacco—A review of demand models.* York: Addiction Research Centre for Health Economics.

Godfrey C. (1989) Factors influencing the consumption of alcohol and tobacco: the use and abuse of economic models. *British Journal of Addiction* 84, 1123–38.

Godfrey C. (1990) Modelling demand. In: Maynard A. and Tether P. (eds.) *Preventing alcohol and tobacco problems*, Vol. 1, pp. 35–53. Aldershot, Avebury.

Grossman M., Coate D., and Arluck G.M. (1987) Price sensitivity of alcoholic beverages in the United States: Youth, alcohol consumption. In: Holder H.D. (ed.) *Advances in substance abuse: Behavioral and biological research. Control issues in alcohol abuse prevention: Strategies for states and communities*, pp. 169–98. Greenwich, CT: JAI Press.

Grossman M., Chaloupka F.J., and Sirtalan I. (1998) An empirical analysis of alcohol addiction: results from the Monitoring the Future panels. *Economic Inquiry* 36, 39–48.

Gruenewald P.J. and Treno A.J. (2000) Local and global alcohol supply: Economic and geographic models of community systems. *Addiction* 95 (Suppl. 4), S537–49.

Gruenewald P.J., Ponicki W.R., and Holder H.D. (1993) The relationship of outlet densities to alcohol consumption: a time series cross-sectional analysis. *Alcoholism: Clinical and Experimental Research* 17, 38–47.

Holder H.D., Kühlhorn E., Nordlund S., *et al.* (1998) *European integration and Nordic alcohol policies: Changes in alcohol controls and consequences in Finland, Norway and Sweden, 1980–1997.* Aldershot, Hampshire, UK: Ashgate Publishing Ltd.

Huitfeldt B. and Jorner U. (1972) *Efterfrågan på rusdrycker i Sverige* (The demand for alcoholic beverages in Sweden). Rapport från alkoholpolitiska utredningen (Report from the Alcohol Policy Commission). Stockholm, Sweden: Government Official Reports.

Hurst W., Gregory E., and Gussman T. (1997) *International survey: Alcoholic beverage taxation and control policies*, 9th edn. Ottawa: Brewers Association of Canada.

Jernigan D.H. (1997) *Thirsting for markets: The global impact of corporate alcohol.* San Rafael, CA: Marin Institute for the Prevention of Alcohol and Other Drug Problems.

Karlsson T. and Österberg E. (2001) A scale of formal alcohol control policy in 15 European Countries. *Nordic Studies on Alcohol and Drugs* 18 (English Suppl.), 117–31.

Kenkel D.S. (1993) Driving, driving and deterrence: the effectiveness and social costs of alternative policies. *Journal of Law and Economics* 36, 877–913.

Kenkel D. and Manning W. (1996) Perspectives on alcohol taxation. *Alcohol Health and Research World* 20, 230–8.

Kortteinen T. (ed.) (1989) *State monopolies and alcohol prevention: Report and working papers of a collaborative international study.* Helsinki, Finland: Social Research Institute of Alcohol Studies.

Laixuthai A. and Chaloupka F. (1993) Youth alcohol use and public policy. *Contemporary Policy Issues* 11 (4), 70–81.

Landis B.Y. (1945) Some economic aspects of inebriety. In: *Alcohol, science and society*, pp. 201–21. New Haven: Quarterly Journal of Studies on Alcohol.

Lau H.H. (1975) Cost of alcoholic beverages as a determinant of alcohol consumption. In: Gibbins R.J., Israel Y., and Kalant H. (eds.) *Research advances in alcohol and drug problems*, Vol. 2, pp. 211–45. New York: John Wiley and Sons, Inc.

Leppänen K., Sullström R., and Suoniemi I. (2001) *The consumption of alcohol in fourteen European countries: A comparative econometric analysis.* Helsinki: STAKES.

Mäkelä K. (1983) The uses of alcohol and their cultural regulation. *Acta Sociologica* 26, 21–31.

Manning W.G., Blumberg L., and Moulton L.H. (1995) Demand for alcohol: The differential response to price. *Journal of Health Economics* 14, 123–48.

Markowitz S. and Grossman M. (1998) Alcohol regulation and domestic violence towards children. *Contemporary Economic Policy* 16, 309–20.

Markowitz S. and Grossman M. (2000) The effects of beer taxes on physical child abuse. *Journal of Health Economics* 19, 271–82.

McCarthy S. (1992) Ontario will defy GATT on beer. *Toronto Star*, Toronto, Ontario, February 14.

Nordlund S. and Österberg E. (2000) Unrecorded alcohol consumption: its economics and its effects in Nordic countries. *Addiction* 95 (Suppl.), 551–64S.

Olsson O. (1991) *Prisets och inkomstens betydelse för alkoholbruk, missbruk och skador* (The effect of prices and income on alcohol consumption and related problems). Stockholm, Sweden: Swedish Council for Information on Alcohol and other Drugs (CAN).

Ornstein S.I. (1980) Control of alcohol consumption through price increases. *Journal of Studies on Alcohol* 41, 807–18.

Ornstein S.I. and Levy D. (1983) Price and income elasticities and the demand for alcoholic beverages. In: Galanter M. (ed.) *Recent developments in alcoholism*, Vol. 1, pp. 303–45. New York: Plenum.

Österberg E. (1995) Do alcohol prices affect consumption and related problems? In: Holder H.D. and Edwards G. (eds.) *Alcohol and public policy: Evidence and issues*, pp. 145–63. Oxford: Oxford University Press.

Österberg E. (2000) Unrecorded alcohol consumption in Finland in the 1990s. *Contemporary Drug Problems* 27, 271–99.

Österberg E. and Karlsson T. (eds.) (2002) *Alcohol policies in EU member states and Norway. A collection of country reports*. Helsinki: STAKES.

Partanen J. (1991) *Sociability and intoxication. Alcohol and drinking in Kenya, Africa and the modern world*, Vol. 39. Helsinki: Finnish Foundation for Alcohol Studies.

Pindyck, R.S. and Rubinfeld, D.L. (1989) *Microeconomics*. New York: Macmillan.

Ponicki W.R., Holder H.D., Gruenewald P.J., *et al.* (1997) Altering the price spectrum in Sweden for alcoholic beverages according to ethanol content. *Addiction* 92, 859–70.

Room R., Jernigan D., Carlini Cotrim B., *et al.* (2002) *Alcohol in developing societies: A public health approach*. Helsinki: Finnish Foundation for Alcohol Studies.

Saffer H. and Grossman M. (1987a) Beer taxes, the legal drinking age, and youth motor vehicle fatalities. *Journal of Legal Studies* 16, 351–74.

Saffer H. and Grossman M. (1987b) Drinking age laws and highway mortality rates: cause and effect. *Economic Inquire* 25, 403–17.

Sloan F.A., Reilly B.A., and Schenzler C. (1994) Effects of prices, civil and criminal sanctions, and law enforcement on alcohol-related mortality. *Journal of Studies on Alcohol* 55, 454–65.

Treno A.J., Nephew T.M., Ponicki W.R., *et al.* (1993) Alcohol beverage price spectra: opportunities for substitution. *Alcoholism: Clinical and Experimental Research* 17, 675–80.

Vuchinich R.E. and Simpson C.A. (1999) Delayed-reward discounting in alcohol abuse. In: Chaloupka F.J., Grossman M., Bickel W.K., *et al.* (eds.) *The economic analysis of substance use and abuse: An integration of econometric and behavioral economic research*, pp. 103–22. Chicago, IL: University of Chicago Press.

WHO. See World Health Organization.

World Health Organization (1999) *Global status report on alcohol*. WHO/HSC/SAB/99.11. Geneva: World Health Organization.

Yen S.T. (1994) Cross-section estimation of US demand for alcoholic beverage. *Applied Economics* 26, 381–92.

Chapter 7

Regulating the physical availability of alcohol

7.1 Introduction

In this chapter we discuss the physical availability of beverage alcohol. Physical availability refers to the accessibility or convenience of the product, which has policy implications for preventing alcohol-related problems through controls on the conditions of sale to the drinker as a retail customer. Such controls extend back at least as far as recorded human history. The Code of Hammurabi, dating from 3800 years ago, included three articles governing the behaviour of tavern-keepers and their customers in Mesopotamia (Hammurabi 2000). A major aim of these measures throughout history and into modern times has been to reduce the harm from drinking.

The retail markets that make alcoholic beverages available can be formal or informal. Formal alcohol markets are regulated by government, whether at the community level or at the regional or national levels. In established market economies, formal retail markets are regulated to ensure purity, safety, and the accurate description of the product. Regulation also enables the collection of taxes. In a number of countries, the special regulation of alcoholic beverage sales reflects social concerns about health, safety, and public order. Thus, there may also be general limits on opening hours or days for retail services, the placement and location of retail markets, how alcohol can be advertised and promoted, and who may purchase alcohol. Special taxes on alcoholic beverages may also be regarded as part of the regulatory regime. Restricting alcohol availability through law has been a key policy in Canada, the United States, the Scandinavian countries, and many other parts of the world (Kortteinen 1989; WHO 1999).

Informal markets provide desired goods and services to consumers, largely through unregulated social and commercial networks (e.g., through home production and distribution of alcohol). Informal alcohol markets are a relatively small part of total consumption in most of the developed world, though their importance has grown in recent years in Europe (Moskalewicz 2000; Leifman 2001). In developing countries, informal markets are often important, accounting in some places for as much as 90% of total consumption (Room *et al.* 2002).

Experience has shown that extreme restrictions on alcohol availability, such as the banning of all alcohol sales, can lower drinking and reduce alcohol problems. Yet these restrictions often have adverse side effects as well, such as the increase in violence and other criminality associated with the illicit markets. These side effects can come to be seen as overbalancing the good effects of the restrictions (Levine 1985; Room *et al.* 2002). The emphasis in this chapter is not on such radical changes. Rather, we consider strategies where the side effects of more modest regulation of alcohol availability can be minimized.

7.2 Changes in general availability

Alcohol retail outlets have been restricted through total or partial bans, restrictions on **hours and days of sale**, and by controlling the number, location, and type of retail premises. In this section, we discuss policies designed to alter the general availability of alcohol. This is based upon the economic principle that supply and demand both affect the consumption of alcohol, with reductions in supply resulting in increases in the full costs of alcohol and concomitant reductions in sales (Chaloupka *et al.* 2002). That is, as availability decreases, its convenience to the consumer decreases, and thus physical availability has the potential to influence the consumer's demand for alcoholic beverages.

7.2.1 Total or partial bans

Total prohibition of alcohol sales on a country-wide basis is uncommon in the modern world. All modern countries with total prohibition, such as Saudi Arabia and Iran, are Islamic. Other countries with strong Moslem majorities, such as Pakistan, allow non-Moslems to purchase alcohol. Still others, such as Indonesia, do not have alcohol prohibition even for Moslems. Modern-day prohibition is much more common in sub-national jurisdictions. For example, one Indian state, Gujarat, has had prohibition since 1947, and has been joined by other states for shorter periods. In Canada and the US, many First Nations and Native American tribes living on designated land (set up as 'reservations' or 'reserves' at the time that Europeans took over the continent) have implemented total prohibition of alcohol within the boundaries of the reservation. Aboriginal groups in Australia have also applied partial and **total bans** on alcohol (d'Abbs and Togni 2000).

Although prohibition is never completely effective, it is easier to enforce in isolated areas, where entries to the 'dry' (i.e., no alcohol) area can be effectively controlled. It is clear from historical evaluations of the prohibition periods in North American and the Nordic countries (e.g., Paulson 1973), and from studies of current more limited prohibitions, that total bans on alcohol production and sales can reduce alcohol-related problems (e.g., Bowerman 1997; Chiu *et al.* 1997). However, where there is a substantial demand for illicit alcohol, it will be filled partly by illegal operators, and there will often be considerable violence associated with their efforts to enforce the illegal market, along with other undesired consequences (Johansen 1994; Österberg and Haavisto 1997).

For most of the developed world, total prohibition is not a politically acceptable option even if the potential for reducing alcohol problems does exist. However, as described later, bans on alcohol sales for specific persons in the population (e.g., children and adolescents), or in specific circumstances, have been applied with demonstrated success. An example of a temporary partial ban in a specific circumstance is shown in Box 7.1.

Box 7.1 **Partial ban on alcohol as a harm reduction measure**

By order of the mayor of Eindhoven, the Netherlands, only half-strength beer (2.5%) was sold in the centre of the town during the Euro 2000 soccer championships. The goal was to minimize the risk of 'trouble' during the tournament. The sale of beer in bottles, which could be used as missiles, was also banned (Millward 2000). Despite the presence of large numbers of English fans, the streets remained largely peaceful. In contrast, there were large-scale riots, primarily involving English fans, the next week in Belgium, where the beer had been left at full strength and was readily available (Randell and Alderson 2000; Whelan 2000).

7.2.2 **Regulating retail outlets for alcohol**

Whether in a formal or an informal market, alcoholic beverages are sold to the retail customer in two ways, called 'off-premise' and 'on-premise' sales, respectively. On-premise sales refer to the purchase of alcoholic beverages for consumption in a designated place such as a bar, café, or restaurant. The purchase of alcohol for consumption elsewhere is called an 'off-premise' or 'take away' sale. For these off-premise alcohol sales, the opportunity to influence the act of drinking, the drinking occasion, and the potential consequences are limited to regulations on the type, strength, and packaging of the alcoholic beverage and the time, costs, and location of alcohol sales.

In 'on-premise' retail outlets, on the other hand, there is an opportunity to directly influence what happens during and after the actual purchase. Regulations may specify drink sizes, disallow discount drink promotions, or require on-premise staff to receive **server training** in responsible beverage service. They may also regulate the design and furnishing of the tavern or restaurant, and include specifications on such matters as food service, availability of entertainment, and other non-alcohol-related matters.

One means to regulate sale of alcohol is through government-owned alcohol outlets. A government monopoly may be operated so as to greatly reduce the **number of outlets**, limit their hours of sale, and remove the private profit motive for increasing sales. The idea of government ownership of alcohol sales outlets in the interest of public order or public health first arose in the 19th century. The original form, known as the 'Gothenburg system', involved municipally-owned taverns, and later became the basis for the Swedish off-premise monopoly stores. Monopoly systems existed at one time or another in parts of Britain, Australia, and New Zealand, and they still operate in parts of the US and much of Canada, as well as in the Nordic countries. In Iceland, Norway, Sweden, and Finland, state monopoly systems were implemented in the early 20th century with substantial powers over the production, sales, and distribution of alcohol. The 1995 membership of Sweden and Finland in the European Union (EU), and Iceland and Norway's special treaty relationship to the EU, caused a substantial weakening of these integrated monopoly systems (Holder *et al.* 1998), although the off-premise retail monopolies have been retained in all four countries. The majority of the North American wholesale and retail monopolies still exist. Government monopolies also operate in Eastern Europe (e.g., Russia), southern Africa, and Costa Rica as well as a number of Indian states (Room 2000). Municipally- or village-owned on-premise outlets can be found in some places, although the most common kind of government-owned on-premise outlets are probably now in such forms as military canteens.

The evidence is quite strong that off-premise monopoly systems limit alcohol consumption and alcohol-related problems, and that elimination of government off-premise monopolies can increase total alcohol consumption. A summary of seven time–series analyses found a consistent increase in total consumption when government-owned off-premise outlets were replaced with privately-owned outlets (Wagenaar and Holder 1995). When Finland changed in 1968 from selling beer only in government monopoly stores to selling it also in grocery stores, alcohol consumption rose by 46% in the next year, and alcohol problem rates also increased (Mäkelä *et al.* 2002). Noval and

Nilsson (1984) found that total alcohol consumption in Sweden was substantially higher when medium strength beer could be purchased in grocery stores between 1965 and 1977, rather than only in state monopoly stores. When medium strength beer was made available in grocery stores in a township in Finland, drinking among 13- to 17-year-olds increased (Valli 1998). Minors were more able to purchase alcohol than when sales had been restricted to state stores. Typically, the network of stores in such a government-operated system is sparse, and the opening hours limited. Elimination of a private profit interest also typically facilitates the enforcement of rules against selling to minors or persons already intoxicated (Her *et al.* 1999).

Regulation of on-premise alcohol outlets has a rich and detailed history in many societies. Within the on-premise category, restaurants are often differentiated from taverns, according to whether dining or drinking is the primary activity. Recognizing that taverns, as places of public accommodation, were frequently gathering places for illegal and undesired activities, authorities in many countries have long restricted what else is going on in the drinking place. Common bans have included prohibition of card playing, gambling, music, dancing, and sexually explicit entertainment. On the other hand, authorities have often required that food be served along with alcohol, and have favoured alcohol licenses for 'restaurants' over those for taverns. Studies have found that drinking–driving is associated with bars and restaurants (Stockwell *et al.* 1993) and in some countries with bars serving high alcohol content beverages (Gruenewald *et al.* 1999, 2000). Violence is associated with bars in particular, but connections have also been found with off-premise outlets (Stevenson *et al.* 1999; Gorman *et al.* 2001; Lipton and Gruenewald 2002).

7.2.3 Outlet location and 'bunching'

The location of alcohol sales outlets may be limited by a number of provisions at local, state, or national levels. For instance, typically the outlet cannot be located in an area that is in violation of local zoning laws, which limit outlets to particular kinds of commercial sites. Other provisions, common in many US states, forbid location near a school or place of worship. The density of outlets may be limited by requiring a minimum distance between them, or by limiting the number of outlets. Sales may also be forbidden at such locations as highway rest stops. Little evidence is available to indicate whether these provisions affect alcohol-related problems, though one study suggests that locating an outlet near a highway system may affect alcohol-related crashes more than locating the same outlet in a dense downtown area (Gruenewald and Treno 2000).

The bunching of bars, restaurants, and off-premise establishments in a particular location has often been seen as a problem in itself. Densities have been found to reach the level of one outlet for every 75 feet (23 metres) of roadway in many California cities (Gruenewald and Treno 2000). Cross-sectional studies suggest that alcohol-related problems, especially motor vehicle crashes, are more likely to occur where drinking places are more densely packed (Jewell and Brown 1995; Gruenewald *et al.* 1996). These results appear to extend to other pedestrian injury collisions (LaScala *et al.* 2001) and violent assaults (Alaniz *et al.* 1998; Stevenson *et al.* 1999). However, while these studies are consistent with the argument that the bunching of outlets may concentrate harmful effects related to alcohol in specific community areas, they have not demonstrated that changes in densities over time affect rates of problem outcomes (Gorman *et al.* 2001).

7.2.4 Hours and days of retail sale

Restricting the days and times of alcohol sales restricts opportunities for alcohol purchasing and may reduce heavy consumption. Although this has in the past been a common strategy for reducing alcohol-related problems, in recent years there has been a trend to remove such restrictions in many countries (e.g., Drummond 2000). In most societies, there is a regular rhythm to drinking, often tied to the end of the work week. Many societies have festivals or 'carnival' times particularly associated with drinking. What is the evidence that changes in hours or days of retail sale can be an effective way to prevent or reduce alcohol-related problems?

A number of studies have indicated that changing either hours or days of alcohol sale can redistribute the times at which many alcohol-related crashes and violent events take place, and may reduce the overall numbers of alcohol-related problems (e.g., Nordlund 1985; Smith 1988). More recent studies in Western Australia (Chikritzhs and Stockwell 2002) and Iceland (Ragnarsdottir *et al.* 2002) have found direct evidence of an overall increase in such problems as injuries and drinking–driving incidents with longer hours of sale.

A study in Sweden (Norström and Skog 2001) found a net 3.2% increase in alcohol sales with Saturday opening of liquor stores. There is also evidence of changes in the opposite direction. In the 1980s, Sweden re-instituted Saturday closing for liquor and wine off-premise sales after studies showed that Saturday sales were associated with increased rates of domestic violence and public drunkenness (Olsson and Wikström 1982). However, a Sunday sales ban in Athens, Georgia, USA, produced effects on drinking–driving arrests that were not reversed when the ban was removed (Ligon and Thyer 1993; Ligon *et al.* 1996). Mixed results have also been found in studies of the effects of extended tavern closing hours in Britain on health and drinking–driving statistics (Raistrick *et al.* 1999, pp. 134–6).

Restrictions on hours and days of sale have also been evaluated in less developed areas. In recent years, there have been new restrictions on opening times or days in some developing countries and in Aboriginal communities within developed countries (see Box 7.2 for an example of a successful approach).

The evidence that such changes can affect young people is limited, as most evaluations have focused on the total drinking population. In one of the few studies focusing on youth and restricted sales, it was found that temporary bans on the sale of alcohol from midnight Friday through 10 am Monday (because of federal elections in Mexico) reduced cross-border drinking by young Americans (Baker *et al.* 2000). In particular, the early closing on Friday night was associated with a 35% reduction in the number of pedestrians crossing the border and a reduction in the number of persons with BACs of 0.08% or higher.

In summary, the evidence of the impact of changes in hours of sale is not entirely consistent, perhaps because of the difficulty in conducting controlled evaluations (Stockwell 1994). However, allowing for methodological weaknesses, it appears that restrictions on hours of alcohol sales and service, if used strategically, have the potential to reduce drinking and alcohol-related problems.

Box 7.2 'Feed the children first!' The impact of Thirsty Thursday in Tennant's Creek

In Tennant's Creek, an outback community in Australia, an Aboriginal community group mounted a long and eventually successful campaign to close the local pubs and off-premise outlets on the day pay checks arrived. On Thursdays, off-premise alcohol sales were banned, and on other days take-away sales were limited to the hours of noon to 9 pm. In addition, bars were closed until noon on Thursdays and Fridays. 'Feed the children first' was the slogan of the campaign. Evaluations of the effects of this much-contested change found a 19.4% decrease in drinking over a two-year period, with a concomitant reduction in arrests, hospital admissions, and women's refuge admissions (Brady 2000; Gray *et al.* 2000). d'Abbs and Togni (2000) found a 34% reduction in alcohol-related hospital admissions and a 46% decline in women's refuge admissions in the first and more stringent phase of the restrictions.

Restricted hours or days of sale for off-premise outlets are likely to have the greatest impact on persons who do not keep a ready supply of alcohol, either because they cannot afford to or because they do not plan ahead. A decrease in violence resulting from Norway's 1984 Saturday closing suggests that the people most affected by this temporary unavailability were more likely to be involved in domestic violence and disruptive intoxication (Nordlund 1985). Those drinking late in taverns, particularly on weekdays, are an especially heavy-drinking segment of the population. Therefore, policies regulating closing hours need to take into account the collective nature of much on-premise drinking, and the problems connected with public order and safety that commonly occur in and around drinking places in many societies. For example, to set closing hours at a time later than local public transport systems operate may invite unsafe journeys home. Overall, studies of specific types of alcohol outlets suggest that reduced hours and days of sale can reduce alcohol consumption and problem levels, with the effects concentrated during the time of closure but not matched by counterbalancing changes at other times of the week.

7.2.5 Densities of retail outlets

As with restrictions on hours and days of sale, restricting the number of outlets may affect levels of drinking and alcohol-related problems (Gruenewald *et al.* 1993). The smaller the number of outlets for alcoholic beverages, the greater the opportunity costs (e.g., time, inconvenience) for obtaining alcohol, a situation that is likely to deter alcohol use and problems.

A series of five Norwegian studies of the effects of opening wine and liquor outlets in places where beer was already available found a shift away from other beverages, including moonshine, with little effect on overall consumption (see Mäkelä *et al.* 2002 for a summary of these reports). In one study from the early 1990s, however, there was evidence of increased consumption and intoxication among women and the elderly—segments of the population that drink less and that previously had less access. Introduction of local beer monopolies, which greatly reduced the number of outlets, was studied in two other Norwegian studies. While beer sales decreased, at least in the first year, sales of wine and spirits increased. Overall, the Norwegian studies suggest that, where there is already some availability of alcohol, the effects on total consumption of changes in the number of off-sale stores selling one or another type of beverage are minor (Mäkelä *et al.* 2002). A time–series study of changes in the number of on-premise outlets in Norway as a whole in 1960–1995 found a significant relation to changes in the number of crimes of violence that were investigated by the police (Norström 2000).

Studies in Finland have more often found some net effect from changes in number of off-sale outlets. One study found that there was an increase in consumption when state liquor stores were opened in rural villages (Kuusi 1957). An econometric study (Lehtonen 1978) estimated that half of the increase in on-premise sales in Finland between 1962 and 1978 was attributable to a rise in the number of restaurants and bars. A case study of five municipalities that withdrew permission for grocery stores to sell beer estimated that overall consumption fell by about 8% (Mäkinen 1978). The most dramatic change was observed in 1969, when beer with up to 4.7% alcohol was allowed to be sold by grocery stores, and it also became easier to get a restaurant license. The number of off-premise sales outlets increased from 132 to about 17 600, and on-premise sales points grew from 940 to over 4000 (Österberg 1979). The overall consumption of alcohol increased by 46%. In the following five years, mortality from liver cirrhosis increased by 50%, hospital admissions for alcoholic psychosis increased by 110% for men and 130% for women, and arrests for drunkenness increased by 80% for men and 160% for women (Poikolainen 1980).

In Sweden, research has been conducted on the effects of allowing the sale of beer (up to 4.5% alcohol) in grocery stores in 1965, and reversing this change in 1977. The change greatly increased the number of outlets for 4.5% beer, although beer up to 3.5% remained available in the groceries both before and after the change. An analysis by Noval and Nilsson (1984) concluded that introducing 4.5% beer to the grocery stores raised total consumption by about 15%, and that removing it reduced total consumption by about the same amount. There is some evidence that the effect was greatest among young people (Hibell 1984). A recent time–series analysis found that motor vehicle accidents were significantly reduced in three of four age groups when the right to sell 4.5% beer was retracted; there was also a significant drop in hospital admissions for alcohol-specific diagnoses among those aged under 20. On the other hand, no significant effects were found for assaults, suicides, and falls (Ramstedt 2002).

Few studies have been conducted outside the Nordic countries to evaluate the effects of increases or decreases in number of outlets. Using US data from 24 to 38 states (with observation periods ranging from three to ten years), Gruenewald et al. (1993) found that variations in numbers of outlets significantly predicted alcohol sales in five of eight analyses (Gruenewald et al. 1993). In contrast to the cross-sectional nature of most studies on this topic, this study employed a time–series cross-sectional panel design, which increases the confidence that can be placed in the findings. Blose and Holder (1987) found that allowing sales of distilled spirits in restaurants in North Carolina, USA (thus increasing the density of on-premises availability) was associated with a 16–24% increase in night-time traffic crashes for male drivers.

In general, it is clear that dramatic changes in the number of outlets can have a substantial influence on consumption and problem levels. But the overall effects of marginal changes where there are already a substantial number of outlets are much less clear. These findings suggest the potential value of regulation at the local level for the prevention of alcohol-related problems (Gruenewald et al. 1996; Holder et al. 2000). Depending on the division of government responsibilities in a given society, it is often at the local level that planning and zoning laws can be used to regulate over-densities of outlets. However, it should be kept in mind that reductions in the physical availability of alcohol can create an opportunity for alternative sources to fill the gap (Österberg and Haavisto 1997; Mäkelä et al. 2002). A Norwegian study (Rossow 2000) found that less physical availability was associated with greater consumption of moonshine, but not with smuggled spirits. Yet, the fact that reductions in physical availability tend to reduce alcohol-related harm indicates that alternative sources of alcohol do not fully compensate for the effect of reduced availability.

7.3 Restrictions on eligibility to purchase and sell alcohol

At various times throughout the world restrictions have been placed on who may buy and sell alcohol. These restrictions are generally intended to exclude one group or another from purchasing alcoholic beverages and to regulate the clerks and sellers of alcohol. For instance, sales of alcoholic beverages to Aboriginal populations were forbidden in many European settler societies (Brady 2000). The most common restrictions on sales in effect throughout the world at the beginning of the 21st century are the prohibition of alcohol sales to children and youths and the denial of sale to persons who are intoxicated.

7.3.1 Limiting alcohol sales on an individual basis

Fifty years ago, broad restrictions on who could purchase alcohol were fairly common. The most elaborate example of such controls was the Bratt system in Sweden, in effect until 1955, where a **rationing** scheme assigned a limit to each adult on how much spirits could be purchased (Norström 1987). There was also a list of those barred altogether from purchasing. Such lists were also maintained in Finland and Norway (Tigerstedt 2000), and this procedure was included in laws in some English-speaking jurisdictions. These individual banning orders were abolished in the Nordic countries in the 1970s, and until recently had also fallen out of favour in English-speaking jurisdictions as impermissible intrusions on civil liberties. Now there are signs of a revival of such approaches, at least in Britain. The government's proposals in 2000 for an end to national restrictions on opening hours for alcohol sales were accompanied by a proposal that 'habitual drunkards' and others convicted of violent assaults should be banned from taverns (Travis 2000).

There is clear evidence that general alcohol rationing schemes, such as Sweden's Bratt system and a similar system in effect in Greenland from 1979 to 1982 (Norström 1987; Schechter 1986) were responsible for reducing liver cirrhosis mortality, violence, and other consequences of heavy drinking. During a political crisis situation in Poland in 1981–1982, alcohol rationing limiting each adult to half a litre of spirits per month was introduced. Heavy drinkers were affected most. Periods of binge drinking became much shorter. Along with a 60% drop in mental hospital admissions for alcoholic psychosis, deaths from liver diseases dropped by one-quarter, and deaths from injuries by 15% (Moskalewicz and Swiatkiewicz 2000, p. 151).

Many countries ban alcohol sales to persons who are already intoxicated. All 50 US states have criminal or civil laws against such sales (Holder et al. 1993). There has been no evaluation of these particular legislative bans, but there are studies on increased enforcement of such bans (see Chapter 8).

7.3.2 Minimum alcohol purchasing age laws

Although legal restrictions on the age at which young people may purchase alcohol vary widely from country to country, ranging typically from 16 to 21 years of age, almost all countries legally restrict these sales. Changes in **minimum alcohol purchasing age** laws can have substantial effects on youth drinking. O'Malley and Wagenaar (1991) found that raising the minimum age reduced alcohol use among young Americans and reduced traffic crashes. Indeed the effect on car crashes continued well after young people reached the legal drinking age. Klepp et al. (1996) found that implementation of the uniform minimum legal drinking age of 21 in the US reduced the overall prevalence of drinking and driving. Other evaluations (Wagenaar 1981, 1986; Wagenaar and Maybee 1986; Saffer and Grossman 1987a, b) indicate that raising the minimum legal drinking age from 18 to 21 years decreased single vehicle night-time crashes involving young drivers by 11% to 16% at all levels of crash severity. Voas and Tippetts (1999), using data from all 50 US states and the District of Columbia for the years 1982 through 1997, concluded that the enactment of the national uniform age 21 minimum drinking age law was responsible for a 19% net decrease in fatal crashes involving young drinking drivers, after controlling for driving exposure, beer consumption, enactment of zero tolerance laws, and other relevant changes in state laws during that time period. Additional studies have shown that changes in the minimum purchasing age are related to changes in alcohol-related injury admissions to hospitals (Smith 1988) and injury fatalities (Jones *et al.* 1992).

In the most comprehensive review to date, Wagenaar and Toomey (2000) analysed all identified published studies on the drinking age from 1960 to 1999, a total of 132 documents. Their analysis led them to conclude that, compared to a wide range of other programs and efforts to reduce drinking among high school students, college students, and other teenagers, increasing the legal age for purchase and consumption of alcohol to 21 appears to have been the most effective strategy. The US National Highway Traffic Safety Administration (NHTSA) estimated that a drinking age of 21 reduced traffic fatalities by 846 deaths in 1997 and prevented a total of 17 359 deaths since 1975 (NHTSA 1998).

The literature on the effectiveness of drinking age restrictions is almost all from North America. How well do these restrictions apply in societies where alcoholic beverages have a different cultural position? One study from Denmark (Møller 2002) evaluated the effect of introducing a minimum 15 year age limit for off-premise purchases. The imposition of the law was found to be associated with a 36% drop in alcohol consumption among teenagers under age 15. In addition, there was also a 17% decline in drinking in students 15 and older. The author hypothesized that the debate around the legislation may have sensitized parents of teenagers to pay more attention to their children's drinking.

However, even in the US, it is clear that the benefits of a higher drinking age are only realized if the law is enforced. Despite higher minimum drinking age laws, young people do succeed in purchasing alcohol (e.g., Preusser and Williams 1992; Forster *et al.* 1994, 1995; Grube 1997). Such sales result from low and inconsistent levels of enforcement, especially when there is little community support for enforcement of age restrictions (Wagenaar and Wolfson 1994, 1995). Even moderate increases in enforcement can reduce sales to minors by as much as 35% to 40%, especially when combined with media and other community activities (Grube 1997; Wagenaar *et al.* 2000). This is illustrated in Box 7.3 in an evaluation of the communities mobilizing for change on alcohol (CMCA) project.

7.3.3 Controls on who is selling

Alcohol control agencies typically spend a considerable part of their time checking the credentials of those seeking licenses to sell alcoholic beverages. Typically, there is a concern to keep those with criminal records or associations out of the trade. The minimum age of alcohol sellers that is set in some countries could affect whether underage sales might occur. Younger sellers, for example, may be more willing to sell to underage buyers. Treno *et al.* (2000) report that among a community-based sample of alcohol establishments,

Box 7.3 **The CMCA project—USA**

The Communities Mobilizing for Change on Alcohol (CMCA) was designed to reduce the accessibility of alcohol to youth under the legal drinking age of 21. Communities ranging in population from 8000 to 65 000 were matched and randomly assigned to the intervention or control condition, resulting in seven intervention sites and eight comparison sites.

The project employed a part-time local organizer within each community to implement interventions designed to reduce underage access to alcohol. Such interventions could include decoy operations with alcohol outlets (in which police typically have underage buyers purchase alcohol at selected outlets), citizen monitoring of outlets selling to youth, keg registration (which requires that purchasers of kegs of beer provide identifying information, thus establishing liability for resulting problems at parties where minors are drinking), developing alcohol-free events for youth, shortening hours of sale for alcohol, responsible beverage service training, and developing educational programs for youth and adults.

Evaluation data collected $2\frac{1}{2}$ years after the initiation of the intervention activities revealed that merchants increased checking for age identification and reported more care in controlling sales to youth (Wagenaar *et al.* 1996). Research using young-looking purchasers confirmed that alcohol merchants increased age-identification checks and reduced their propensity to sell to minors. A telephone survey indicated that 18- to 20-year-olds were less likely to consume alcohol themselves and less likely to provide it to other underage persons (Wagenaar *et al.* 2000). Finally, the project found a statistically significant decline (intervention compared to control communities) in drinking–driving arrests among 18- to 20-year-olds and disorderly conduct violations among 15- to17-year-olds (Wagenaar *et al.* 2000).

off-premise sales were more likely from younger than older sales people. There has, however, been no evaluation of minimum age-of-seller restrictions.

7.4 **Strength of alcoholic beverages**

Lower alcohol content beverages have been encouraged in many countries in recent years. Lower alcohol beverages often have a reduced rate of taxation, resulting in reduced retail prices. This lower taxation has been used in many Scandinavian countries, which have defined several classes of beer, and at least two classes of wine, according to their alcohol content. Allowing 4.7% beer to be sold in grocery stores in Finland in 1969, and allowing and then recinding such sales in Sweden, can be seen as natural experiments in changing the relative availability of different strength beverages. Part of the motivation of the Finnish change was to wean Finns from their traditional preference for strong spirits (Tigerstedt 2000). In the long run, both Finland and Sweden changed from spirits-drinking to beer-drinking nations (Leifman 2001). But as we have seen, the result of the Finnish change was the addition of a new beverage and new drinking occasions to existing ones, rather than the intended substitution.

On the other hand, some success has been reported with the promotion of lighter beers. Skog (1988), analysing the effect of the introduction of light beer in Norway in March 1985, found a substitution of lower for higher alcohol content beer, although the effect was not statistically significant. He concluded that the data do not permit unequivocal evidence of substitution or addition. Another small-scale study conducted in Perth, Western Australia, indicates that changes in sales of high vs. low strength beers are strongly related to rates of alcohol-related crashes over time (Gruenewald *et al.* 1999).

Overall, the evidence is suggestive but not conclusive that making available and promoting beverages of low alcohol content can be an effective strategy. With no tax on 2.7% beer in Sweden, it often costs half as much as the 3.5% beer also available in the grocery stores, with the result that it has captured half the grocery sales market. Such a strategy does, on the face of it, have the potential to reduce the level of absolute alcohol consumed and associated intoxication and impairment.

7.5 **Promoting alcohol-free activities and events**

Promoting alcohol-free events may be seen as a means of diminishing alcohol availability, although in many such cases no alcohol control legislation or authorities may be involved.

The idea of preventing alcohol problems by providing alternatives to drinking has a long history. Temperance movements of the 19th and early 20th centuries put considerable effort into promoting 'temperance beverages'. In late 19th century Norway, coffee drinking substituted for alcoholic beverages to a considerable degree in a period of rising temperance sentiment (Skog 1985). Carbonated beverages such as Coca Cola were originally introduced as temperance drinks. From the 1920s on, the French anti-alcohol movement emphasized the promotion of apple and grape juice as more healthful alternatives to wine and cider (Prestwich 1988, pp. 233–5). How to provide 'substitutes for the saloon' that would effectively compete for the workingman's leisure time was the subject of detailed studies by social reformers (Calkins 1919). However, in the longer run, alcoholic beverages have often combined well with these beverages or activities originally conceived of as alternatives.

In recent years in the US, a number of alternatives to teenage drinking and drug use have been developed, including alternative events programming such as Sober Graduation parties and alcohol-free New Year celebrations; athletic and other recreational alternatives; adventure-oriented activities; and involvement in cultural heritage (e.g., among Native American teenagers), entrepreneurial ventures, community service projects, and creative or artistic endeavours (Carmona and Stewart 1996). Behind each of these approaches is an inherent assumption about why the target population is likely to drink (e.g., because of too much unsupervised free time, because of alienation from an ancestral culture, or because of anxiety or low self-esteem). Systematic evaluations of alternatives programs are rare (Paglia and Room 1999). An early review of this literature (Schaps *et al.* 1981) found that only two of 12 alternatives programs had substantial positive effects, and both of those also employed at least one other prevention strategy. A meta-analysis found substantial effects only for high intensity alternative programs directed at high-risk youth (Tobler 1986). Some well-designed evaluations of alternatives programs found little or no effects on alcohol use (e.g., Schaps *et al.* 1986), and there is one example of an alternatives program being associated with an increased frequency of drunkenness (Stein *et al.* 1984). Norman *et al.* (1997) comment that, 'in general, the preponderance of negative outcomes has influenced professionals in the field to almost entirely discount the Alternatives strategy as effective in substance use prevention'. Despite these conclusions, the alternatives strategy remains a highly popular and prevalent approach (Kumpfer 1999). One form of alternative programming that shows some promise is the promotion of alcohol-free festivals, such as First Night (see Box 7.4), to replace what have become heavily alcoholized celebrations on such occasions as New Year's Eve.

Box 7.4 **'First Night'**

First Night has become a program that changes the way New Year's Eve is celebrated in many cities by promoting alcohol-free community street festivals of the arts (Kerstetter and Mowrer 1998). Although no formal evaluations have been conducted, the mayor of Boston commented that 'First Night has transformed what was once a holiday marked by excessive drinking and casualties into a time of wholesome celebration' (First Night 2000). First Night is now celebrated in more than 200 cities in the US, Canada, England, and Australia.

7.6 Cost-effectiveness, and potential for adverse effects

The cost of restricting physical availability of alcohol is cheap relative to the costs of health consequences related to drinking, especially heavy drinking. The most obvious case in point is the minimum drinking age for alcohol. The increased minimum drinking age in the US was estimated to have saved thousands of lives over the past decade (Wagenaar et al. 1998). Thus, some policies can be very cost-effective in their implementation. When such regulation encounters resistance, however, the costs of enforcing or administering these policies increase. Planning and zoning ordinances and other regulations on the geographical distribution of alcohol outlets will also interact with business demand to determine the local conditions of physical availability.

The most notable adverse effect that may arise from imposing greater restrictions on the physical availability of alcohol is the increase in informal market activities (e.g., home production, illegal imports). While this has been observed in response to reductions in the number of alcohol outlets, informal market activities do not appear sufficient to replace formal production and have not produced equivalent levels of alcohol-related problems (Rossow 2000). An increase in the minimum drinking age may shift underage buyers to informal means of accessing alcohol, but the overall effect of increasing the minimum drinking age is to reduce overall harm (Forster et al. 1994). Lower densities of alcohol outlets may cause some drivers to travel greater distances for alcohol, but the increased risk may not outweigh the benefit. Reductions in outlet densities were found in one study to be unrelated to alcohol-related motor vehicle crashes (Gruenewald and Ponicki 1995).

Formal cost-effectiveness analyses of alcohol policy measures are a relatively new phenomenon. An analysis of a local policy to enforce laws against service to intoxicated customers showed a positive return on program investment (Levy and Miller 1995). A WHO generalized cost-effectiveness analysis included a 'restricted access' option, choosing Saturday closing as its exemplary alcohol control measure. It was estimated that Saturday closing would have considerable effectiveness and cost-effectiveness in most parts of the world, though clearly less than a substantial rise in alcohol taxation (Chisholm et al. 2003). Such methodologies need to be further developed and applied more broadly to alcohol availability controls.

7.7 Summarizing the impact of regulating physical availability

Most of the research on limiting availability of alcohol comes from the US and Nordic countries. There is, however, a little research from other European countries and developing countries. With regard to developing countries, the likely change in physical availability as these countries develop will be both an opportunity for research and a challenge for policy-makers to translate the current research into policy initiatives.

Studies demonstrate that controlling alcohol availability can contribute to the reduction of alcohol problems. Reductions in the hours and days of sale, numbers of alcohol outlets, and restrictions on access to alcohol, are associated with reductions in both alcohol use and alcohol-related problems.

For young people, laws that lower the minimum legal drinking age reduce alcohol sales and problems among young drinkers. This strategy has the strongest empirical support (Grube and Nygaard 2001).

Where there is popular support for these measures, changes in availability can have large effects. But even where the regulations impose only a mild inconvenience, as when there is a limited number of outlets or there are restrictions on opening hours, there may be significant effects on rates of alcohol-related problems.

The strategies considered in this chapter are all measures that affect the drinker's environment. A consistent theme in the literature is that prevention regulations directed toward commercial sellers of alcohol and backed-up with enforcement are more effective than prevention programs relying solely on education or persuasion directed toward individual drinkers. Behind enforcement may lie a variety of threats: for instance, criminal prosecution, or civil liability for damages. The most direct and immediate enforcement mechanism in many jurisdictions is the requirement that the seller hold a specific license to sell alcoholic beverages. If the system has effective power to suspend or revoke a license in the case of selling infractions, it can be an effective and flexible instrument for holding down rates of alcohol-related problems.

References

Alaniz M.L., Cartmill, R.S., and Parker R.N. (1998) Immigrants and violence: the importance of neighborhood context. *Hispanic Journal of Behavioral Sciences* 20, 155–74.

Baker T.K., Johnson M.B., Voas R.B., *et al.* (2000) Reduce youthful binge drinking: Call an election in Mexico. *Journal of Safety Research* 31, 61–9.

Blose J.O. and Holder H.D. (1987) Liquor-by-the-drink and alcohol-related traffic crashes: a natural experiment using time-series analysis. *Journal of Studies on Alcohol* 48, 52–60.

Bowerman R.J. (1997) Effect of a community-supported alcohol ban on prenatal and other substance abuse. *American Journal of Public Health* 87, 1378–9.

Brady M. (2000) Alcohol policy issues for indigenous people in the United States, Canada, Australia and New Zealand. *Contemporary Drug Problems* 27, 435–509.

Calkins R. (1919) *Substitutes for the saloon: An investigation originally made for the committee of fifty*, 2nd edn (revised). Boston: Mifflin Company.

Carmona M. and Stewart K. (1996) *Review of alternative activities and alternative programs in youth-oriented prevention.* CSAP Technical Report 13. Rockville, MD: Center for Substance Abuse Prevention.

Chaloupka F.J, Grossman M., and Saffer H. (2002) The effects of price on alcohol consumption and alcohol-related problems. *Alcohol Research and Health* 26, 22–34.

Chikritzhs T. and Stockwell T.R. (2002) The impact of later trading hours for Australian public houses (hotels) on levels of violence. *Journal of Studies on Alcohol* 63, 591–9.

Chisholm D., Rehm J., Van Ommeren M., *et al.* (2003) Choosing interventions to reduce heavy alcohol use: a generalized cost-effectiveness analysis (WHO-CHOICE). Geneva: WHO CHOICE Project.

Chiu A.Y., Perez P.E., and Parker R.N. (1997) Impact of banning alcohol on outpatient visits in Barrow, Alaska. *Journal of the American Medical Association* 278, 1775–7.

d'Abbs P. and Togni S. (2000) Liquor licensing and community action in regional and remote Australia: a review of recent initiatives. *Australian and New Zealand Journal of Public Health* 24, 45–53.

Drummond, D.C. (2000) UK Government announces first major relaxation in the alcohol licensing laws for nearly a century: Drinking in the UK goes 24–7. *Addiction* 95, 997–8.

Forster J.L., McGovern P.G., Wagenaar A.C., *et al.* (1994) Ability of young people to purchase alcohol without age identification in northeastern Minnesota, USA. *Addiction* 89, 699–705.

Forster J.L., Murray D.M., Wolfson M., *et al.* (1995) Commercial availability of alcohol to young people: Results of alcohol purchase attempts. *Preventive Medicine* 24, 342–7.

Gorman D., Speer P.W., Gruenewald P.J., *et al.* (2001) Spatial dynamics of alcohol availability, neighborhood structure and violent crime. *Journal of Studies on Alcohol* 62, 628–36.

Gray D., Saggers S., Sputore B., *et al.* (2000) What works? A review of evaluated alcohol misuse interventions among Aboriginal Australians. *Addiction* 95, 11–22.

Grube J.W. (1997) Preventing sales of alcohol to minors: Results from a community trial. *Addiction* 92 (Suppl. 2), S251–60.

Grube J.W. and Nygaard P. (2001) Adolescent drinking and alcohol policy. *Contemporary Drug Problems* 28, 87–132.

Gruenewald P.J. and Treno A.J. (2000) Local and global alcohol supply: Economic and geographic models of community systems. *Addiction* 95 (Suppl. 4), S537–49.

Gruenewald P.J. and Ponicki W.R. (1995) Relationship of the retail availability of alcohol and alcohol sales to alcohol-related traffic crashes. *Accident Analysis and Prevention* 27, 249–59.

Gruenewald P.J., Ponicki W.R., and Holder H.D. (1993) The relationship of outlet densities to alcohol consumption: a time series cross-sectional analysis. *Alcoholism: Clinical and Experimental Research* 17, 38–47.

Gruenewald P.J., Millar A.B., and Roeper P. (1996) Access to alcohol: geography and prevention for local communities. *Alcohol Health and Research World* 20, 244–51.

Gruenewald P.J., Stockwell T., Beel A., *et al.* (1999) Beverage sales and drinking and driving: The role of on-premise drinking places. *Journal of Studies on Alcohol* 60, 47–53.

Gruenewald P.J., Johnson F.W., Millar A., *et al.* (2000) Drinking and driving: Explaining beverage-specific risks. *Journal of Studies on Alcohol* 61, 515–23.

Hammurabi (2000) *Code of Hammurabi*, translated by L.W. King. Website: http://www.fordham.edu/halsall/ancient/hamcode.html

Her M., Giesbrecht N., Room R., *et al.* (1999) Privatizing alcohol sales and alcohol consumption: evidence and implications. *Addiction* 94, 1125–39.

Hibell B. (1984) Mellanölets borttagande och indikationer på alkoholskadeutvecklingen (The withdrawal of medium beer and indications on alcohol damages). In: Nilsson T. (ed.) *När Mellanölet Försvann* (When the medium beer was withdrawn), pp. 121–72. Linköping: Samhällsvetenskapliga institutionen, Universitetet i Linköping.

Holder H.D., Janes K., Mosher J., *et al.* (1993). Alcoholic beverage server liability and the reduction of alcohol-involved problems. *Journal of Studies on Alcohol* 54, 23–36.

Holder H.D., Kühlhorn E., Nordlund S., *et al.* (1998) *European integration and Nordic alcohol policies. Changes in alcohol controls and consequences in Finland, Norway and Sweden, 1980–1997.* Aldershot, UK: Ashgate.

Holder H.D., Gruenwald P.J., Ponicki W.R., *et al.* (2000) Effect of community-based interventions on high-risk drinking and alcohol-related injuries. *Journal of the American Medical Association* 248, 2341–7.

Jewell R.T. and Brown R.W. (1995) Alcohol availability and alcohol-related motor vehicle accidents. *Applied Economics* 27, 759–65.

Johansen P.O. (1994) *Markedet som Ikke Ville Døslash. Forbudstiden og de Illegale Alkoholmarkedene i Norge og USA* (The market that would not die. Times of prohibition and the illegal alcohol markets in Norway and the US). Oslo, Norway: National Directorate for Prevention of Alcohol and Drug Use.

Jones N.E., Pieper C.F., and Robertson L.S. (1992) Effect of legal drinking age on fatal injuries of adolescents and young adults. *American Journal of Public Health* 82, 112–15.

Klepp K.I., Schmid L.A., and Murray D.M. (1996) Effects of the increased minimum drinking age law on drinking and driving behavior among adolescents. *Addiction Research* 4, 237–44.

Kortteinen T. (ed.) (1989) *State monopolies and alcohol prevention: Report and working papers of a collaborative international study.* Helsinki, Finland: Social Research Institute of Alcohol Studies.

Kumpfer K.L. (1999) *Identification of drug abuse prevention programs: Literature review*, part B. Rockville, MD: NIDA Resource Center for Health Services Research.

Kuusi P. (1957) *Alcohol sales experiment in rural Finland*, Vol. 3A. Helsinki: Finnish Foundation for Alcohol Studies.

LaScala E.A., Johnson F., and Gruenewald P.J. (2001) Neighborhood characteristics of alcohol-related pedestrian injury collisions: A geostatistical analysis. *Prevention Science* 2, 123–34.

Lehtonon O. (1978) Anniskeluravintoloiden kehityspiirteitä ja näkymiä 1962–1980 (Development and prospects of the restaurant industry, 1962–1980). *Alkoholipolitiikka* 43, 290–8.

Leifman H. (2001) Homogenization in alcohol consumption in the European Union. *Nordic Studies on Alcohol and Drugs* 18 (English Suppl.), 15–30.

Levine H.G. (1985) The birth of American alcohol control: prohibition, the power elite, and the problem of lawlessness. *Contemporary Drug Problems* 12, 63–115.

Levy D.T. and Miller T.R. (1995) A cost–benefit analysis of enforcement efforts to reduce serving intoxicated patrons. *Journal of Studies on Alcohol* 56, 240–7.

Ligon J. and Thyer B.A. (1993) Effects of a Sunday liquor ban on DUI arrests. *Journal of Alcohol and Drug Education* 38, 33–40.

Ligon J., Thyer B.A., and Lund R. (1996) Drinking, eating, and driving: evaluating the effects of partially removing a Sunday liquor sales ban. *Journal of Alcohol and Drug Education* 42, 15–24.

Lipton R. and Gruenewald P.J. (2002) The spatial dynamics of violence and alcohol outlets. *Journal of Studies on Alcohol* 63, 187–95.

Mäkelä P., Tryggvesson K., and Rossow I. (2002) Who drinks more or less when policies change? The evidence from 50 years of Nordic studies. In: Room R. (ed.) *The effects of Nordic alcohol policies: What happens to drinking and harm when control systems change?* Publication No. 42, pp. 17–70. Helsinki: Nordic Council for Alcohol and Drug Research.

Mäkinen H. (1978) *Kunnallisten keskiolutkieltojen vaikutukset. Tapaustutkimus viidessä kunnassa* (Effects of banning medium beer in municipalities. Case study in five municipalities). Helsinki: Alkoholipoliittisen tutkimuslaitoksen tutkimusseloste 122.

Møller L. (2002) Legal restrictions resulted in a reduction of alcohol consumption among young people in Denmark. In: Room R. (ed.) *The effects of Nordic alcohol policies: What happens to drinking and harm when control systems change?* Publication No. 42, pp. 155–66. Helsinki: Nordic Council for Alcohol and Drug Research.

Moskalewicz J. (2000) Alcohol in the countries in transition: the Polish experience and the wider context. *Contemporary Drug Problems* 27, 561–92.

Moskalewicz J. and Swiatkiewicz G. (2000) Alcohol consumption and its consequences in Poland in the light of official statistics. In: Leifman H. and Edgren Henrichsen N. (eds.) *Statistics on alcohol, drugs and crime in the Baltic Sea region.* Publication No. 37, pp. 143–61. Helsinki: Nordic Council for Alcohol and Drug Research.

National Highway Traffic Safety Administration (1998) *Traffic safety facts, 1997.* Washington, DC: US Government Printing Office.

NHTSA. See National Highway Traffic Safety Administration.

Nordlund S. (1985) *Effects of Saturday closing of wine and spirits shops in Norway.* SIFA Mimeograph No. 5/85. Oslo: National Institute of Alcohol Research.

Norman E., Turner S., Zunz S.J., *et al.* (1997) Prevention programs reviewed: what works? In: Norman E. (ed.) *Drug-free youth: A compendium for prevention specialists*, pp. 22–45. New York and London: Garland Publishing.

Norström T. (1987) Abolition of the Swedish rationing system: effects on consumption distribution and cirrhosis mortality. *British Journal of Addiction* 82, 633–41.

Norström T. (2000) Outlet density and criminal violence in Norway, 1960–1995. *Journal of Studies on Alcohol* 61, 907–11.

Norström T. and Skog O.-J. (2001) *Effekter av lördagsöppna Systembolagsbutiker: uppföljning av de först tio månaderna* (Effects of Saturday opening of the alcohol monopoly shops: follow-up of the first 10 months). Stockholm: Social and Health Ministry. Web address: http://social.regeringen.se/pressinfo/pdf/folkhalsa/ rapport_lordagsoppet.pdf

Noval S. and Nilsson T. (1984) Mellanölets effekt på konsumtionsnivån och tillväxten hos den totala alkoholkonsumtionen (The effects of medium beer on consumption levels and the rise in overall alcohol consumption). In: Nilsson T. (ed.) *När Mellanölet Försvann* (When the medium beer was withdrawn), pp. 77–93. Linköping: Samhällsvetenskapliga institutionen, Universitetet i Linköping.

Olsson O. and Wikström P.H. (1982) Effects of the experimental Saturday closing of liquor retail stores in Sweden. *Contemporary Drug Problems* 11, 325–53.

Österberg E. (1979) *Recorded consumption of alcohol in Finland, 1950–1975*. Report No. 125. Helsinki: Social Research Institute of Alcohol Studies.

Österberg E. and Haavisto K. (1997) Alkoholsmugglingen till Finland under 1990-talet (Smuggling of alcoholic beverages into Finland in the 1990s). *Nordisk Alkohol- and Narkotikatidskrift* 14, 290–303.

O'Malley P.M. and Wagenaar A.C. (1991) Effects of minimum drinking age laws on alcohol use, related behaviors and traffic crash involvement among American youth: 1976–1987. *Journal of Studies on Alcohol* 52, 478–91.

Paglia A. and Room R. (1999) Preventing substance use problems among youth: A literature review and recommendations. *Journal of Primary Prevention* 20, 3–50.

Paulson R.E. (1973) *Women's suffrage and prohibition: A comparative study of equality and social control*. Glenview, IL: Scott, Foresman.

Poikolainen K. (1980) Increase in alcohol-related hospitalizations in Finland 1969–1975. *British Journal of Addiction* 75, 281–91.

Prestwich P.E. (1988) *Drink and the politics of social reform: Antialcoholism in France since 1870*. Palo Alto, CA: Society for the Promotion of Science and Scholarship.

Preusser D.F. and Williams A.F. (1992) Sales of alcohol to underage purchasers in three New York counties and Washington, DC. *Journal of Public Health Policy* 13, 306–17.

Ragnarsdottir T., Kjartansdottir A., and Davidsdottir S. (2002) Effect of extended alcohol serving-hours in Reykjavik. In: Room R. (ed.) *The effects of Nordic alcohol policies: What happens to drinking and harm when control systems change?* Publication No. 42, pp. 145–54. Helsinki: Nordic Council for Alcohol and Drug Research.

Raistrick D., Hodgson R., and Ritson B. (1999) *Tackling alcohol together: The evidence base for a UK alcohol policy*. London and New York: Free Association Books.

Ramstedt M. (2002) The repeal of medium strength beer in grocery stores in Sweden: the impact on alcohol-related hospitalizations in different age groups. In: Room R. (ed.) *The effects of Nordic alcohol policies: What happens to drinking and harm when control systems change?* Publication No. 42, pp. 117–31. Helsinki: Nordic Council for Alcohol and Drug Research.

Room R. (2000) Alcohol monopolies as instruments for alcohol control policies. In: Österberg E. (ed.) *International seminar on alcohol retail monopolies*, pp. 7–16. Helsinki: National Research and Development Centre for Welfare and Health, Themes 5/2000.

Room R., Jernigan J., Carlini Marlatt B., *et al.* (2002) *Alcohol in developing societies: A public health approach*. Helsinki: Finnish Foundation for Alcohol Studies.

Rossow I. (2000) The validity of political arguments in the Norwegian alcohol policy debate: associations between availability of liquor and consumption of illegal spirits. *Contemporary Drug Problems* 27, 253–69.

Saffer H. and Grossman M. (1987a) Beer taxes, the legal drinking age, and youth motor vehicle fatalities. *Journal of Legal Studies* 16, 351–74.

Saffer H. and Grossman M. (1987b) Drinking age laws and highway mortality rates: Cause and effect. *Economic Inquiry* 25, 403–17.

Schaps E., DiBartolo R., Moskowitz J., *et al.* (1981) A review of 127 drug abuse prevention evaluations. *Journal of Drug Issues* 11, 17–43.

Schaps E., Moskowitz J., Malvin J.H., *et al.* (1986) Evaluation of seven school-based prevention programs: a final report on the Napa project. *International Journal of the Addictions* 21, 1081–112.

Schechter E. (1986) Alcohol rationing and control systems in Greenland. *Contemporary Drug Problems* 13, 587–620.

Skog O.-J. (1985) *Changes in alcohol and coffee consumption in the 19th century: A case of beverage substitution?* SIFA Mimeograph. Oslo: National Institute for Alcohol and Drug Research.

Skog O.-J. (1988) Effect of introducing a new light beer in Norway: substitution or addition? *British Journal of Addiction* 83, 665–8.

Smith D.I. (1988) Effectiveness of restrictions on availability as a means of preventing alcohol-related problems. *Contemporary Drug Problems* 15, 627–84.

Stein J.A., Swisher J.D., Hu T., *et al.* (1984) Cost-effectiveness evaluation of a Channel One program. *Journal of Drug Education* 14, 251–69.

Stevenson R.J., Lind B., and Weatherburn D. (1999) Relationship between alcohol sales and assault in New South Wales, Australia. *Addiction* 94, 397–410.

Stockwell T. (1994) Do controls on the availability of alcohol reduce alcohol problems? In: Stockwell T. (ed.) *An examination of the appropriateness and efficacy of liquor licensing laws across Australia*, Vol. 5, pp. 119–44. Canberra, Australia: Government Publishing Services.

Stockwell T., Lang E., and Rydon P. (1993) High risk drinking settings: the association of serving and promotional practices with harmful drinking. *Addiction* 88, 1519–26.

Tigerstedt C. (2000) Discipline and public health. In: Sulkunen P., Sutton C., Tigerstedt C., *et al.* (eds.) *Broken spirits: Power and ideas in Nordic alcohol control.* NAD Publication No. 39, pp. 93–112. Helsinki: Nordic Council for Alcohol and Drug Research.

Tobler N.S. (1986) Meta-analysis of 143 adolescent drug prevention programs: quantitative outcome results of program participants compared to a control or comparison group. *Journal of Drug Issues* 16, 537–67.

Travis A. (2000) Straw unveils 24-hour pubs revolution. *Guardian* (London), April 11.

Treno A.J., Alaniz M.L., and Gruenewald P.J. (2000) The use of drinking places by gender, age and ethnic groups: An analysis of routine drinking activities. *Addiction* 95, 537–51.

Valli R. (1998) Forandringar i ungdomarnas alkoholvanor nar mellanolet slapptes fritt: Fallet Jakobstad (Changes in young people's alcohol consumption with improved availability of medium strength beer: The case of Pietarsaari). *Nordisk Alkohol- & Narkotikatidskrift* 15, 168–75.

Voas R.B. and Tippetts A.S. (1999) *Relationship of alcohol safety laws to drinking drivers in fatal crashes.* Washington, DC: National Highway Traffic Safety Administration.

Wagenaar A.C. (1981) Effects of the raised legal drinking age on motor vehicle accidents in Michigan. *HSRI Research Review* 11 (4), 1–8.

Wagenaar A.C. (1986) Preventing highway crashes by raising the legal minimum age for drinking: The Michigan experience 6 years later. *Journal of Safety Research* 17, 101–9.

Wagenaar A.C. and Holder H.D. (1995) Changes in alcohol consumption resulting from the elimination of retail wine monopolies: Results from five US states. *Journal of Studies on Alcohol* 56, 566–72.

Wagenaar A.C. and Maybee R.G. (1986) Legal minimum drinking age in Texas: Effects of an increase from 18 to 19. *Journal of Safety Research* 17, 165–78.

Wagenaar A.C. and Toomey T.L. (2000) Alcohol policy: gaps between legislative action and current research. *Contemporary Drug Problems* 27, 681–733.

Wagenaar A.C. and Wolfson M. (1994) Enforcement of the legal minimum drinking age in the United States. *Journal of Public Health Policy* 15, 37–53.

Wagenaar A.C. and Wolfson M. (1995) Deterring sales and provision of alcohol to minors: a study of enforcement in 295 counties in four states. *Public Health Reports* 110, 419–27.

Wagenaar A.C., Gehan J.P., Jones-Webb R., *et al.* (1998) *Communities mobilizing for change on alcohol: Experiences and outcomes from a randomized community trial.* Minneapolis, MN: University of Minnesota.

Wagenaar A.C., Murray D.M., and Toomey T.L. (2000) Communities Mobilizing for Change on Alcohol (CMCA): effects of a randomized trial on arrest and traffic crashes. *Addiction* 95, 209–17.

World Health Organization (1999) *Global status report on alcohol.* WHO/HSC/SAB/99.11. Geneva: WHO Substance Abuse Department.

Chapter 8

Modifying the drinking context

8.1 Introduction

Alcohol use takes place within a social, cultural, and community context. Therefore, heavy consumption can be modified and problems reduced by using strategies that change this context. Such efforts are considered **harm reduction** measures in that they start from an acceptance that there will be consumption of alcoholic beverages and seek to modify or limit the drinking or the drinking environment so that potential harm is minimized. The measures considered in this chapter generally target the drinking environment, particularly environments where alcohol is sold and consumed. Therefore, their effectiveness does not depend on the support or compliance of individual drinkers, although such support may enhance the measures' effects. Prevention directed at high-risk drinking environments such as **licensed premises** provides an alternative or complement to broadly focused prevention measures such as alcohol pricing and individual approaches such as treatment.

In Western countries, licensed drinking environments have been identified as drinking locations that are especially high risk for alcohol-related intoxication (Snow and Landrum 1986), drinking–driving (O'Donnell 1985; Single and McKenzie 1992; Fahrenkrug and Rehm 1995; Gruenewald *et al.* 1996), and problem behaviours such as aggression and violence (Ireland and Thommeny 1993; Stockwell *et al.* 1993; Rossow 1996). Because of the high rate of problems in licensed premises and the feasibility of controlling these high-risk environments through licensing and other controls, licensed premises are a prime target for alcohol policies aimed at the prevention of alcohol-related problems.

Aggressive behaviour is a major problem associated with drinking in licensed premises in many countries. As discussed in Chapter 4, experimental studies of the effects of alcohol on aggression suggest that alcohol intoxication plays a causal role in aggressive behaviour (Bushman 1997). It is also clear that personality and situational factors play key moderating roles in alcohol's effects (Graham *et al.* 1998). For example, the high rate of problems in bars is at least partly attributable to the types of drinkers who tend to frequent these establishments (i.e., young adult males). Certain aspects of the bar environment also appear to increase the likelihood that drinking will be associated with problems (Graham and Homel 1997), including serving practices that promote intoxication, an aggressive approach taken to closing time by bar staff and local police (Marsh and Kibby 1992; Tomsen 1997), the inability of bar staff to manage problem behaviour (Homel *et al.* 1992; Wells *et al.* 1998), general characteristics of the bar-room environment such as crowding and permissiveness of bar staff (Homel and Clark 1994), and the general type of bar (Stockwell *et al.* 1992; Gruenewald *et al.* 1999).

The focus on high-risk environments such as licensed premises has several advantages. It can have a broader impact than individual approaches on persons who are at high risk, especially young people and subcultures with risky drinking practices. A variety of approaches can be applied at one time (e.g., training, enforcement, reducing environmental risks) to enhance effects. Finally, most approaches targeting high-risk environments are generally perceived as acceptable across cultures and are therefore readily adopted. This chapter focuses primarily on interventions that address problems related to drinking in licensed premises. These include training bar staff in responsible beverage service practices, management of problem behaviour, enforcement of alcohol serving regulations, use of voluntary codes of practices, and community mobilization.

8.2 **Responsible beverage service training and policy**

As described in Box 8.1, **responsible beverage service** (RBS) programs (also referred to as Server Training or Server Intervention programs) focus on attitudes, knowledge, skills, and practices of persons involved in serving alcoholic beverages on licensed premises (see Carvolth 1995; Toomey *et al.* 1998). The primary goal of RBS is to prevent intoxication and underage drinking. Some programs have included separate or extended training for managers on policy development.

Research on RBS programs has occurred mostly in Canada, the US, Australia, and Sweden. Nearly all evaluations have demonstrated improved knowledge and attitudes among participants (see review by Graham 2000). These studies have also shown some effects on serving practices. In particular, servers are usually willing to intervene with customers who are visibly intoxicated (Gliksman *et al.* 1993), but generally will not intervene with individuals solely on the basis of the customer's estimated blood alcohol concentration (BAC) or number of drinks consumed (Howard-Pitney *et al.* 1991; Saltz and Stanghetta 1997). In addition, training tends to decrease bad serving practices

Box 8.1 **Components of responsible beverage service programs**

RBS programs typically include the following four components:

1. **Attitude change**: The benefits of preventing intoxication and not serving underage patrons are stressed so that bar staff and management will take responsibility to prevent intoxication.

2. **Knowledge**: The effects of alcohol, the relationship between alcohol consumption and BAC, the signs of intoxication, the laws and regulations related to serving alcohol, legal liability, strategies for dealing with intoxicated or underage patrons, and refusing service.

3. **Skills**: The ability to recognize intoxication, refuse service, and avoid problems in dealing with an intoxicated person.

4. **Practice**: Checking age identification of young patrons, preventing intoxication, refusing service to someone who is becoming intoxicated, and arranging safe transport for intoxicated patrons.

such as 'pushing' drinks and increase 'soft' interventions such as suggesting food or slowing service. But training is less likely to increase actual refusal of service to intoxicated individuals (McKnight 1991; Gliksman *et al.* 1993). With regard to patron intoxication, several studies have found that server training generally results in lower BAC levels of patrons (Geller *et al.* 1987; Russ and Geller 1987) and fewer patrons with high BAC levels (Saltz 1987; Stockwell *et al.* 1993; Lang *et al.* 1998). Moreover, time–series analyses of mandatory server training suggest that training is associated with fewer visibly intoxicated patrons (Dresser 2000) and fewer single-vehicle night-time injury-producing crashes (Holder and Wagenaar 1994).

There is increasing recognition of the need to focus on house rules and management support for RBS (see Stockwell 2001). Many RBS programs have included training for managers in the implementation of standard house policies or have used a 'risk assessment' approach to policy development (Saltz 1987; Mosher 1990). For example, the Australian 'Freo Respects You' project (Lang *et al.* 1998) included a House Policy Checklist that covered the following topics: providing positive incentives for avoiding intoxication (e.g., food, cheaper prices for low or no alcohol drinks), avoiding incentives for intoxication (e.g., drink specials), policies to minimize harm (e.g., increasing safe transportation options), and policies to minimize intoxication (e.g., slowing then refusing service to intoxicated patrons). A number of studies have found modest effects of interventions focused on house policies (Howard-Pitney *et al.* 1991; Lang *et al.* 1998; Wallin *et al.* 1999; Toomey *et al.* 2001). The findings suggest that RBS training, if supported by actual changes in serving policies of licensed establishments and reinforced by local policing enforcement, can reduce heavy consumption and high-risk drinking.

8.3 Enforcement of alcohol serving practices and potential liability

The greatest impact of government policies regarding alcohol service is likely to occur if the policy is combined with active enforcement (see Homel *et al.* 2001). The importance of enforcement was demonstrated by McKnight and Streff (1994), who evaluated the effect of increased enforcement of laws prohibiting the sale of alcohol to intoxicated patrons in bars and restaurants in one county in the state of Michigan, USA. Their study found a significantly higher rate of refusal of service to pseudo patrons (i.e., actors who appeared to be intoxicated) in the county where enforcement was increased, compared to refusal rates in a comparison county. They also found a significant decrease in Driving While Impaired (DWI) charges in the experimental county compared to no change in DWI charges in three counties for which comparison data were available. Moreover, econometric analyses (Levy and Miller 1995) indicated that the benefits of increased alcohol-related law enforcement greatly exceeded the costs.

Proactive policing, involving regular visits to licensees, is a slightly different enforcement strategy that has been used to reduce offences relating to underage drinking and drunkenness. Although an early study in the UK found this to be an effective strategy (Jeffs and Saunders 1983), a replication in Australia was unable to show a clear positive impact (Burns *et al.* 1995).

Holding servers legally liable for the consequences of providing more alcohol to persons who are already intoxicated or those underage has shown consistent benefits as a policy measure in the US. In particular, states that hold bar owners and staff legally liable for damage attributable to alcohol intoxication have lower rates of traffic fatalities (Chaloupka *et al.* 1993; Sloan *et al.* 1994a; Ruhm 1996) and homicide (Sloan *et al.* 1994b), compared to states that do not have this liability. In addition, Wagenaar and Holder (1991) found that when one state deliberately distributed publicity about the legal liability of servers, there was a 12% decrease in single-vehicle night-time injury-producing traffic crashes, a statistically significant change when compared to trends in other states. Several studies suggest that these changes are mediated by the effects of legal liability on the attitudes and behaviour of bar owners and staff (Holder *et al.* 1993; Sloan *et al.* 2000).

8.4 **Use of voluntary codes of practice**

When problems in bars are concentrated in a specific geographical area, some approaches have involved agreements among bar owners to limit the major risk factors for violence and other alcohol-related problems. A number of communities, most notably in Australia, have implemented voluntary codes of practice among local bar owners.

Although controlled evaluations of voluntary codes have not been done, informal evaluations suggest that the success of voluntary codes depends on a number of factors, including community pressure from the police and the public (Arnold and Laidler 1994). For example, as described in Box 8.2, the apparent effectiveness of the Geelong Accord, one of the most successful voluntary codes, was due largely to the leadership of the police (Lang and Rumbold 1997), suggesting that a bar owners' association provides a useful starting point for raising awareness but that enforcement may be a necessary component for codes to be successful (Homel *et al.* 1997).

Box 8.2 **The Geelong Accord**

The Geelong Accord was initiated by local police in one Australian community to reduce pub-hopping (i.e., moving from one drinking place to another) and associated problems. The Accord also aimed to minimize heavy drinking by underage patrons. Stipulations within the accord included cover charges to enter bars after 11 pm, removal of cover charge exemptions for women, prohibition of unlimited re-entry with cover charge, banning of drink promotions that lead to intoxication, consistent serving policies among bars, and increased enforcement of laws regarding underage drinking and drinking in the streets. Bar owners reported a positive impact of the Accord, which is consistent with an observed decline in the assault rate from 0.8 to 0.5 per day (Felson *et al.* 1997). The Geelong Accord appeared to have a substantial and sustained impact on the local crime rate, although the lack of a controlled evaluation makes this conclusion tentative. Support from the local police seemed to be a key factor in the success of the voluntary code.

8.5 **Managing aggression and other problem behaviour**

Training programs specifically focused on aggressive patrons rather than serving practices have been developed for several reasons.

1. Not all problems arise because patrons are intoxicated. For example, some bar settings attract patrons who may be looking for a fight (Burns 1980; Graham *et al.* 1980; Homel *et al.* 1992; Graham and Wells 2001).

2. Some individuals arrive at the bar already intoxicated, rather than being served to intoxication while there.

3. Sometimes problems in bars are less related to intoxicated patrons and more related to aggressive bar staff, as illustrated in Box 8.3 (Wells *et al.* 1998).

4. When drinks are obtained from a busy serving bar, it is often not possible for staff to monitor consumption levels, regardless of how well trained they are (Kulis 1998).

A number of programs in the UK have been developed specifically to train door staff on relevant laws, the effects of alcohol and drugs, fire safety, first aid, and communication skills in order to keep problem patrons out of the bar (see MCM Research 1993). Training programs for licensees have also been developed in the UK, including one associated with the alcoholic

---

Box 8.3 **A tragedy that could have been avoided**

The following newspaper quotation describes an incident related to alcohol consumption in a licensed premise in Canada. It shows how a rather trivial incident by an intoxicated patron led to violence that dramatically affected the lives of two ordinary young people.

'Former bouncer Patrick John Brownlow sat in the prisoners' box and swallowed hard as a judge sentenced him to 30 months in penitentiary Friday for the crime of aggravated assault. Across the courtroom and surrounded by members of his large family, the victim, Gary Tordoff, sat in the wheelchair he is unable to rise from. . . . The jury was told the incident began when Brownslow, then a 23-year-old nursing student at Fanshawe College, and another bouncer tried to stop Tordoff from leaving the bar with a beer in his hand. In the struggle, Tordoff's head was banged against a wall about four times and he was tossed out of the door where his head apparently hit the sidewalk.'

(London Free Press, June 17, 1995)

beverage industry that deals with establishing order, recognition of early warning signs, controlling angry patrons, understanding frustration, and procedures for reducing risks at closing time (MCM Research 1993). Although these programs seem to be popular, there have been no published evaluations of them.

The *Safer bars* program recently developed in Canada includes a risk assessment (Graham 1999) and a training component (Braun *et al.* 2000) for owners, managers, and all staff. The program is designed to increase early intervention by staff, improve teamwork and staff abilities in managing problem behaviour, and reduce the risk of injury to patrons. The *Safer bars* training has been shown to be highly valued by bar staff and managers, and has demonstrated a significant impact on knowledge and attitudes (Graham *et al.* 2002).

The impact of training on actual behaviour was investigated as part of a multi-component community project in Australia (Homel *et al.* 1997; Hauritz *et al.* 1998a), which implemented a two-day training program in crowd control and security for door staff, as well as security management training for licensees and police that included management skills, staff recruitment, conflict resolution, venue security, civil and criminal law related to the operations of public venues, major incidents and emergencies, and incident reporting (Homel *et al.* 1997). Observational data in bars indicated a number of improvements in staff behaviour and bar management including friendlier bouncers, more systematic checking of identification at the door, an increase in bouncers controlling areas inside the bar as well as at the door (Homel *et al.* 1997; Hauritz *et al.* 1998a), and staff who were less permissive of deviant behaviour and friendlier in their interactions with patrons (Hauritz *et al.* 1998a). Although these projects did not use an experimental design, the ability to replicate the impact on staff behaviour of the initial Surfers Paradise project makes the evidence for this intervention more convincing. However, the effects of the Surfers Paradise intervention quickly 'wore off' in the two years after the intervention ended (Hauritz *et al.* 1998b), suggesting that continuing success of such programs depends on developing methods to maintain the program's initial success.

8.6 Reducing environmental precipitants of aggression and other problem behaviour

Logbooks and other approaches to recording critical incidents have been used as a tool to identify and correct trouble spots and problem issues in bars (Dickson *et al.* 1994). As described in Box 8.4, recent approaches to identifying 'hot' spots have gone beyond logbooks by using research knowledge on

Box 8.4 **The Safer bars risk assessment workbook**

The *Safer bars* program includes a self-administered risk assessment workbook for bar owners and managers (Graham 1999). It is designed to change the bar environment in ways that minimize risk of aggression. The workbook contains 97 self-rated items and explanations covering the following areas:

- risk factors associated with patrons entering the bar
- bar layout
- characteristics of servers and security staff
- closing time
- other aspects of the bar environment

environmental precipitants of aggression to help bar owners reduce risk factors for aggression and other problems.

8.7 **Community mobilization approaches**

Community mobilization has been used to raise awareness of problems associated with on-premise drinking, develop specific solutions to problems, and pressure bar owners to recognize that they have a responsibility to the community in terms of such bar-related issues as noise level and patron behaviour (Homel *et al.* 1992; Putnam *et al.* 1993; Hauritz *et al.* 1998a, b). Evaluation results from community mobilization approaches as well as documentation from grassroots projects (Arnold and Laidler 1994; Cusenza 1998) suggest that community mobilization can be highly successful at reducing aggression and other problems related to drinking in licensed premises. Box 8.5 provides a description of one community mobilization project in the USA.

Other examples of successful community mobilization, training, and policy development efforts include the Surfers Paradise project (Homel *et al.* 1997). The goal of the project was to reduce violence and disorder associated with the high concentration of licensed establishments in the resort town of Surfers Paradise in Queensland, Australia (Homel *et al.* 1997). The project involved three major strategies:

1. The creation of a Community Forum including the development of task groups and a safety audit.

Box 8.5 **Community alcohol abuse/injury prevention project (CAAIPP)—USA (1984–1989)**

The Rhode Island community alcohol abuse/injury prevention project (Putnam *et al.* 1993) utilized community mobilization as a means to reduce alcohol-related injuries. One community was randomly selected for the intervention while two others served as controls. The intervention included a five-hour Responsible Beverage Service training program, policy development for on- and off-premise alcohol sales, enhanced enforcement of liquor and DWI laws, training of police, and mass media campaigns. The RBS program trained 61% of servers in the intervention community. A high rate of adoption of house policies was achieved for both on-premise (79%) and off-premise (100%) licensed establishments. Following the training there were significant improvements in knowledge and self-reported serving behaviour. Effects were mostly sustained over a four-year period (Buka and Birdthistle 1999). Police and emergency room surveillance indicated a 27% increase in alcohol-related assault arrest rates in the intervention community (reflecting increased enforcement), while emergency room visits declined 9% for injuries, 21% for assaults, and 10% for motor vehicle crashes. There were no declines in the control community. Although the project showed immediate success, follow-up data indicated that the increased enforcement stimulated by the project was not maintained after the project ended (Stout *et al.* 1993).

2. The implementation of risk assessments, Model House Policies, and a Code of Practice.

3. Regulation of licensed premises by police and liquor licensing inspectors.

This project and its replications in three North Queensland cities (Cairns, Townsville, and Mackay) (Hauritz *et al.* 1998a) resulted in significant improvements in alcohol policy enforcement in the bar environment, in bar staff practices, and in the frequency of violence. Following the intervention, the number of incidents per 100 hours of observation dropped from 9.8 at pre-test to 4.7 in Surfers Paradise and from 12.2 at pre-test to 3.0 in the replication sites. However, the initial impact of the project was not sustained. Two years following the intervention in Surfers Paradise, the rate had increased to 8.3. This rate change highlighted the need to find ways to maintain gains achieved from community action projects. Therefore, the replication sites attempted to put in place safeguards for maintaining the intervention gains. The long-term effectiveness of these strategies is not known at this time.

As a result of this project, there are a number of community action manuals available to facilitate the process of grassroots mobilization (e.g., Lander 1995; Neves *et al.* 1998). This may increase the future likelihood of systematic implementation and evaluation of grassroots efforts. Overall, community mobilizing approaches appear to have at least a temporary impact on licensed premise policies with associated changes in the bar environment, staff practices, and patron violence. These approaches, however, have not been implemented in a systematic way except through applied research projects, which tend to be expensive and difficult to sustain beyond the project evaluation period (see Graham and Chandler Coutts 2000; Holder and Moore 2000).

8.8 **Other approaches to harm reduction**

Other approaches to reducing the harm while accepting the drinking include general safety measures that have particular relevance to intoxicated persons and modifying the potential behaviour of bystanders or victims. For example, tempered glass has been recommended as an alternative to regular glass in licensed premises in order to prevent cuts and other injuries when glass vessels are used as weapons in bar fights (Alcohol Concern 1996); however, a recent randomized control trial found that injuries to bar staff actually increased when toughened glassware was used (Warburton and Shepherd 2000), suggesting that the only safer alternative at this time would be metal, paper, or plastic drink containers.

Third parties often play a role in controlling aggressive and other problem behaviours in licensed premises (Wells and Graham 1999), at fiestas and other occasions (Perez 2000), and among adults generally (Graham and Wells 2001). Therefore, in addition to prevention interventions focused on bar staff, there have been efforts to enlist friends and potential victims as prevention agents (e.g., the 'friends don't let friends drive drunk' campaign—see Hawkins *et al.* 1977; McKilip *et al.* 1985; McKnight 1990). Although one study (Kennedy *et al.* 1997) found that 55% of a sample of men aged 21–34 reported having received such an intervention, the effect of these programs on drinking–driving has not been demonstrated.

Dealing with alcohol issues in sexual assault prevention programs for women is commonly recommended in the literature (e.g., Abbey *et al.* 1996). An important issue in discussing the prevention of sexual victimization or aggression is that victims are themselves frequently intoxicated when such incidents occur. For example, a study on a university campus found that approximately one-third of the victims of sexual assault were incapacitated because of alcohol consumption (Meilman and Haygood-Jackson 1996). Training programs must also face the issue of whether it is appropriate to suggest to potential victims that some of the responsibility for avoiding victimization is theirs. In some cultures a potential victim's intoxication might be regarded as making the victim partly responsible (e.g., Miers 1978; Aramburu and Leigh 1991). De Crespigny *et al.* (1998) noted that female bar patrons rely on girlfriends to assist them with safety issues. Therefore, prevention programs aimed at friends rather than potential victims may prove efficacious. However, while training potential victims or bystanders in methods of reducing the harm from someone else's intoxication appears to have some promise, there have been no studies of the effectiveness of this strategy.

8.9 **Conclusion**

Increasingly, interventions focusing on reducing the harm from alcohol when drinking is occurring are being developed and implemented, especially in societies and settings where drinking is widely accepted. This approach to prevention is relatively new, however, and many of the interventions currently in practice have not been adequately evaluated. The most effective options to date have involved enhanced enforcement of regulations around serving and legal liability of bar staff and owners for the actions of those they serve. Training programs for bar staff and managers have also demonstrated reductions in high-risk drinking and drinking problems, although these effects tend to be fairly modest and have not been found in all evaluations. In addition, a small body of research has shown that interventions that result in the adoption and enforcement of policies to make licensed premises safer have also been associated with lower levels of intoxication and problems. Community mobilization focused on licensed premises has proven to be a powerful strategy in reducing problem behaviour; however, the long-term sustainability of these efforts remains to be demonstrated.

Environmentally-directed measures, when appropriately designed and implemented, can have substantial effects on the occurrence of alcohol-related problems. However, some of these interventions may require substantial resources, and such approaches are unlikely to be as cost-effective as general alcohol control and tax measures.

Measures to reduce the harm in the drinking situation are thus a useful option in the mix of strategies for preventing alcohol-related problems. The less the political process is willing to support general alcohol control and tax measures, the more important local harm reduction measures become. However, given the limited current evidence of effectiveness of these approaches, they should not be considered as substitutes for other alcohol policy strategies that have well documented evidence of effectiveness.

References

Abbey A., Ross L.T., McDuffie D., *et al.* (1996) Alcohol and dating risk factors for sexual assault among college women, *Psychology of Women Quarterly* 20, 147–69.

Alcohol Concern (1996) Toughen rules on toughened glasses, in light of 5000 serious bar injuries. Press release (July 5). Website: http://www.alcoholconcern.org.uk/information/pressrel/1996/05–07–96.htm

Aramburu B. and Leigh B.C. (1991) For better or worse: attributions about drunken aggression toward male and female victims. *Violence and Victimization* 6, 31–41.

Arnold M.J. and Laidler T.J. (1994) *Situational and environmental factors in alcohol-related violence*, Vol. 7. Canberra, Australia: Government Publishing Services.

Braun K. and Graham K., with Bois C., *et al.* (2000) *Safer bars trainer's guide*. Toronto, Ontario, Canada: Centre for Addiction and Mental Health.

Buka S.L. and Birdthistle I.J. (1999) Long-term effects of a community-wide alcohol server training intervention. *Journal of Studies on Alcohol* 60, 27–36.

Burns L., Flaherty B., Ireland S., *et al.* (1995) Policing pubs: What happens to crime? *Drug and Alcohol Review* 14, 369–75.

Burns T.F. (1980) Getting rowdy with the boys. *Journal of Drug Issues* 10, 273–86.

Bushman B.J. (1997) Effects of alcohol on human aggression: validity of proposed mechanisms. In: Galanter M. (ed.) *Recent developments in alcoholism*, Vol. 13, *Alcohol and violence*, pp. 227–44. New York: Plenum Press.

Carvolth R. (1995) *The contribution of risk assessment to harm reduction through the Queensland safety action approach*. Proceedings of the 'Window of Opportunity Congress', Brisbane, Australia.

Chaloupka F.J., Saffer H., and Grossman M. (1993) Alcohol-control policies and motor-vehicle fatalities. *Journal of Legal Studies* 22, 161–86.

Cusenza S. (1998) Organizing to reduce neighborhood alcohol problems: A frontline account. *Contemporary Drug Problems* 25, 99–111.

De Crespigny C., Vincent N., and Ask A. (1998) *Young women and drinking*, Vol. 1. Adelaide, South Australia: The Flinders University of South Australia School of Nursing.

Dickson R., Leather P., Beale D., *et al.* (1994) Intervention strategies to manage workplace violence. *Occupational Health Review* (August), 15–18.

Dresser J. (2000) *Comparing statewide alcohol server training systems*. (Unpublished manuscript)

Fahrenkrug H. and Rehm J. (1995) Drinking contexts and leisure-time activities in the prephase of alcohol-related road accidents by young Swiss residents. *Sucht* 41, 169–80.

Felson M., Berends R., Richardson B., *et al.* (1997) Reducing pub hopping and related crime. In: Homel R. (ed.) *Policing for prevention: Reducing crime, public intoxication and injury*, Vol. 7, pp. 115–32. Monsey, New York: Criminal Justice Press.

Geller E.S., Russ N.W., and Delphos W.A. (1987) Does server intervention training make a difference? An empirical field evaluation. *Alcohol, Health and Research World* 11, 64–9.

Gliksman L., Single E., McKenzie D., *et al.* (1993) The role of alcohol providers in prevention: An evaluation of a server intervention programme. *Addiction* 88, 1189–97.

Graham K. (1999) *Safer bars: Assessing and reducing risks of violence.* Toronto, Canada: Centre for Addiction and Mental Health.

Graham K. (2000) Preventive interventions for on-premise drinking: A promising but underresearched area of prevention. *Contemporary Drug Problems* 27, 593–668.

Graham K. and Chandler Coutts M. (2000) Community action research: Who does what to whom and why? Lessons learned from local prevention efforts (international experiences). *Substance Use and Misuse* 35, 87–110.

Graham K. and Homel R. (1997) Creating safer bars. In: Plant M., Single E., and Stockwell T. (eds.) *Alcohol: Minimizing the harm*, pp. 171–92. London, UK: Free Association Press.

Graham K. and Wells S. (2001) Aggression among young adults in the social context of the bar. *Addiction Research* 9, 193–219.

Graham K., LaRocque L., Yetman R., *et al.* (1980) Aggression and barroom environments. *Journal of Studies on Alcohol* 41, 277–92.

Graham K., Leonard K.E., Room R., *et al.* (1998) Current directions in research in understanding and preventing intoxicated aggression. *Addiction* 93, 659–76.

Graham K., Jelley J., and Purcell J. (2002) *Evaluation of the safer bars training program.* Paper presented at an International Experts Forum: Setting the agenda for correctional research in substance abuse, Charlottetown, Prince Edward Island, Canada.

Gruenewald P., Mitchell P., and Treno A.J. (1996) Drinking and driving: drinking patterns and drinking problems. *Addiction* 91, 1637–49.

Gruenewald P.J., Stockwell T., Beel A., *et al.* (1999) Beverage sales and drinking and driving: The role of on-premise drinking places. *Journal of Studies on Alcohol* 60, 47–53.

Hauritz M., Homel R., Townsley M., *et al.* (eds.) (1998a) *An evaluation of the local government safety action projects in Cairns, Townsville and Mackay: A report to the Queensland Department of Health, the Queensland Police Service and the Criminology Research Council.* Australia: Griffith University, Centre for Crime Policy and Public Safety; School of Justice Administration.

Hauritz M., Homel R., McIlwain G., *et al.* (1998b) Reducing violence in licensed venues through community safety action projects: the Queensland experience. *Contemporary Drug Problems* 25, 511–51.

Hawkins T.E., Dreyer C.B., and Cooper E.J. (1977) *Analysis of public information and education 1975–1976.* San Antonio, TX: San Antonio Alcohol Safety Action Project, Analytic Study No. 7.

Holder H.D. and Moore R.S. (2000) Institutionalization of community action projects to reduce alcohol-use related problems: Systematic facilitators. *Substance Use and Misuse*, 35, 75–86.

Holder H.D. and Wagenaar A.C. (1994) Mandated server training and reduced alcohol-involved traffic crashes: A time series analysis of the Oregon experience. *Accident Analysis and Prevention* 26, 89–97.

Holder H.D., Janes K., Mosher J., *et al.* (1993) Alcoholic beverage server liability and the reduction of alcohol-involved problems. *Journal of Studies on Alcohol* 54, 23–36.

Homel R. and Clark J. (1994) The prediction and prevention of violence in pubs and clubs. *Crime Prevention Studies* 3, 1–46.

Homel R., Tomsen S., and Thommeny J. (1992) Public drinking and violence: Not just an alcohol problem. *Journal of Drug Issues* 22, 679–97.

Homel R., Hauritz M., Wortley R., *et al.* (1997) Preventing alcohol-related crime through community action: The Surfers Paradise safety action project. *Crime Prevention Studies* 7, 35–90.

Homel R., McIlwain, G., and Carvolth R. (2001) Creating safer drinking environments. In: Heather N., Peters T.J., and Stockwell T. (eds.) *Handbook of alcohol dependence and alcohol-related problems*, pp. 721–40. Chichester, UK: John Wiley and Sons.

Howard-Pitney B., Johnson M.D., Altman D.G., *et al.* (1991) Responsible alcohol service: A study of server, manager, and environmental impact. *American Journal of Public Health* 81, 197–9.

Ireland C.S. and Thommeny J.L. (1993) The crime cocktail: Licensed premises, alcohol and street offences. *Drug and Alcohol Review* 12, 143–50.

Jeffs B.W. and Saunders W.M. (1983) Minimizing alcohol related offences by enforcement of the existing licensing legislation. *British Journal of Addiction* 78, 67–77.

Kennedy B.P., Isaac N.E., Nelson T.F., *et al.* (1997) Young male drinkers and impaired driving intervention: results of a US telephone survey. *Accident Analysis and Prevention* 29, 707–13.

Kulis R.E. (1998) The public interest and liquor licenses in Ontario. *Contemporary Drug Problems* 25, 85–97.

Lander A. (1995) *Preventing alcohol-related violence: A community action manual.* Darlinghurst, NSW, Australia: St. Vincent's Alcohol and Drug Service.

Lang E. and Rumbold G. (1997) The effectiveness of community-based interventions to reduce violence in and around licensed premises: A comparison of three Australian models. *Contemporary Drug Problems* 24, 805–26.

Lang E., Stockwell T., Rydon P., *et al.* (1998) Can training bar staff in responsible serving practices reduce alcohol-related harm? *Drug and Alcohol Review* 17, 39–50.

Levy D.T. and Miller T.R. (1995) A cost-benefit analysis of enforcement efforts to reduce serving intoxicated patrons. *Journal of Studies on Alcohol* 56, 240–7.

Marsh P. and Kibby K. (1992) *Drinking and public disorder.* London, UK: Portman Group.

McKilip J., Lockhart D.C., Eckert P.S., *et al.* (1985) Evaluation of a responsible alcohol use media campaign on a college campus. *Journal of Alcohol and Drug Education* 30, 88–97.

McKnight A.J. (1990) Intervention with alcohol-impaired drivers by peers, parents and purveyors of alcohol. *Health Education Research: Theory and Practice* 5, 225–36.

McKnight A.J. (1991) Factors influencing the effectiveness of server-intervention education. *Journal of Studies on Alcohol* 52, 389–97.

McKnight A.J. and Streff F.M. (1994) The effect of enforcement upon service of alcohol to intoxicated patrons of bars and restaurants. *Accident Analysis and Prevention* 26, 79–88.

MCM Research (1993) *Keeping the peace: A guide to the prevention of alcohol-related disorder.* London, UK: Portman Group.

Meilman P.W. and Haygood-Jackson D. (1996) Data on sexual assault from the first 2 years of a comprehensive campus prevention program. *Journal of American College Health* 44, 157–65.

Miers D. (1978) *Responses to victimization: A comparative study of compensation for criminal violence in Great Britain and Ontario.* Abingdon, UK: Professional Books.

Mosher J.F. (1990) *Community responsible beverage service programs: An implementation handbook.* San Rafael, CA: Marin Institute for Prevention of Alcohol and Other Drug-Related Problems.

Neves P., De Pape D., Giesbrecht N., *et al.* (1998) *Communities take action!* Toronto, Canada: Centre for Addiction and Mental Health.

O'Donnell M. (1985) Research on drinking locations of alcohol-impaired drivers: Implications for prevention policies. *Journal of Public Health Policy* 6, 510–25.

Perez R.L. (2000) Fiesta as tradition, fiesta as change: Ritual, alcohol and violence in a Mexican community. *Addiction* 95, 365–73.

Putnam S.L., Rockett I.R.H., and Campbell M.K. (1993) Methodological issues in community-based alcohol-related injury prevention projects: Attribution of program effects. In: Greenfield T.K. and Zimmerman R. (eds.) *Experiences with community action projects: New research in the prevention of alcohol and other drug problems,* pp. 31–9. Rockville, MD: Center for Substance Abuse Prevention.

Rossow I. (1996) Alcohol related violence: The impact of drinking pattern and drinking context. *Addiction* 91, 1651–61.

Ruhm C.J. (1996) Alcohol policies and highway vehicle fatalities. *Journal of Health Economics* 15, 435–54.

Russ N.W. and Geller E.S. (1987) Training bar personnel to prevent drunken driving: A field evaluation. *American Journal of Public Health* 77, 952–4.

Saltz R.F. (1987) The roles of bars and restaurants in preventing alcohol-impaired driving: An evaluation of server intervention. *Evaluation and the Health Professions* 10, 5–27.

Saltz R.F. and Stanghetta P. (1997) A community-wide responsible beverage service program in three communities: early findings. *Addiction* 92 (Suppl. 2), 237–49S.

Single E. and McKenzie D. (1992) *The epidemiology of impaired driving stemming from licensed establishments.* Presented at 18th Annual Alcohol Epidemiology Symposium, Toronto, June 1–5.

Sloan F.A., Reilly B.A., and Schenzler C.M. (1994a) Tort liability versus other approaches for deterring careless driving. *International Review of Law and Economics* 14, 53–71.

Sloan F.A., Reilly B.A., and Schenzler C. (1994b) Effects of prices, civil and criminal sanctions and law enforcement on alcohol-related mortality. *Journal of Studies on Alcohol* 55, 454–65.

Sloan F.A., Stout E.M., Whetten-Goldsteing K., *et al.* (2000) *Drinkers, drivers and bartenders: Balancing private choices and public accountability.* Chicago, Illinois: The University of Chicago Press.

Snow R.W. and Landrum J.W. (1986) Drinking locations and frequency of drunkenness among Mississippi DUI offenders. *American Journal of Drug and Alcohol Abuse* 12, 389–402.

Stockwell T. (2001) Editor's introduction to prevention of alcohol problems. In: Heather N., Peters T.J., and Stockwell T. (eds.) *Handbook of alcohol dependence and alcohol-related problems,* pp. 680–3. Chichester, UK: John Wiley and Sons.

Stockwell T., Somerford P., and Lang E. (1992) The relationship between license type and alcohol-related problems attributed to licensed premises in Perth, Western Australia. *Journal of Studies on Alcohol* 53, 495–8.

Stockwell T., Lang E., and Rydon P. (1993) High risk drinking settings: the association of serving and promotional practices with harmful drinking. *Addiction* 88, 1519–26.

Stout R.L., Rose J.S., Speare M.C., *et al.* (1993) Sustaining interventions in communities: The Rhode Island community-based prevention trial. In: Greenfield T.K. and Zimmerman R. (eds.) *Experiences with community action projects: New research in the prevention of alcohol and other drug problems*, pp. 253–61. Rockville, MD: US Department of Health and Human Services.

Tomsen S. (1997) A top night out: social protest, masculinity and the culture of drinking violence. *British Journal of Criminology* 37, 990–1002.

Toomey T.L., Kilian G.R., Gehan J.P., *et al.* (1998) Qualitative assessment of training programs for alcohol servers and establishment managers. *Public Health Reports* 113, 162–9.

Toomey T.L., Wagenaar A.C., Gehan J.P., *et al.* (2001) Project ARM: Alcohol risk management to prevent sales to underage and intoxicated patrons. *Health Education and Behavior* 28, 186–99.

Wagenaar A.C. and Holder H.D. (1991) Effects of alcoholic beverage server liability on traffic crash injuries. *Alcoholism: Clinical and Experimental Research* 15, 942–7.

Wallin E., Hjalmarsson K., Lindewald B., *et al.* (1999) *Effects of RBS training: A focus group study*. Paper presented at the 25th annual meeting of the Kettil Bruun Society for Social and Epidemiological Research on Alcohol, Montreal, Canada.

Warburton A.L. and Shepherd J.P. (2000) Effectiveness of toughened glassware in terms of reducing injury in bars: a randomized controlled trial. *Injury Prevention* 6, 36–40.

Wells S. and Graham K. (1999) The frequency of third party involvement in incidents of barroom aggression. *Contemporary Drug Problems* 26, 457–80.

Wells S., Graham K., and West P. (1998) 'The good, the bad, and the ugly': Responses by security staff to aggressive incidents in public drinking settings. *Journal of Drug Issues* 28, 817–36.

Chapter 9

Drinking–driving countermeasures

9.1 Introduction

The automobile age has brought with it unprecedented prosperity and freedom of movement, but at a great cost. Motor vehicles have directly caused the death and injury of millions of people. When the driver of a motor vehicle has been drinking alcohol, the risk of injury and death is substantially increased. The generally favoured term for the criminal action of driving a vehicle under the influence of alcohol is 'drinking–driving' (WHO 1994). Drinking–driving accidents are a problem in any country that makes substantial use of motor vehicles for transportation. For this reason a variety of drinking–driving countermeasures have been developed, and many of them have been systematically evaluated.

This chapter first discusses general enforcement and the deterrence effect of drinking–driving laws, then turns to the impact of other prevention policies. Programs for convicted offenders fall somewhere between these domains, since their aim is not punishment or deterrence but reform. The chapter concludes by examining specific strategies to reduce the risk of drinking–driving among young people and the general population, such as designated driver and ride share programs.

9.2 BAC and driving performance

The level of alcohol in a person's blood is called the blood alcohol concentration or BAC. In addition to the amount consumed, BAC depends on such factors as an individual's weight, rate of drinking, and presence of food in the stomach. Laboratory research has demonstrated that tasks related to driving performance are affected at BAC levels much lower than those normally associated with legal intoxication (Moskowitz and Robinson 1988). Deterioration in performance becomes quite marked between BACs of 0.05% and 0.08%, but there can be impaired performance even when a driver has a BAC lower than 0.05%.

Studies have also found that the relative crash risk of drivers with BACs of 0.05% is double the crash risk for a person with a zero BAC. When BACs are at 0.08%, the risk is multiplied by ten. BACs of 0.15% or higher have a relative crash risk in the hundreds (Borkenstein *et al.* 1974). The risk curve is even steeper for serious and fatal crashes, for single-vehicle crashes, and for young people (Mayhew *et al.* 1981; Jonah 1986). Given the strong relationship between BAC and crash risk, countries have established *per se* laws concerning specific BAC levels (usually 0.05 or 0.08%, but varying between 0.00 and 0.15%; WHO 1999) above which a driver could be arrested (Andenaes 1988). BAC can be measured by taking a blood sample from a driver but also via an analysis of the exhaled breath. The invention of the Breathalyzer and other portable devices for collecting samples of driver breaths, combined with *per se* legislation, have revolutionized law enforcement of drinking–driving countermeasures in the developed countries.

9.3 **Patterns of drinking–driving**

A number of countries carry out breath tests from a random sample of motorists, usually during nights and weekends, when drinking–drivers are more numerous. Two groups of countries emerge from these studies. In the first group, which includes the Scandinavian countries, there are relatively few drinking–drivers on the roads (Andenaes 1988; Ross 1993). Moderate-to-high levels of blood alcohol are found among less than 1% of drivers in these countries, even at peak driving times. The second group includes the United States, Canada, France, and the Netherlands, where between 5% and 10% of drivers have moderate-to-high blood alcohol levels during night-time leisure hours. These patterns are broadly consistent with overall road fatality rates for different countries. When drivers are asked at random about their personal behaviour, a considerable percentage acknowledge driving after drinking. For example, a 1988 study found that 28% of Australians, 24% of Americans, but only 2% of Norwegians admitted to driving in the past year after four or more drinks (Berger *et al.* 1990).

However, analyses of the blood alcohol levels of drivers killed indicate that even in the Scandinavian countries more than a quarter of drivers had been drinking (Andenaes 1988). More generally, all countries have the problem of hard-core drinking–drivers, characterized by persistent heavy drinking before driving. A recent Canadian report estimates that such drivers account for only 1% of all drivers on the road at night during the weekend, but they represent nearly half of all the fatal crashes at that time (ICADTS Reporter 1997). A surprisingly high percentage of these heavy drinking–drivers have no prior drinking–driving convictions. Only one-quarter to one-third of all drinking–drivers or riders killed in Canada, the United States, Australia, and New Zealand had prior offences (Ross 1992; Mayhew 2002).

In the last two decades there has been a general decline in the incidence of drinking–driving across the developed world, where dramatic reductions were experienced in most countries especially during the 1980s. The drinking–driving indicators reversed direction in the early 1990s, but then continued in modest decline in the second half of the decade (Sweedler 2000). Thus prevention of drinking–driving is one of the big public health success stories from the last quarter of the 20th century.

9.4 General deterrence as prevention

Traditionally, law enforcement directed at drinking–driving has been designed to catch offenders, on the assumption that such practices will prevent or deter people from driving after drinking. Deterrence is essentially a means to increase the perceived probability or likelihood of apprehension for drinking–driving (see Box 9.1). However, deterrence is also influenced by such factors as severity and swiftness of punishment (Ross 1992).

9.4.1 Lowering BAC limits

Certainty policies depend on laws that clearly define drinking–driving with a BAC at or above a prescribed level for the whole population (e.g., 0.08 or 0.05%) or for young drivers (usually zero or 0.02%). The evidence for the general deterrent impact of such *per se* laws is strong, although the effects tend to erode over time (Ross 1982). This success has led many countries to set increasingly stringent BAC levels.

Jonah *et al.* (2000) reviewed the international evidence for the impact of lower BAC laws. They found that lower BAC limits consistently produce

---

Box 9.1 **Classical doctrine of deterrence**

In the 18th century, the Italian intellectual Cesare Beccaria offered the following observation on the doctrine of deterrence:

'One of the greatest curbs on crime is not the cruelty of punishments, but their infallibility . . . The certainty of a punishment, even if it be moderate, will always make a stronger impression than the fear of another which is more terrible but combined with the hope of impunity; even the least evils, when they are certain, always terrify men's minds . . . Let the laws, therefore, be inexorable, and inexorable their executors in particular cases, but let the legislator be tender, indulgent, and humane.'

(Beccaria 1963, pp. 58–9).

positive results on drinking–driving accidents, and other indicators such as positive BACs. The impact for Sweden of the 0.02 law that was introduced in 1990 was estimated at 6% (Norström 1997). Henstridge *et al.* (1997) analysed daily accident data for four Australian states between 1976 and 1992, controlling for seasonal effects, daily weather patterns, economic and road use activity, alcohol consumption, the day of the week, and other legal interventions. They concluded that the impact of the 0.05 BAC limit on fatal accidents ranged from 8% in New South Wales to 18% in Queensland. Using roadside survey data in South Australia, Kloeden and McLean (1994) observed a 14% decline in drivers with a positive BAC. The final major initiative involving BAC levels has been the establishment of very low BACs (usually 0.02) for young or inexperienced drivers. Shults *et al.* (2001) reviewed six well-designed studies of the effect of these laws in the US and Australia. Estimated declines in fatal crashes ranged from 24% to 9%. Although further evaluative work is required, the research to date suggests that the effects of BAC laws are mostly positive, long-term, and cost-effective (Mann *et al.* 2001).

Nevertheless, at least some of the impact of measures to increase perceived certainty appear to erode over time. Ross (1982) hypothesized that the deterrent impact wears off because initially drivers grossly exaggerate the certainty of apprehension in response to the publicity, but gradually become used to the new law and realize that their chances of detection are in fact not very high. Despite the evidence for the positive impact of laws that target certainty, making motorists uncertain about the real risk of detection may paradoxically be the key to cost-effective deterrence (Homel 1988a; Nagin 1998).

9.4.2 Enforcement: random versus selective breath testing

One strategy for increasing certainty of apprehension and punishment is to increase the frequency and visibility of drinking–driving enforcement. Ross (1992) estimated that the objective probability of apprehension for an impaired driver in the United States is one in a thousand. Therefore, increasing this probability may translate into a higher perceived probability of detection, and fewer accidents. The traditional way of producing a higher perceived probability of apprehension is simply to intensify police enforcement. Short-term campaigns do generally reduce accidents, but their effects are generally temporary (Ross 1982).

One approach to strengthening enforcement is to use **sobriety or selective checkpoints**. However, at sobriety checkpoints, only motorists who are judged by police to have been drinking are asked to take a breath test. This approach greatly weakens the deterrent potential since experienced offenders believe (with some justification) that they can avoid detection. In Australia, alcohol-impaired drivers comprised fewer than 10% of those pulled over (Watson and Fraine 1994); moreover, there is reliable evidence from the US that police miss as many as 50% of drivers with a BAC over 0.10% (McKnight and Voas 2001).

An alternative to such selective testing of drivers is **random breath testing** (**RBT**) or compulsory breath testing as it is practiced in Australia, New Zealand, and some European countries. Motorists are stopped at random by police and required to take a preliminary breath test, even if they are in no way suspected of having committed an offence or of being involved in an accident. The defining feature of RBT is that any motorist at any time may be required to take a test, and there is nothing he or she can do to influence the chances of being tested. Testing varies from day-to-day and from week-to-week, and is not announced publicly in advance. Nevertheless, it is always highly visible and publicized in the news media. Refusal to submit to a breath test is equivalent to failing. By the mid-1990s, millions of motorists in Australia were being tested each year, at a rate of about 0.6 tests per license holder per year (Henstridge *et al.* 1997). In 1999, 82% of Australian motorists reported having been stopped at some time, compared with 16% in the UK and 29% in the US (Williams *et al.* 2000).

Shults *et al.* (2001) reviewed 23 studies of RBT and selective testing. They found a decline of 22% (range 13–36%) in fatal crashes, with slightly lower decreases for non-injury and other accidents for such enforcement strategies. Henstridge *et al.* (1997), in a time–series analysis of accidents in four Australian states, found that RBT was twice as effective as selective checkpoints. For example, in Queensland, RBT resulted in a 35% reduction in fatal accidents, compared with 15% for selective checkpoints. Henstridge *et al.* (1997) estimated that every increase of 1000 in the daily testing rate corresponded to a decline of 6% in all serious accidents and 19% in single-vehicle night-time accidents. Moreover, analyses revealed a measurable deterrent effect of RBT on the whole population of motorists ten years later. This effect was periodically boosted for individual motorists by exposure to RBT operations, whose presence was remembered and acted upon up to 18 months later (Sherman 1990). Homel (1988b) showed that the deterrent impact of RBT also provided heavy drinkers with a legitimate excuse to drink less when drinking with friends.

The research evidence is quite strong that highly visible, non-selective testing can have a sustained and significant effect in reducing drinking–driving and the associated crashes, injuries, and deaths. Box 9.2 provides an illustration of a community prevention program utilizing such strategies.

Box 9.2 **New Zealand rural drinking–driving project dates (1996–1998)**

The Waikato rural drink–driving project was begun in 1996 as a community action effort to implement strategies to reduce drinking–driving crashes in a large rural district with no cities. The district had the highest fatal road toll in New Zealand. As a community action effort, project governance was in the hands of a coordinating group with representatives from each of the seven local government regions within the district.

A major strategy focused on increasing police enforcement of drinking–driving through adoption of random breath testing (RBT) and mobile patrols to better fit the rural setting. Activities included increasing the element of surprise (unexpected testing of drivers on the road) and actually encouraging the 'bush telegraph' (i.e., local informal communication) to deter potential drinking–drivers. In addition to highly visible and frequent enforcement, especially on Thursday through Saturdays from 7 pm to 3 am, the project disseminated current information to police and licensees on premises that had been identified from a survey of drivers as 'problem establishments'. These premises were monitored as part of the project intervention. In addition, news coverage of local enforcement was increased through efforts by the project staff. During the time of this local action project, there was a reduction in fatal traffic crashes from 22% to 14%. In addition, alcohol positive breath test results by the police decreased from 1 in 35 tests to 1 in 216 tests, prosecutions for drinking–driving increased by 23%, and local news coverage of drinking–driving and enforcement increased (Stewart and Conway 1999).

9.4.3 **Severity of punishment**

Punishment for a drinking–driving conviction has typically been increased either by changing the maximum penalties or by introducing mandatory minimum penalties. There is limited evidence to support the positive impact of these laws (Ross and Voas 1989). Indeed, their effects could be counterproductive if the judicial system is overburdened, or if prosecutors fail to pursue these cases (Little 1975; Ross and Voas 1989). Severe punishments do not lead to fewer accidents than less severe penalties (Homel 1988b; Ross 1992). However, McKnight and Voas (2001) observed that tough penalties such as imprisonment can have beneficial indirect effects. They provided a sanction of last resort to motivate repeat offenders to participate in more constructive programs such as probation or residential treatment.

The one punishment that seems to have a consistent impact is license disqualification. License loss can be effective for both alcohol-involved and non-alcohol-involved accidents. Offenders with no license suspension recidivate more (Peck *et al.* 1985; Ross 1992; Siskind 1996; McKnight and Voas 2001). Conversely, those offenders receiving longer periods of suspension tend to recidivate less, at least for non-alcohol offences (Homel 1981). One study found that as many as three-quarters of disqualified drivers continue to drive while unlicensed (Ross and Gonzales 1988), but they tend to drive less frequently and to be more cautious, at least for the period of suspension.

9.4.4 Swiftness of punishment

'Celerity' or swiftness of punishment is the proximity of punishment to the drinking–driving event. One example is **administrative license suspension**, or revocation for drinking–driving. With an administrative suspension, licensing authorities can suspend licenses without a court hearing, quickly and closer in time to the actual offence. Administrative suspension is permitted in 40 of the 50 states in the USA, and the impact on drinking–driving accidents is consistently positive. The mechanism seems to be general deterrence, with an average reduction of 5% in alcohol-involved crashes and a reduction in fatal crashes of 26% associated with administrative licensing revocation (Ross 1992; McKnight and Voas 2001). Miller *et al.* (1998), in a study on novice drivers, concluded that the benefit-to-cost ratio was $11 per dollar invested, when violators receive a six month license suspension. Thus evidence supports a conclusion that setting a reasonably low level of BAC, undertaking highly frequent and visible enforcement of existing BAC limits, threatening and actually suspending driving privileges, and establishing certainty of punishment especially through randomized enforcement, form a combined strategy with the strongest potential for prevention success.

9.5 Preventing recidivism: treatment and victim impact panels

Some convicted offenders continue drinking–driving and are re-arrested or involved in further traffic crashes. The impact of routine punishments for these repeat offenders can be enhanced when combined with alcohol treatment (Deyoung 1997). From a policy perspective, well-designed treatment programs are probably worth the investment if a reduction in alcohol-involved crashes is the goal. Successful programs are well structured, go beyond information provision to address alcohol abuse, are conducted for more than ten weeks, and have rules of attendance enforced by a court (Wells-Parker 2000).

Wells-Parker *et al.* (1995) carried out a meta-analysis of 215 evaluations of drinking–driving remediation programs, and concluded that treatment without license suspension is generally ineffective. License suspension plus education, psychotherapy counselling, or follow-up contact probation (preferably in combination), produced an additional 7–9% reduction in drinking–driving recidivism and alcohol-involved accidents, when compared with control groups that largely received license restrictions only (sometimes more severe than for the treatment groups).

A relatively new type of intervention is **victim impact panels** (Shinar and Compton 1995), or more generally, restorative justice conferences, where several people representing victims of drinking–driving meet with the offender in a structured situation controlled by a trained facilitator. The conferences collectively determine a penalty. A meta-analysis of 35 randomized studies of restorative programs, most not involving drinking–drivers (Latimer *et al.* 2001), found that this process decreased the recidivism of offenders (72% of 32 studies yielded a reduction in recidivism) when compared to more traditional criminal justice responses (i.e., incarceration, probation, court-ordered restitution). One large-scale randomized experiment in the Australian Capital Territory with drinking–drivers (typically not involving license loss) showed a slight increase in recidivism for drinking–drivers compared with those assigned to court (Sherman *et al.* 2000). This is consistent with the mixed but mostly null results obtained by victim impact panels for drinking–drivers (Shinar and Compton 1995).

Another approach for high-risk repeat offenders is to use ignition interlock devices that prevent a vehicle from being started until the driver passes a breath test. These devices have been shown to be very effective for many alcohol-impaired offenders in eight studies in the United States (McKnight and Voas 2001). However, the effects tend to be limited to the period of the court order, unless combined with treatment in a case management framework to deal with the underlying problems.

Overall, evidence supports the effectiveness of comprehensive treatment including counselling or therapy plus license suspension in reducing recidivism. These approaches, while promising if they incorporate license loss, require further evaluation. The application of ignition interlock devices has shown positive results, but has not been widely tested in countries other than the USA.

9.6 **Restrictions on young or inexperienced drivers**

Young drivers (adolescents between 16–20) are at risk for traffic crashes, especially alcohol-involved crashes, as a result of their limited driving experience and their tendency to experiment with heavy or binge drinking. Traditional countermeasures such as driver training and school-based education programs are either ineffective or have yielded mixed results, with the possible exception of peer intervention, which does seem to produce enduring improvements in intervention behaviours (Stewart and Klitzner 1990; McKnight and Voas 2001). Special policy strategies have been formulated to prevent drinking–driving among this age group.

9.6.1 **Low BAC limits for young drivers**

Lower BAC limits for young drivers (sometimes called 'zero tolerance laws') set BAC limits at the minimum that can be reliably detected by breath testing equipment (i.e., 0.01–0.02). Zero tolerance laws also commonly invoke other penalties such as automatic confiscation of the driving license. An analysis of the effect of zero tolerance laws in the first 12 US states to enact them found a 20% relative reduction in the proportion of single-vehicle night-time fatal crashes among drivers under 21, compared with nearby states that did not pass zero tolerance laws (Hingson *et al.* 1994; Martin *et al.* 1996). In a review of six studies on the effects of zero tolerance, Zwerling and Jones (1999) concluded that all of the studies showed a reduction in injuries and crashes, but three were not statistically significant due to lack of statistical power. A national study of US states found a net decrease of 24% in the number of young drivers with positive BACs as a result of zero tolerance laws (Voas *et al.* 1999). Similarly, a 19% reduction in self-reported driving after any drinking, and a 24% reduction in driving after five or more drinks, was found using survey data from 30 states (Wagenaar *et al.* 2001). While all of these studies were conducted in the US, evidence of the effectiveness of lower BAC limits for young drivers is quite strong, and has been reinforced by a Shults *et al.* (2001) review of both US and Australian studies, which found reductions of between 9% and 24% in fatal crashes.

9.6.2 **Licensing restrictions**

While the minimum driving age in Sweden and some other European countries is 18, minimum ages for drivers' licenses have traditionally been lower in most English-speaking countries, sometimes as low as 14. On the basis of careful comparisons of US states with differing ages of licensing (Williams *et al.* 1983; Williams 1985), it was estimated that between 65% and 85% reductions in 16-year-old driver fatal crash involvement could be achieved by raising the legal age of driving to 17. However, such laws are unpopular. As an alternative to raising the driving age, parts of the US have implemented night-time curfews for teenage drivers in order to achieve some of the benefits of delayed licensing. Williams (1985) and his colleagues (Preusser *et al.* 1984) have explored the impact of such policies by comparing crash rates for young teenagers (15-, 16-, or 17-year-olds, depending on the state) in states with curfew laws with rates in states without such laws. The researchers estimated reductions in the crash involvement of 16-year-old drivers during curfew hours ranging from 25% to 69%, and concluded that the laws had very beneficial effects relative to their costs.

In short, the scientific evidence shows that lower BAC limits, delayed access to a full license, and curfews for young drivers can be effective strategies for reducing drinking–driving among the young. **Graduated licensing** schemes can incorporate all of these strategies within one system, by controlling the rate and manner in which young drivers gain access to full driving privileges. These schemes have been well-accepted where implemented, and the small number of evaluations all show safety benefits (Begg *et al.* 2000; Mayhew 2000; Ulmer *et al.* 2000).

9.7 Designated driver and ride service programs

Many drinking–drivers consume alcohol in locations other than their homes, such as licensed establishments and social events. Two strategies have been designed to provide safe transport following a drinking event: designated drivers and ride service programs.

9.7.1 Designated drivers

Designated driver programs encourage one person in a group of drinkers to abstain in order to provide safe transport for the group. Simons-Morton and Cummings (1997) evaluated the effect of a retraining program for bar staff in six bars and restaurants. Despite changes in staff activities, promotion of the designated driver program was low, and use of the program by patrons did not increase. Several studies (Brigham *et al.* 1995; Meier *et al.* 1998) evaluated the effect of increased advertising on the use of the designated driver program in selected bars. A small but consistent increase in use of the program was observed. One study showed an increase from 3 users at baseline to 7.5 during the intervention. Results from a general population survey and bar-room surveys indicated that younger respondents, and those who reached higher BACs when drinking outside the home, were most likely to use designated drivers (Caudill and Harding 1997). There is no evidence that designated driver programs have negative effects. On the other hand, the impact of on-premise designated driver programs appears to be small. Even intensive promotions produce only modest increases.

9.7.2 Ride service programs

Ride service programs provide transportation to intoxicated persons who would otherwise drive. Unlike designated driver programs, they apply to all intoxicated persons who are potential drivers, not just to groups, and they do not require planning prior to the social event. Molof et al. (1995) evaluated two long-standing, well functioning US-based ride service programs, one serving primarily bar patrons and persons attending corporate or social host parties (providing 2500 free rides per year) and the other program operating over the Christmas and New Year season (providing 700 free taxi rides home). Although the programs in both communities were well established and popular, there was no identifiable impact of either program on annual crash rates. The 'Operation Nez Rouge' (Operation Red Nose) program in Switzerland uses volunteer drivers to drive people home. A survey of past users found that about half planned on using the service before they were drinking, while the other half decided at the time. Almost 75% thought it was a good prevention program, while 7.5% thought it encouraged people to drink. About two-thirds of respondents reported that the program made them more aware of possible impairment due to alcohol (Ayer et al. 1994).

In summary, designated drivers and ride services appear to be popular among people who presumably would otherwise drive while intoxicated. They are able to reach high-risk groups for drinking–driving (young, male heavier drinkers), and may generally increase awareness of the risks of drinking–driving (Ayer et al. 1994; Molof et al. 1995). However, because these services account for a relatively small per cent of drivers, no overall impact on alcohol-involved accidents has been demonstrated to date.

9.8 Conclusion

The assertion early in this chapter that the drinking–driving field is one of the great public health success stories of the late 20th century seems justified by the evidence assembled and reviewed here. The evidence suggests that drinking–driving countermeasures consistently produce population-wide long-term problem reductions of between 5% and 30%. Recognition of the great problems remaining, such as the persistent delinquency of high-risk impaired drivers and their consistent contribution to the fatality statistics, should not detract from the enormous achievements of recent decades.

Most of what has been accomplished has been done through new laws or more imaginative enforcement of existing laws. Deterrence-based approaches, using innovations such as random breath testing that yield few arrests but big accident reductions, have taught police and society the power of deterrence. However, despite progress, much more can be accomplished by intensifying the policies of the past. Deterrence programs in particular should not be scaled back, but should build on the evidence.

Sweedler (2000) observed that evidence-based strategies adapted to local conditions will differ from country to country, but that the overall results of the mixture of countermeasures may ultimately be similar. Box 9.3 provides an example of a mixed strategy community prevention program. By examining the strengths and weaknesses of different program mixtures across countries, much can be learned about how all countries could improve performance.

Box 9.3 **The saving lives project, USA 1984 to 1993**

The saving lives project conducted in six communities in Massachusetts, USA, was designed to reduce alcohol-impaired driving and related problems such as speeding (Hingson *et al.* 1996). In each community a full-time coordinator from the local government organized a task force representing various city departments. Programs were designed locally and involved a host of activities including media campaigns, business information programs, speeding and drunk–driving awareness days, speed watch telephone hotlines, police training, high school peer-led education, Students Against Drunk Driving chapters, college prevention programs, and other activities. During the five years that the program was in operation, sites that received the Saving Lives intervention produced a 25% greater decline in fatal crashes than the rest of Massachusetts, a 47% reduction in the number of fatally injured drivers who were positive for alcohol as well as a 5% decline in visible crash injuries, and an 8% decline in crash injuries affecting 16- to 25-year-olds. In addition, there was a decline in self-reported driving after drinking (specifically among youth) as well as observed speeding. The greatest fatal and injury crash reductions occurred in the 16- to 25-year-old age group (Hingson *et al.* 1996).

References

Andenaes J. (1988) The Scandinavian experience. In: Laurence M.D., Snortum J.R., and Zimring F.E. (eds.) *Social control of the drinking driver*, pp. 43–63. Chicago, IL: University of Chicago Press.

Ayer S., FranHois Y., and Rehm J. (1994) *Opération Nez Rouge, Hiver 1993–1994: Evaluation Auprés des Usagers.* Lausanne, Switzerland: Insitut suisse de prévention de l'alcoolisme et autres toxicomainies.

Beccaria C. (1963) *On crimes and punishments* (translated by Henry Paolucci). Indianapolis, IN: Bobbs-Merrill.

Begg D.J., Alsop J., and Langley J.D. (2000) The impact of graduated driver licensing restrictions on young driver crashes in New Zealand. In: *Proceedings of the 15th International Conference on Alcohol, Drugs and Traffic Safety.* Stockholm, Sweden. www.icadts.com

Berger D.E., Snortum J.R., Homel R.J., *et al.* (1990) Deterrence and prevention of alcohol-impaired driving in Australia, the United States and Norway. *Justice Quarterly* 7, 453–65.

Borkenstein R.F., Crowther R.F., Shumate R.P., *et al.* (1974) The role of the drinking driver in traffic accidents. *Blutalkohol* 11 (Suppl. 1), 1–134.

Brigham T.A., Meier S.M., and Goodner V. (1995) Increasing designated driving with a program of prompts and incentives. *Journal of Applied Behavior Analysis* 28, 83–4.

Caudill B.D. and Harding W.M. (1997) *Designated drivers: Who are they and do at-risk drinkers use them?* Paper presented at the annual meeting of the Research Society on Alcoholism, San Francisco, CA.

Deyoung D.J. (1997) An evaluation of the effectiveness of alcohol treatment, driver license actions and jail terms in reducing drunk driving recidivism in California. *Addiction* 92, 989–97.

Henstridge J., Homel R., and Mackay P. (1997) *The long-term effects of random breath testing in four Australian states: A time series analysis.* Canberra, Australia: Federal Office of Road Safety.

Hingson R.W., Heeren T., and Winter M. (1994) Effects of lower legal blood alcohol limits for young and adult drivers. *Alcohol, Drugs and Driving* 10, 243–52.

Hingson R.W., McGovern T., Howland J., *et al.* (1996) Reducing alcohol-impaired driving in Massachusetts: The Saving Lives Program. *American Journal of Public Health* 86, 791–7.

Homel R. (1981) Penalties and the drink-driver: A study of one thousand offenders. *Australian and New Zealand Journal of Criminology* 14, 225–41.

Homel R. (1988a) Random breath testing in Australia: A complex deterrent. *Australian Drug and Alcohol Review* 7, 231–41.

Homel R. (1988b) *Policing and punishing the drinking driver: A study of general and specific deterrence.* New York, NY: Springer–Verlag.

ICADTS Reporter (1997) Dealing with the hard core drinking driver. *The Newsletter of the International Council on Alcohol, Drugs and Traffic Safety* 8, 1–2.

Jonah B.A. (1986) Accident risk and risk-taking behavior among young drivers. *Accident Analysis and Prevention* 18, 255–71.

Jonah B., Mann R., Macdonald S., *et al.* (2000) The effects of lowering legal blood alcohol limits: A review. In: *Proceedings of the 15th International Conference on Alcohol, Drugs and Traffic Safety.* Stockholm, Sweden. www.icadts.com

Kloeden C.N. and McLean A.J. (1994) *Late night drink driving in Adelaide two years after the introduction of the .05 limit.* Adelaide, SA: NHMRC Road Accident Research Unit.

Latimer J., Dowden C., and Muise D. (2001) *The effectiveness of restorative justice practices: A meta-analysis.* Ottawa, Ontario, Canada: Research and Statistics Division, Department of Justice.

Little J.W. (1975) *Administration of justice in drunk driving cases.* Gainesville, FL: The University Presses of Florida.

Mann R.E., Macdonald S., Stoduto G., *et al.* (2001) The effects of introducing or lowering legal per se blood alcohol limits for driving: an international review. *Accident Analysis and Prevention* 33, 569–83.

Martin S., Grube J.W., Voas R.B., *et al.* (1996) Zero tolerance laws: Effective policy? *Alcoholism: Clinical and Experimental Research* 20 (Nov. Suppl.), 147a–50a.

Mayhew D.R. (2000) Effectiveness of graduated driver licensing. In: Kursius T., Bullock W., Edwards N., *et al.* (eds.) *Proceedings of Conference: Road safety—research, policing and education, November 26–28, 2000,* pp. 5–10. Brisbane, Queensland, Australia.

Mayhew D.R. (2002) Personal e-mail communication to Ross Homel (January 25).

Mayhew D.R., Warren R.A., Simpson H.M., *et al.* (1981) *Young driver accidents: Magnitude and characteristics of the problem.* Ottawa: Traffic Injury Research Foundation of Canada.

McKnight A.J. and Voas R.B. (2001) Prevention of alcohol-related road crashes. In: Heather N., Peters T.J., and Stockwell T. (eds.) *International handbook of alcohol dependence and problems,* pp. 741–70. Chichester, UK: John Wiley and Sons.

Meier S.E., Brigham T.A., and Gilbert B.J. (1998) Analyzing methods for increasing designated driving. *Journal of Prevention and Intervention in the Community* 17, 1–14.

Miller T.R., Lestina D.C., and Spicer R.S. (1998) Highway crash costs in the United States by driver age, blood alcohol level, victim age, and restraint use. *Accident Analysis and Prevention* 30, 137–50.

Molof J.J., Dresser J., Ungerleider S., *et al.* (1995) *Assessment of year-round and holiday ride service programs.* DOT HS 808 203. Springfield, Virginia: National Technical Information Service.

Moskowitz H. and Robinson C. (1988) *Effects of low doses of alcohol on driving-related skills: A review of the evidence* (Technical report). Washington, DC: National Highway Traffic Safety Administration.

Nagin D.S. (1998) Criminal deterrence research at the outset of the twenty-first century. In: Tonry M. (ed.) *Crime and justice: A review of research,* Vol. 23, pp. 1–42. Chicago, IL: University of Chicago Press.

Norström T. (1997). Assessment of the impact of the 0.02% BAC-limit in Sweden. *Studies on Crime and Crime Prevention* 6, 245–58.

Peck R.C., Sadler D.D., and Perrine M.W. (1985) The comparative effectiveness of alcohol rehabilitation and licensing control actions for drunk driving offenders: a review of the literature. *Alcohol, Drugs and Driving: Abstracts and Reviews* 1, 15–40.

Preusser D.F., Williams A.F., Zador P.L., *et al.* (1984) The effect of curfew laws on motor vehicle crashes. *Law and Policy* 6, 115–28.

Ross H.L. (1982) *Deterring the drinking driver: Legal policy and social control.* Lexington, MA: Lexington Books.

Ross H.L. (1992) *Confronting drunk driving: Social policy for saving lives.* New Haven, CT: Yale University Press.

Ross H.L. (1993) Prevalence of alcohol-impaired driving: an international comparison. *Accident Analysis and Prevention* 25, 777–9.

Ross H.L. and Gonzales P. (1988) The effect of license revocation on drunk-driving offenders. *Accident Analysis and Prevention* 20, 379–91.

Ross H.L. and Voas R.B. (1989) *The New Philadelphia story: The effects of severe penalties for drunk driving.* Washington, DC: AAA Foundation for Traffic Safety.

Sherman L.W. (1990) Police crackdowns: Initial and residual deterrence. In: Tonry M. and Morris N. (eds.) *Crime and justice. An annual review of research,* Vol. 12, pp. 1–48. Chicago, IL: University of Chicago Press.

Sherman L.W., Strang H., and Woods D.J. (2000) *Recidivism patterns in the Canberra reintegrative shaming experiment (RISE).* Canberra, ACT: Centre for Restorative Justice, Research School of Social Sciences, Australian National University.

Shinar D. and Compton R.P. (1995) Victim impact panels: their impact on DWI recidivism. *Alcohol, Drugs and Driving* 11, 73–87.

Shults R.A., Elder R.W., Sleet D.A., *et al.* and the Task Force on Community Preventive Services (2001) Reviews of evidence regarding interventions to reduce alcohol-impaired driving. *American Journal of Preventive Medicine* 21 (Suppl. 1), 66–88.

Simons-Morton B.G. and Cummings S.S. (1997) Evaluation of a local designated driver and responsible server program to prevent drinking and driving. *Journal of Drug Education* 27, 321–33.

Siskind V. (1996) Does license disqualification reduce reoffense rates? *Accident Analysis and Prevention* 28, 519–24.

Stewart L. and Conway K. (1999) Community action to reduce rural drink driving crashes: Encouraging sustainable efforts in changing environments. In: Casswell S., Holder H., Holmila M., *et al.* (eds.) *Fourth symposium on community action research and the prevention of alcohol and other drug problems: Based upon Kettil Bruun Society Thematic Meeting,* pp. 233–46. Auckland, NZ: Alcohol and Public Health Research Unit, University of Auckland.

Stewart K. and Klitzner M. (1990) Youth anti-drinking-driving programs. In: Wilson R.J. and Mann R.E. (eds.) *Drinking and driving: Advances in research and prevention,* pp. 226–49. New York: The Guilford Press.

Sweedler B.M. (2000) The worldwide decline in drinking and driving: Has it continued? In: *Proceedings of the 15th International Conference on Alcohol, Drugs and Traffic Safety.* Stockholm, Sweden. www.icadts.com

Ulmer R.G., Preusser D.F., Williams A.F., *et al.* (2000) Effects of Florida's graduated licensing program on the crash rate of teenage drivers. *Accident Analysis and Prevention* 32, 527–32.

Voas R.B., Tippetts A.S., and Fell J. (1999) *United States limits drinking by youth under age 21: Does this reduce fatal crash involvements?* Paper presented at the annual meeting of the Association for the Advancement of Automotive Medicine, Barcelona, Spain.

Wagenaar A.C., O'Malley P.M., and LaFond C. (2001) Very low legal BAC limits for young drivers: Effects on drinking, driving, and driving-after-drinking behaviors in 30 states. *American Journal of Public Health* **91**, 801–4.

Watson B. and Fraine G. (1994) Enhancing the effectiveness of RBT in Queensland. In: Homel R. (ed.) *Proceedings of the Conference on alcohol-related road crashes: Social and legal approaches*, pp. 31–49. Brisbane, Queensland, Australia: Centre for Crime Policy and Public Safety, Griffith University.

Wells-Parker E. (2000) Assessment and screening of impaired driving offenders: An analysis of underlying hypotheses as a guide for development of validation strategies. In: *Proceedings of the 15th International Conference on Alcohol, Drugs and Traffic Safety*. Stockholm, Sweden. www.icadts.com

Wells-Parker E., Bangert-Drowns R., McMillen R., *et al.* (1995) Final results from a meta-analysis of remedial interventions with drink/drive offenders. *Addiction* **90**, 907–26.

Williams A.F. (1985) Laws and regulations applicable to teenagers or new drivers: Their potential for reducing motor vehicle injuries. In: Mayhew D.R., Simpson H.M., and Donalsen A.C. (eds.) *Young driver accidents: In search of solutions*, pp. 43–62. Ottawa, Canada: The Traffic Injury Research Foundation.

Williams A.F., Karpf R.S., and Zador P.L. (1983) Variations in minimum licensing age and fatal motor vehicle crashes. *American Journal of Public Health* **73**, 1401–3.

Williams A.F., Ferguson S.A., and Cammisa M.X. (2000) *Self-reported drinking and driving practices and attitudes in four countries and perceptions of enforcement.* Arlington, VA: Insurance Institute for Highway Safety.

WHO. See World Health Organization.

World Health Organization (1994) *Lexicon of alcohol and drug terms.* Geneva: World Health Organization.

World Health Organization (1999) *Global status report on alcohol.* WHO/HSC/SAB/99.11. Geneva: Substance Abuse Department, World Health Organization.

Zwerling C. and Jones M.P. (1999) Evaluation of the effectiveness of low blood alcohol concentration laws for younger drivers. *American Journal of Preventive Medicine* **16** (Suppl. 1), 76–80.

Chapter 10

Regulating alcohol promotion

10.1 Introduction

Alcohol marketing is now a global industry, in which the largest corporations have an international reach across industrialized countries and into new markets in developing nations (Jernigan 1997; Walsh 1997; Parry 1998; Riley and Marshal 1999; WHO 1999). The resulting coherence of marketing strategies is contributing to convergence between traditional patterns of drinking in different countries (Gual and Colom 1997). Alcohol brands marketed world-wide and those targeted to local markets are promoted through an integrated mix of strategies: television, radio and print advertisements, point of sale promotions, and the internet. Niche markets are developed by associating these brands with a range of different sports, lifestyles, and consumer identities.

A central question is whether this varied, dynamic, and widespread promotional activity is likely to have adverse consequences for public health. A major question facing policy-makers is whether the promotion of alcohol should be regulated in the public interest or left to industry self-regulation. As discussed in this chapter, a considerable body of research has now been accumulated to inform the answers to these questions.

10.2 Measuring the impact of alcohol advertising

Econometric studies, including some funded by the alcoholic beverage industry (Strickland 1982; Calfee and Scherega 1994), have investigated whether there is a discernible link between advertising and alcohol consumption. These studies involved analyses of data on advertising expenditure and aggregate consumption. Consumption was taken as a proxy for alcohol-related harm and expenditure as a proxy for exposure and response to advertising. Studies in Britain, Canada, and the US in the 1980s showed mixed results. Annual advertising expenditure showed little impact on total alcohol consumption, but some effect was seen where alcoholic beverages were analysed separately, usually for wine or spirits (Bourgeois and Barnes 1979; McGuiness 1980, 1983; Duffy 1981; Strickland 1983; Lee and Tremblay 1992). One US study compared data from states with different policies on non-broadcast advertising and showed that spirits consumption was increased by price advertising and novelty give-aways, and beer consumption was increased by outdoor price advertising (Ornstein and Hanssens 1985).

Among more recent econometric studies, analyses of annual advertising expenditure and aggregate all-beverage consumption in France, Germany, the Netherlands, the UK, and Sweden over the 1970s and 1980s found that, in each of these countries, advertising did nothing to counter the more general trend toward reduced consumption (Calfee and Scherega 1994). A study using US annual data for 1964–1990 found no impact of advertising expenditure on *per capita* alcohol consumption and little impact by beverage for beer and spirits. However, wine advertising increased consumption, with some displacement between wine and spirits from increased advertising for each of these (Nelson and Moran 1995). An analysis of US data for 16 spirits brands between 1976 and 1989 concluded that expenditure on advertising increased demand for the brand advertised with insignificant secondary benefits for rival brands (Gius 1995). A UK study, testing six econometric models, used quarterly 1963–1992 expenditures on television, radio, and print advertising. Small or statistically non-significant positive impacts on sales of wine and spirits, and negative results for beer, were found (Duffy 1995).

Saffer (1995, 1996, 1997, 1998) has challenged the methodology used in most econometric studies on a number of counts. Most studies have used annual data on advertising expenditure. Saffer argued that using local-level data measured at points through the year would better reflect the 'pulsing' and seasonal variation used by advertisers to overcome audience saturation effects. In addition, many of the studies were conducted within jurisdictions with a mature alcohol market and heavy advertising, and were therefore unlikely to find an effect of advertising, as the marginal benefit of additional spending was close to zero. Expenditure on advertising as a proxy for marketing effects is also problematic, as these 'above the line' costs represent only a fraction of the total marketing effort (Stewart and Rice 1995).

10.3 **Effects on individuals of exposure to alcohol advertising**

A further body of research, described below, has focused on responses to advertising by children and young people. Experimental studies measuring consumption after exposure to alcohol advertisements show mixed results. Studies using more sophisticated research designs, with participants unaware of the purpose of the study, show an impact on drinking behaviour.

Both econometric and experimental studies hypothesize an immediate impact of advertising on drinking. However, the cumulative effect of exposure to thousands of advertisements might be to reinforce positive attitudes towards alcohol and drinking practices. Such a continuous flow of messages, images, and values, for which television is a prime source, constitutes a system of 'cultural cultivation' that influences both mainstream attitudes and responses to advertising by different social groups (Gerbner *et al.* 1986). The impact of advertising can therefore be measured in terms of cognitive responses in processing advertising messages (Petty and Cacioppo 1981), and the links between these responses and drinking behaviour.

In the US, fifth- and eighth-grade children (aged 10 and 13 years) showed no increase in expectations of drinking after viewing television beer advertisements (Lipsitz *et al.* 1993). However, teenage students rated alcohol as more beneficial and less risky after repeated exposure to magazine alcohol advertisements (Snyder and Blood 1992). After viewing televised beer advertisements, college students had increased confidence in positive assessments of the benefits of beer. These positive beliefs were linked to plans about future alcohol use (Slater and Domenech 1995; Slater *et al.* 1995).

The effect of repeated exposure to alcohol advertising in real life is measured by the many surveys that compare participants with higher than average awareness or more positive responses to alcohol advertisements with participants with lower awareness or less positive responses. Cross-sectional analyses of such survey data have linked self-reported awareness or positive responses to advertising to positive beliefs about alcohol and higher consumption. The US research that first took this approach showed that both exposure to alcohol advertising and the attention paid to it (awareness) increased through the teenage years. Those who reported seeing the most advertisements tended to perceive the typical drinker as more fun-loving, happy, and good-looking, and in turn this was associated with more favourable attitudes regarding amounts, situations, and benefits of drinking. The cumulative effect of the advertisements was to shape young people's perceptions, encouraging pro-drinking attitudes, and greater consumption (Atkin and Block 1981, 1984).

A number of other studies have explored relationships with consumption and also expectations about future drinking. Interviews with 433 Glasgow children aged 10–17 found that they were very aware of alcohol advertising, which became increasingly salient and attractive between the ages of 10 and 14. Underage drinkers were more adept than non-drinkers at recognizing and identifying brand imagery in television advertisements (Aitken *et al.* 1988). A survey of Californian children aged 10–12 found that awareness of alcohol advertisements was linked with increased knowledge of beer brands and slogans and led to more positive beliefs about drinking and a higher expectation of drinking as an adult. The beliefs most linked to future expectations were that beer drinking was a good way to relax, to get to know people, and to unwind with friends and that drinking beer was cool and 'manly'. One-third of the respondents believed alcohol was not a substantial health risk (Wallack *et al.* 1990; Grube 1995).

Alcohol advertising also shapes perceptions about how much other people drink. In Atkin and Block's (1981) study of 12- to 22-year-olds, participants who saw the most advertisements tended to perceive drinking as pervasive in society. Their estimations of the amount consumed by a typical drinker were two drinks a week higher than the estimations of participants with less exposure (Atkin and Block 1981). In a New Zealand survey of 500 boys and girls aged 10–17, those with the best recall of alcohol advertisements were more likely to say their friends would think it acceptable for young people of their age and gender to 'drink alcohol at least once a week', and to 'get drunk at least once every few weeks'. The more advertisements they recalled seeing, the more frequently they thought their friends drank. Perceived frequency of drinking by friends was strongly and consistently associated with the respondent's own drinking, although this perceived frequency was much higher than actual drinking among participants (Wyllie and Zhang 1994; Wyllie 1997; Wyllie *et al.* 1998). Through this cognitive process, exposure to alcohol advertising may normalize heavier drinking.

Liking an advertisement is a more important variable in drinking behaviour than advertising recall. Those 14- to 17-year-old boys who liked the advertisements (as distinct from having high recall) were more likely to be drinkers and to drink larger quantities. This was partly because liking the ads was linked with feelings that 'drinking makes life more fun and exciting' and 'people get on better together when they've had a few drinks'. Boys and girls who liked the advertisements more than other participants were more likely to say that they would drink at least weekly at age 20, the legal age of purchase at the time of study. Half of the 10- to 13-year-old boys said that they knew more about drinking from watching alcohol advertisements, and this was the age group most likely to think the advertisements were realistic (Wyllie and Zhang 1994; Wyllie *et al.* 1998).

A longitudinal study of New Zealand young people also demonstrated an impact of both exposure to and liking for advertisements (Connolly *et al.* 1994; Casswell and Zhang 1998). The longitudinal design was able to address the issue of causal links. It found that those who at age 18 gave more positive responses to alcohol advertising were heavier drinkers and reported more alcohol-related aggression at age 21. Furthermore, this was independent of the amount study members were drinking at age 18 (Casswell and Zhang 1998). A subsequent follow-up with the same cohort has shown a continued impact of advertising on frequency of drinking at age 26 (Casswell *et al.* 2002).

10.4 **Effects of alcohol advertisement content on young people**

Researchers have also investigated how alcohol advertising content, as distinct from repeated exposure, works to influence young people. Atkin and Block (1981) identified two major appeals relevant to alcohol attitudes: social interaction and psychological escape.

Social camaraderie and peer acceptance are important to young people. In New Zealand television advertisements during the 1990s, the key images for spirits were escapist, such as island parties or swirling psychedelic imagery. The preferred drink of young males was beer, and beer advertisements focused strongly on masculinity themes: friendship between males, male sports, and national pride (Thomson *et al.* 1994; Wyllie *et al.* 1997; Hill 1999). In interviews with heavy drinking young adults and with 12- to 13- and 15- to 16-year-olds, all groups identified similar appeals: fun and good times, 'macho' imagery, and associations between group acceptance and drinking (Wyllie *et al.* 1997). Content analyses of US beer advertising identified a similar focus on masculinity myths, promoting not just beer but 'a particular view of what it means to be a man' (Postman *et al.* 1988; Buchanan and Lev 1989). This use of alcohol as a symbol of masculinity was explicit in a recent New Zealand beer campaign: 'Lion Red—What it means to be a man' (Hill 1999). Extreme stereotypes of masculinity are presented through humour, allowing the drinker some psychological distance (Abrahamson 1998) while he or she responds to the brand and purchases the product.

The advertisements most likely to appeal to teenagers are stylish and colourful with lively action, music, and humour (Aitken *et al.* 1988). Brand characters, such as Budweiser frogs, and celebrity endorsements are particularly effective with the young (Atkin and Block 1983; Garretson and Bruton 1998). Research shows that advertisements do not need to show heavy drinking and intoxication for this to be assumed by young viewers to be occurring, even in situations of risk (Atkin *et al.* 1983; Wyllie *et al.* 1997). Harmful consequences of drinking are not shown, supporting an inference that drinking is non-problematic.

Image advertising meets an especially positive response from younger teenagers (Covell 1992; Covell *et al.* 1994; Kelly and Edwards 1998). Attractive young adults are shown enjoying the lifestyles to which teenagers aspire (Atkin and Block 1981; Hill and Casswell 2001). Effective advertising increasingly operates at the symbolic, intuitive level of consciousness, and alcohol advertisements can use a minimum of information to evoke cultural meanings in the minds of viewers. Embedded life themes of the target market enable young drinkers to relate masculinity myths and fantasy advertising to personal daily experiences (Strate 1991; Parker 1998; Treise *et al.* 1999).

10.5 Sponsorship

By the early 1990s, more than half of all alcohol advertising expenditure was on other forms of promotion, such as sponsorship of sports events and teams (Stewart and Rice 1995). These are particularly important where broadcast alcohol advertising is banned or partially banned, but their use increased greatly over the 1990s in the US (Cornwell and Maignan 1998) and other countries, as marketing delivered through integrated packages of promotions. Among these promotion packages is marketing that associates alcohol with sporting activities that attract young males, the group most likely to be heavier drinkers.

The effectiveness of linking alcohol, masculinity, and sports was demonstrated in a US study in which male teenagers consistently preferred televised beer advertisements with sports content, and correlations were found between liking these advertisements, levels of drinking, and future drinking intentions (Slater *et al.* 1996, 1997). In US sampling in 1990–1992, alcohol ads appeared in major professional sports coverage twice as often as in college sports coverage and eight times as often as in fictional programming (Madden and Grube 1994; Grube 1995). Televised alcohol sponsorship has an effect similar to actual advertising. A sample of boys aged between 9 and 14 years responded positively to sports sponsorship carrying an alcohol company logo; 81% said their friends would take notice of this form of marketing, and 36% said beer or alcohol was being advertised, rather than the team or company (Wyllie *et al.* 1989).

Alcohol sports sponsorship provides promotional opportunities that go beyond passive absorption of images to embed the product in the everyday activities of consumers and potential consumers, tapping into social processes that establish and reinforce cultural identity (Buchanan and Lev 1989). Alcohol 'impressions' are made on many people well below the drinking age, helping form in adolescence the attitudes and preferences of later life (Kelder *et al.* 1994).

The association between beer and sports in English-speaking countries is longstanding, but from the 1970s was reinforced by marketing strategies borrowed from the tobacco industry (Buchanan and Lev 1989; Vaidya *et al.* 1996; Collins and Vamplew 2002). Alcohol sponsorship deals for sports events, teams, and clubs routinely involve event-naming rights and mentions in sports commentaries, signage on clothing, sports grounds, and products retailed to fans, and opportunities for direct marketing through product donations and the right to be the only brand available on site (Alkokutt 2002). Market-driven sponsorship has replaced philanthropic sponsorship, with costs set off against company taxation (Cornwell and Maignan 1998). As well as mass audiences for football and motor sports, more diverse consumer identities are targeted through athletics, ice hockey, basketball, skiing, snowboarding, and also rock music and cultural events. Events, activities, and venues are used by alcohol marketers to target particular demographic or psychographic segments of the market. Global communications now take sports and associated alcohol logos into the homes of millions of potential customers. International sports coverage enables alcohol advertising to reach across and infringe national laws in Scandinavia and France (Rekve 1997).

Less attention has, as yet, been paid to sponsorship of music and cultural events but these are also common strategies employed by alcohol companies. Klein (2000) cites the case of the Canadian beer, Molson, which through the 1990s had its name promoted almost every time a rock or pop star got on a stage in Canada. It then went a step further, pioneering the concept of concerts staged by Molson in which the name of the band was not released until the concert happened, in this way ensuring that the brand was bigger than the stars.

10.6 Internet marketing

The internet has provided an opportunity for global marketing with particular relevance to the young (Center for Media Education 1997, 1999). A 1998 analysis of beer, wine, and spirits marketing on the internet looked for website features that suggested targeting of the young. These features included the use of cartoons, personalities, language, music, or branded merchandise popular in youth culture, and whether the site offered interactive games, online magazines geared to youth, chat rooms, or sponsorship of music or sports events. The majority of beer (82%) and spirits (72%) sites had at least one of these features and most had about three. Wine sites were less targeted at the young (Center for Media Education 1997). An analysis of the content of several alcohol sites in terms of the Australian voluntary code of advertising content found that the internet provided an opportunity for alcohol marketing targeted at underage consumers and that some web pages were in breach of the code (Carroll and Donovan 2002). The visual and interactive nature of the internet puts unprecedented power in the hands of alcohol marketers, especially in reaching and influencing the young (Montgomery 1997).

10.7 **Policy interventions**

10.7.1 **Industry self-regulation of alcohol advertising standards**

Research on other industries has shown the limitations of self-regulation at both firm and industry levels. The greater the number of players and activities involved, the less likely it is that voluntary codes will be sufficient to restrain unacceptable practices (Ayres and Braithwaite 1992). Self-regulation is most commonly adopted by industries under threat of government regulation but, being against self-interest, tends towards under-regulation and under-enforcement (Baggott 1989). A review of media self-regulation in the US concluded that, although sometimes a useful supplement to government regulation, it rarely lived up to its claims (Campbell 1999).

Experiences in different countries show that these codes may work best where the media, advertising, and alcohol industries are all involved, and an independent body has powers to approve or veto advertisements, rule on complaints, and impose sanctions. Few countries currently have all these components. The effectiveness of codes in developed countries is often under-cut by their vagueness, while in developing countries and the transitional markets of Eastern Europe codes are unlikely to be well-enforced. The voluntary nature of codes also makes them inherently susceptible to collapse, as demonstrated in Australia in the early 1990s and with voluntary bans on spirits advertising in the US and UK in 1996 (Saunders and Yap 1991; Campbell 1999; Hill and Casswell 2001).

The US provides an example of weak self-regulation through separate beer, wine, and spirits codes administered by the alcohol industries themselves. Public controversies have arisen over the use of cartoons and Halloween imagery by major beer brands, alcohol billboard advertising near playgrounds, and depictions of violence against women in alcohol advertisements. A Federal Trade Commission (1999) inquiry into the advertising practices of eight large beer and spirits companies found that half were in violation of their codes and two were targeting underage audiences in a quarter of their ads.

A possible consequence of industry self-regulation through voluntary codes is that attention is diverted from policy questions about whether it serves the public interest to allow promotion of products that have a considerable adverse impact on public health. Instead, energy is focused on refinement of the codes, and reaction to unacceptable practices.

Moreover, codes are largely irrelevant to the way most alcohol advertising actually works. Much alcohol advertising and sports marketing does not show the product or drinking at all, but rather a simple logo. A successful mix of marketing promotions means that the media advertising to which the codes are applied can be restricted to association of the brand with images, lifestyles, and events that are attractive and relevant to target audiences, particularly the young.

10.7.2 Legislation against alcohol advertising on broadcast media

Internationally, legislation restricting alcohol advertising is a well-established, if contested, reality. Some current bans are partial, applying only to spirits, to certain hours of television viewing, or to state-owned media. These bans often operate alongside codes of self-regulation that govern permitted forms of alcohol advertising. In Europe, the overall policy trend by the mid-1990s was towards tighter control over alcohol advertising, through regulation or self-regulation.

The mix of regulation and self-regulation in industrialized countries often reflects unsuccessful efforts to secure more restrictive legislation, and systems remain in flux as decisions continue to be contested. One example is the Netherlands. A bill to ban all alcohol advertising was defeated in 1997, but by 2000 the Ministry of Health was threatening to revoke self-regulation because of the industry's unsatisfactory performance (NIGZ 2000; Sheldon 2000).

Many US states have regulated against alcohol advertising or against certain content in advertisements. For some time, the US spirits and broadcasting industries maintained voluntary bans on spirits advertising that date back to the repeal of prohibition. However, one major brand broke ranks in 1996, and the spirits industry retracted its ban, partly due to spirits' falling share of US alcohol sales. Public outcry has kept spirits advertising off the television networks, but there is now much spirits advertising on cable television. Efforts to pass federal legislation foundered on freedom of speech protections under the US Constitution. Community efforts to ban alcohol billboards through city ordinances also encountered this Constitutional block, which undermines any credible threat of regulation. Although legal debate continues on the extent to which commercial speech is protected, US advocacy efforts now focus on the need to protect children and young people under the legal age of purchase.

Arguments about the protection of commercial speech are considerably less relevant in systems based on parliamentary sovereignty, where legislation restricting alcohol advertising is common. The most comprehensive legislation to date has been in France and Norway. This legislation addressed both alcohol advertising and sports sponsorship. In 1991, television alcohol advertising and most sports sponsorship were banned, and the content of all alcohol advertisements was severely restricted through the Loi Evin. Since the ban, however, these national policies have been undermined by cross-border transmissions of sports coverage and circumvented by some of the major advertisers. Within the European Union (EU), national legislation must now comply with EU directives. In February 2001 at a conference on Young People and Alcohol in Stockholm, European Ministers called for national-level measures to minimize the pressures on young people to drink, including the pressures of alcohol advertising and sponsorship.

There have been some attempts to evaluate the effectiveness of legislative responses. Saffer (1991) evaluated the effectiveness of bans on broadcast alcohol advertising by comparing countries with different policy regimes. Using a time–series of 1970–1983 data, he compared 17 countries with full bans, partial bans, or no bans on alcohol advertising in terms of consumption levels and motor vehicle fatalities. Countries with a ban on spirits advertising had 16% lower alcohol consumption levels and 10% fewer motor vehicle fatalities than countries with no such ban. Countries with bans on beer, wine, *and* spirits advertising had 11% lower alcohol consumption levels and 23% fewer motor vehicle fatalities than countries with spirits advertising bans alone (Saffer 1991). Nelson and Young (2001) evaluated the effectiveness of bans using a similar database but a different time period (1977–1995). They found no effect of advertising bans on alcohol consumption or measures of related harm. A number of earlier studies of short-term or partial bans in single jurisdictions also indicated no effect on alcohol consumption (Smart and Cutler 1976; Ogborne and Smart 1980; Schweitzer *et al.* 1983; Makowsky and Whitehead 1991). The most recent study of the impact of bans has used a pooled time series of data from 20 countries over 26 years. This study concluded that alcohol advertising bans decreased alcohol consumption (Saffer and Dave 2002).

Another study by Saffer (1997) compared regions in the US in order to explore associations between advertising expenditure and alcohol-related harm. Regression analysis of 1986–1989 quarterly data, controlling for numerous variables, indicated that local alcohol advertising was a significant factor in motor vehicle fatalities, although it had a smaller effect than alcohol pricing. Saffer concluded that if the US ban at that time on broadcast spirits advertising had been extended to beer and wine advertising, road fatalities could have been reduced by 2000–3000 lives per year. To be effective, bans should be sufficiently inclusive to reduce opportunities for substitution, although displacement and increased saturation effects in other advertising media would reduce the effectiveness of these bans (Saffer 1997, 1998).

10.8 Conclusion

Alcohol advertising and other forms of promotion have increased dramatically over recent decades, as television and other electronic communications, including internet marketing, extend into homes where they can easily reach young adults. The promotion of alcohol is an enormously well-funded, ingenious and pervasive aspect of modern life. Standing back from the research detail, there are two conclusions that can justifiably be drawn from the research presented in this chapter.

First, the research provides information about increasingly sophisticated marketing mixtures that aim to attract, influence, and recruit new generations of potential drinkers. Exposure to repeated high level alcohol promotion inculcates pro-drinking attitudes and increases the likelihood of heavier drinking. Research has indicated the cumulative influence of alcohol advertising in shaping young people's perceptions of alcohol and drinking norms. Alcohol advertising predisposes minors to drinking well before the legal age of purchase. Marketing strategies such as alcohol sports sponsorships embed images and messages about alcohol into young people's everyday lives.

Secondly, the range and sophistication of marketing influences are not adequately addressed by industry codes of self-regulation. Self-regulation has been shown to be fragile and largely ineffective. In addition, although many countries have restricted alcohol advertising to various degrees, the findings from evaluations of legislative responses are inconsistent. Despite the difficulties inherent in disentangling cause and effect, the evaluation findings suggest that the restrictions which were feasible in the 1980s and 1990s have not achieved a major reduction in drinking and related harms in the short-term. Instead, the climate created by sophisticated alcohol marketing has facilitated the recruitment of new cohorts of young people to the ranks of heavier drinkers, and has worked against health promotion messages.

While the research in the area of alcohol advertising is likely to remain hotly contested, there is some evidence that marketing may have an impact on our youth. Advertising has been found to promote and reinforce perceptions of drinking as positive, glamorous, and relatively risk free. It is imperative that alcohol advertising research influence policy-makers to create a more level playing field for the reception of health promotion messages by the young.

References

Abrahamson M. (1998) Humour and mundane reason about alcohol drinking. *Nordic Studies on Alcohol and Drugs (English Supplement)* 15, 24–39.

Aitken P.P., Eadie D.R., Leathar D., *et al.* (1988) Television advertisements for alcoholic drinks do reinforce under-age drinking. *British Journal of Addiction* 83, 1399–419.

Alkokutt (2002) *Holdninger til salgs.* Oslo: Alkokutt.

Atkin C. and Block M. (1981) *Content and effects of alcohol advertising.* Springfield, VA: US National Technical Information Service.

Atkin C. and Block M. (1983) Effectiveness of celebrity endorsers. *Journal of Advertising Research* 23, 57–61.

Atkin C. K. and Block M. (1984) The effects of alcohol advertising. In: Kinnear T.C. (ed.) *Advances in consumer research*, pp. 688–93. Provo, Utah: Association for Consumer Research.

Atkin C., Neuendorf K., and McDermott S. (1983) The role of alcohol advertising in excessive and hazardous drinking. *Journal of Drug Education* 13, 313–23.

Ayres I. and Braithwaite J. (1992) *Responsive regulation: Transcending the deregulation debate.* New York: Oxford University Press.

Baggott R. (1989) Regulatory reform in Britain: The changing face of self-regulation. *Public Administration* 67, 435–54.

Bourgeois J.C. and Barnes J.G. (1979) Does advertising increase consumption? *Journal of Advertising Research* 19, 19–29.

Buchanan D. and Lev J. (1989) *Beer and fast cars: How brewers targets blue-collar youth through motor sports sponsorship.* Washington, DC: AAA Foundation for Traffic Safety.

Calfee J.E. and Scherega C. (1994) The influence of advertising on alcohol consumption: A literature review and an econometric analysis of four European nations. *International Journal of Advertising* 13, 287–310.

Campbell A.J. (1999) Self-regulation and the media. *Federal Communications Law Journal* 51, 711–46.

Carroll T.E. and Donovan R.J. (2002) Alcohol marketing on the internet: new challenges for harm reduction. *Drug and Alcohol Review* 21, 83–91.

Casswell S. and Zhang J.-F. (1998) Impact of liking for advertising and brand allegiance on drinking and alcohol-related aggression: A longitudinal study. *Addiction* 93, 1209–17.

Casswell S., Pledger M., and Pratap S. (2002) Trajectories of drinking from 18 to 26: Identification and prediction. *Addiction* 97, 1427–37.

Center for Media Education (1997) *Alcohol and tobacco on the web: New threats to youth.* Washington, DC: Center for Media Education.

Center for Media Education (1999) *Youth access to alcohol and tobacco web marketing. The filtering and rating debate.* Washington, DC: Center for Media Education.

Collins T. and Vamplew W. (2002) *Mud, sweat and beers: A cultural history of sport and alcohol.* Oxford and New York: Berg.

Connolly G., Casswell S., Zhang J.F., *et al.* (1994) Alcohol in the mass media and drinking by adolescents: A longitudinal study. *Addiction* 89, 1255–63.

Cornwell, T.B. and Maignan, I. (1998) An international review of sponsorship research. *Journal of Advertising* 27, 1–22.

Covell K. (1992) The appeal of image advertisements: Age, gender, and product differences. *Journal of Early Adolescence* 12, 46–60.

Covell K., Dion K.L., and Dion K.K. (1994) Gender differences in evaluations of tobacco and alcohol advertisements. *Canadian Journal of Behavioural Sciences* 26, 404–30.

Duffy M. (1981) The influence of prices, consumer incomes and advertising upon the demand for alcoholic drink in the United Kingdom: An econometric study. *British Journal on Alcohol and Alcoholism* 16, 200–8.

Duffy M. (1995) Advertising in demand systems for alcoholic drinks and tobacco: A comparative study. *Journal of Policy Modeling* 17, 557–77.

Federal Trade Commission (1999) *Self-regulation in the alcohol industry: A review of industry efforts to avoid promoting alcohol to underage consumers* (WWW document). URL: http://www.ftc.gov/reports/alcohol/alcoholreport.htm

Garretson J.A. and Bruton S. (1998) Alcoholic beverage sales promotion: An initial investigation of the role of warning messages and brand characters among consumers over and under the legal drinking age. *Journal of Public Policy and Marketing* 17, 35–47.

Gerbner G., Gross L., Morgan M., *et al.* (1986) Living with television: The dynamics of the cultivation process. In: Bryant J. and Zillman D. (eds.) *Perspectives on media effects*, pp. 17–40. Hillsdale, NJ: Lawrence Erlbaum.

Gius M.P. (1995) Using panel data to determine the effect of advertising on brand-level distilled spirits sales. *Journal for Studies on Alcohol* 56, 73–6.

Grube J.W. (1995) Television alcohol portrayals, alcohol advertising and alcohol expectancies among children and adolescents. In: Martin S.E. (ed.) *The effects of the mass media on the use and abuse of alcohol*, pp. 105–121. Bethesda, MD: US Dept of Health and Human Sciences.

Gual A. and Colom J. (1997) Why has alcohol consumption declined in countries of southern Europe. *Addiction* 92, S21–S32.

Hill L. (1999) What it means to be a Lion Red man: Alcohol advertising and Kiwi masculinity. *Women's Studies Journal* 15, 65–85.

Hill L. and Casswell S. (2001) Alcohol advertising and sponsorship: Commercial freedom or control in the public interest? In: Heather N.P., Peters T.J., and Stockwell T. (eds.) *Handbook on alcohol dependence and related problems*, pp. 821–46. Chichester: John Wiley and Sons.

Jernigan D. (1997) *Thirsting for markets*. San Rafael: Marin Institute.

Kelder S., Perry C., and Klepp K.-I. (1994) Longitudinal tracing of adolescent smoking, physical activity and food choice behaviours. *American Journal of Public Health* 84, 1121–6.

Kelly K. and Edwards R. (1998) Image advertisements for alcohol products: Is their appeal associated with adolescents' intention to consume alcohol? *Adolescence* 33, 47–59.

Klein N. (2000) *No space, no choice, no jobs, no logo: Taking aim at the brand bullies*. New York: Picador USA.

Lee B. and Tremblay V.J. (1992) Advertising and the US market demand for beer. *Applied Economics* 24, 69–77.

Lipsitz A., Brake G., Vincent E.J., *et al.* (1993) Another round for the brewers: Television ads and children's alcohol expectancies. *Journal of Applied Social Psychology* 23, 439–50.

Madden P.A. and Grube J.W. (1994) The frequency and nature of alcohol and tobacco advertising in televised sports, 1990 through 1992. *American Journal of Public Health* 84, 297–9.

Makowsky C. and Whitehead P.C. (1991) Advertising and alcohol studies: A legal impact study. *Journal of Studies on Alcohol* 52, 555–67.

McGuiness T. (1980) An econometric analysis of total demand for alcoholic beverages in the UK, 1956–1975. *Journal of Industrial Economics* 29, 85–109.

McGuiness T. (1983) The demand for beer, wine and spirits in the UK: 1956–1979. In: Grant M., Plant M., and Williams A. (eds.) *Economics and alcohol: Consumption and controls*. London: Croom Helm.

Montgomery K. (1997) *Alcohol and tobacco on the web: New threats to young* (Executive summary). Washington, DC: Center for Media Education. http://www.cme.org/children/marketing/execsum.html

National Instituut voor Gezondheidsbevorderung en Ziektepreventie (2000) *Some things only happen after dark . . .* Woerden, Netherlands: NIGZ.

Nelson J.P. and Moran J.R. (1995) Advertising and US alcohol beverage demand: System-wide estimates. *Applied Economics* 27, 1225–36.

Nelson J.P. and Young D.J. (2001) Do advertising bans work? An international comparison. *International Journal of Advertising* 20, 273–96.

NIGZ. See National Instituut voor Gezondheidsbevorderung en Ziektepreventie.

Ogborne A.C. and Smart R.G. (1980) Will restrictions on alcohol advertising reduce alcohol consumption? *British Journal of Addiction* 75, 293–329.

Ornstein S.I. and Hanssens D.M. (1985) Alcohol control laws and the consumption of distilled spirits and beer. *Journal of Consumer Research* 12, 200–13.

Parker B.J. (1998) Exploring life themes and myths in alcohol advertisements through a meaning-based model of advertising experiences. *Journal of Advertising* 27, 97–112.

Parry C.D.H. (1998) *Alcohol policy and public health in South Africa.* Cape Town: Oxford University Press.

Petty R.E. and Cacioppo J.T. (1981) *Attitudes and persuasion: Classic and contemporary approaches.* Dubrique, IA, USA: Wm. C. Brown.

Postman N., Nystrom C., Strate L., *et al.* (1988) *Myths, men and beer: An analysis of beer commercials on broadcast television, 1987.* Falls Church: AAA Foundation for Traffic Safety.

Rekve D. (1997) *Status report from a joint project between Alkokutt and the Norwegian Football Association.* Oslo: Alkokutt.

Riley L. and Marshal M. (1999) *Alcohol and public health in 8 developing countries.* Geneva: Substance Abuse Department, World Health Organization.

Saffer H. (1991) Alcohol advertising bans and alcohol abuse: An international perspective. *Journal of Health Economics* 10, 65–79.

Saffer H. (1995) Alcohol advertising and alcohol consumption: econometric studies. In: Martin S.E. (ed.) *The effects of the mass media on the use and abuse of alcohol,* pp. 83–100. Bethesda, MD: US Dept of Health and Human Sciences.

Saffer H. (1996) Studying the effects of alcohol advertising on consumption. *Alcohol Health and Research World* 20, 266–73.

Saffer H. (1997) Alcohol advertising and motor vehicle fatalities. *Review of Economics and Statistics* 79, 431–42.

Saffer H. (1998) Economic issues in cigarette and alcohol advertising. *Journal of Drug Issues* 28, 781–93.

Saffer H. and Dave D. (2002) Alcohol consumption and alcohol advertising bans. *Applied Economics* 30, 1325–34.

Saunders B. and Yap E. (1991) Do our guardians need guarding? An examination of the Australian system of self-regulation of alcohol advertising. *Drug and Alcohol Review* 10, 15–17.

Schweitzer S.O., Intriligator M.D., and Salehi H. (1983) Alcoholism: An econometric model of its causes, its effects and its control. In: Grant M., Plant M., and Williams A. (eds.) *Economics and alcohol: Consumption and controls,* pp. 107–27. London: Croom Helm.

Sheldon T. (2000) Dutch tighten their rules on advertising of alcohol. *British Medical Journal* 320, 1094.

Slater M. and Domenech M.M. (1995) Alcohol warnings in TV beer advertisements. *Journal of Studies on Alcohol* 56, 361–7.

Slater M., Murphy K., Beauvais F., *et al.* (1995) Modeling predictors of alcohol use and use intentions among adolescent Anglo males: Social, psychological, and advertising influences. Presented: *Annual Conference of the Research Society on Alcoholism* (June 1995), Steamboat Springs, CO.

Slater M.D., Rouner D., Murphy K., *et al.* (1996) Male adolescents' reactions to TV beer advertisements: The effects of sports content and programming context. *Journal of Studies on Alcohol* 57, 425–33.

Slater M.D., Rouner D., Domenech-Rodriguez M., *et al.* (1997) Adolescent responses to TV beer ads and sports content/context: Gender and ethnic differences. *Journal and Mass Communications Quarterly* 74, 108 22.

Smart R.G. and Cutler R.E. (1976) The alcohol advertising ban in British Colombia: Problems and effects on beverage consumption. *British Journal of Addiction* 71, 13–21.

Snyder L.B. and Blood D.J. (1992) Caution: Alcohol advertising and the Surgeon General's alcohol warnings may have adverse effects on young adults. *Journal of Applied Communication Research* 20, 53–7.

Stewart D.W. and Rice R. (1995) Non-traditional media and promotions in the marketing of alcoholic beverages. In: Martin S.E. (ed.) *The effects of the mass media on the use and abuse of alcohol*, pp. 209–38. Bethesda, MD: US Dept of Health and Human Services.

Strate L. (1991) The cultural meaning of beer commercials. *Advances in Consumer Research* 18, 115–19.

Strickland D.E. (1982) Alcohol advertising: Orientations and influence. *International Journal of Advertising* 1, 307–19.

Strickland D.E. (1983) Advertising exposure, alcohol consumption and misuse of alcohol. In: Grant M., Plant M., and Williams A. (eds.) *Economics and alcohol: Consumption and controls*. London: Croom Helm.

Thomson A., Casswell S., and Stewart L. (1994) Communication experts' opinions on alcohol advertising in the electronic media. *Health Promotion International* 9, 145–52.

Treise D., Wolburg J.M., and Otnes C.C. (1999) Understanding the 'social gifts' of drinking rituals: An alternative framework for PSA developers. *Journal of Advertising* 28, 17–42.

Vaidya S.G., Naik U.C., and Vaidya J.S. (1996) Effect of sports sponsorship by tobacco companies on children's experimentation with tobacco. *British Medical Journal* 313, 400.

Wallack L., Cassady D., and Grube J. (1990) *TV beer commercials and children: Exposure, attention, beliefs and expectations about drinking as an adult.* Washington DC: AAA Foundation for Traffic Safety.

Walsh B. (1997) Trends in alcohol production, trade and consumption. *Addiction* 92 (Suppl. 1), 61–6S.

WHO. See World Health Organization.

World Health Organization (1999) *Global status report on alcohol.* Geneva: Substance Abuse Department, World Health Organization.

Wyllie A. (1997) *Love the ads—love the beer: Young people's responses to televised alcohol advertising* (Doctoral Thesis). Auckland: Alcohol and Public Research Unit, University of Auckland.

Wyllie A. and Zhang J.-F. (1994) *Responses of 10 to 17 year olds to alcohol and host responsibility advertising on television: Survey data.* Auckland: Alcohol and Public Health Research Unit.

Wyllie A., Casswell S., and Stewart J. (1989) The response of New Zealand boys to corporate and sponsorship alcohol advertising on television. *British Journal of Addiction* **84**, 639–46.

Wyllie A., Holibar F., Casswell S., *et al.* (1997) A qualitative investigation of responses to televised alcohol advertisements. *Contemporary Drug Problems* **24**, 103–32.

Wyllie A., Zhang J.F., and Casswell S. (1998) Responses to televised alcohol advertisements associated with drinking behaviour of 10 to 17 year olds. *Addiction* **93**, 361–71.

Chapter 11

Education and persuasion strategies

11.1 Introduction

Education and persuasion strategies are among the most popular approaches to the prevention of alcohol-related problems. In this chapter, these strategies are examined in several contexts and settings, including schools, colleges, and communities. Both individual- and population-level orientations are evident in these strategies, which have the following objectives:

1. Changing knowledge about alcohol and risks related to drinking.
2. Changing attitudes with regard to drinking in order to lower risks.
3. Changing drinking behaviour itself.
4. Lowering the frequency or seriousness of problems related to drinking.
5. Increasing resources and support for alcohol policies.

As with other chapters in this book, the goal is to derive policy-relevant conclusions from an objective review of the research evidence. However, this chapter differs from the others in that the research leads to rather negative conclusions. These conclusions were also made in an earlier review (Edwards *et al.* 1994). Updating the evidence only confirms earlier findings. For the most part, the behavioural objectives listed above have not been realized. Nevertheless, it is important to examine the available research in order to understand the relative ineffectiveness of education and persuasion strategies, and to see how they compare with other evidence-based policy choices.

11.2 Initiatives involving the media

11.2.1 Mass media and counter-advertising

Although the most sophisticated and expensive media portrayals are advertisements that favour the use of alcohol, public health and safety perspectives are also portrayed in the mass media. Public service announcements on television or radio, paid counter-advertisements, billboards, magazine and newspaper pieces, and news or feature stories on television and radio, all attempt to provide information about the risks and complications associated with drinking. While it is expected that these public service messages have a direct effect on the target audience, this is seldom the case.

Public service announcements (PSAs) are messages prepared by non-governmental organizations, health agencies, and media organizations for the purpose of providing important information for the benefit of a particular audience. As opposed to paid advertising, PSAs depend upon donated time or space for distribution to the public. When applied to alcohol, PSAs usually deal with **responsible drinking,** the hazards of drinking–driving, and related topics. Despite their good intentions, PSAs are an ineffective antidote to the high quality pro-drinking messages that appear much more frequently as paid advertisements in the mass media (see Ludwig 1994; Murray *et al.* 1996).

In many cases, PSA messages are intended to be particularly relevant to drinking by youth (Connolly *et al.* 1994; Holder 1994). Gorman (1995) pointed out the limited impact that mass media interventions using a **universal strategy** have on alcohol use and alcohol-related problems. Nevertheless, a Canadian study (Casiro *et al.* 1994) found that after a TV campaign was broadcast on the dangers of alcohol consumption during pregnancy, more women concluded that drinking would put their baby at risk, and attributed this information to 'television'. In general, there is a need for more research about what audiences perceive and understand from mass media campaigns (Martin 1995). However, exploring the ways in which different media set the public and policy agenda is potentially more fruitful (Casswell 1997). For example, portrayal of alcohol issues in the news media (print, TV, and radio) tends to be simplistic, sensational, and dramatic (Gusfield 1995). The news media focus on stories about individual people rather than alcohol in its social perspective. These portrayals raise interesting questions about the way news reporting may shape public attitudes and policy about alcohol, but this area has not been extensively researched.

In response to the extensive promotion of alcoholic beverages in many countries, governments and private organizations have sponsored **counter-advertising**. This has taken several forms, including PSAs and placement of warning messages on actual advertisements.

Counter-advertising involves disseminating information about a product, its effects, and the industry that promotes it, in order to decrease its appeal and use. It is distinct from other types of informational campaigns in that it directly addresses the fact that the particular commodity is promoted through advertising (Agostinelli and Grube 2002). Tactics include health-warning labels on product packaging and media literacy efforts to raise public awareness of the advertising tactics of an industry, as well as prevention messages in magazines and on television (see Barlow and Wogalter 1993). Counter-advertising may also be included in community or school prevention programs (e.g., Giesbrecht *et al.* 1990; Greenfield and Zimmerman 1993), and be used as part of government liquor board retail systems (Goodstadt and Flynn 1993).

In most countries, the number of PSAs and counter-advertisements concerning alcohol are at best a small fraction of the total volume of alcohol advertisements (see Fedler *et al.* 1994; Wyllie *et al.* 1996), and are rarely seen on television. Moreover, the quality of counter-advertising is often poor. For example, a study of high school students in the Moselle region in France (Pissochet *et al.* 1999) found that respondents considered alcohol risk prevention advertising to be less effective than alcohol advertising, and daily drinkers were more critical than intermittent and non-drinkers. Although public acceptance of counter-advertising is high (e.g., Giesbrecht and Greenfield 1999), legislative initiatives to place warnings directly on alcohol advertisements, particularly electronic messages, have not succeeded in the United States (Greenfield *et al.* 1999; Giesbrecht 2000). In some countries, however, such warnings are required; billboard advertisements in Mexico, for instance, carry general warnings to use alcohol with caution.

Other developments related to counter-advertising include media literacy efforts to teach young people to resist the persuasive appeals of alcohol advertising. Some small positive effects have been observed in media literacy programs with children (Austin and Johnson 1997). Slater *et al.* (1996) found that recency of exposure to alcohol education classes and discussion of alcohol advertising predicted cognitive resistance to such advertising for several months or even years after exposure. Canzer (1996) exposed college students to educational videos about the alcohol industry, its advertising efforts, and health-related information. A general reduction in drinking was observed. Nearly two-thirds of the participants reduced the number of times they went to social environments where risky alcohol consumption was likely.

Given the relatively low frequency of broadcast counter-advertising, and typical placement of such messages at either unattractive times or in connection with unpopular programming, it is surprising that any impact has been found (Saffer 1996). In order to counter the ubiquitous and glamorized images of alcohol portrayed in many advertisements, Gerber (1995) advocates the development of alternative strategies. These alternatives include the production of more diverse images, the portrayal of better role models, and the saturation of communities with health information. Recent developments in tobacco counter-advertising in some parts of the US suggest that intensive and hard-hitting counter-advertising can have significant effects, at least in the short run. Florida teenagers were impressed by the spectacle of a government agency sponsoring advertisements attacking the tobacco industry as 'not in business for your health'. At the end of a year these teenagers had stronger anti-tobacco attitudes and smoked less than a comparison population (Sly *et al.* 2001). However, such an effort could not be sustained. The state program was undermined by political pressure after one year (Givel and Glantz 2000).

From a public health perspective, counter-advertising has intuitive appeal, and may be a more realistic political option than seeking a ban on alcohol advertising (Saffer 2002). While there is nothing in the research to suggest that counter-advertising offers powerful outcomes within realistically available budgets, the recent US tobacco experience suggests that a hard-hitting counter-advertising program can be effective as part of a comprehensive prevention strategy (Rohrbach *et al.* 2002).

11.2.2 Warning labels

A fairly extensive amount of research has been conducted on US-mandated alcoholic beverage container **warning labels**, which were introduced in 1989 (Kaskutas 1995). Emphasis has been placed on the potential for birth defects when alcohol is consumed during pregnancy, the danger of alcohol impairment when driving or operating machinery, and general health risks. Some states require posted warnings of alcohol risks in establishments that serve or sell alcohol.

A significant proportion of the population has reported seeing these warning labels (Kaskutas and Greenfield 1992; Graves 1993; Greenfield *et al.* 1993). There is some survey evidence (Kaskutas and Greenfield 1992; Greenfield 1997; Greenfield and Kaskutas 1998; Greenfield *et al.* 1999) that warning labels may increase knowledge regarding the risks of drinking–driving and drinking during pregnancy among some sub-groups (e.g., light drinkers). A series of national surveys found that awareness, as indicated by conversations about risks, was greater among the more frequent drinkers, including young adults (Kaskutas and Greenfield 1997; Greenfield and Kaskutas 1998). Kaskutas and Greenfield (1997) conducted a US national telephone survey to explore recall of warning messages on alcohol container labels, signs at point-of-sale, and warning messages in media advertisements. Recall was good for all three types of messages. For warning labels, recall was especially high for young people, males, and heavy drinkers. There was a dose–response relationship between pregnancy-related conversations about drinking while pregnant and the number of types of messages seen (e.g., point-of-sale signage, advertisements, magazine stories, and warning labels) (Kaskutas *et al.* 1998). Pregnant women who saw more messages reported more conversations about their drinking. No direct impacts of warning labels on consumption or alcohol-related problems have been reported.

Several warning label studies have focused on youth. The first year after warning labels were introduced, MacKinnon *et al.* (1993) found that 12th graders (about 17-years-old) reported increases in awareness of, exposure to, and recognition of warning labels. However, there were no substantial changes in alcohol use or beliefs about the risks described in the labels. An experimental study by Snyder and Blood (1992) involved a sample of 159 college students who viewed six different advertisements for alcohol products, some with the US Surgeon General's warning and some without. The warnings did not increase perceptions of alcohol risk, and may even have made products more attractive to both drinkers and non-drinkers.

In summary, the warning label research does not demonstrate that exposure produces a change in drinking behaviour *per se*. Andrews (1995) concludes that warning labels are not significantly effective in preventing alcohol consumption by heavy drinkers. Other reviews (Grube and Nygaard 2001; Agostinelli and Grube 2002) conclude that there is little evidence that alcohol warning labels have measurable effects on drinking behaviours. However, there is evidence that some intervening variables are affected, such as intention to change drinking patterns (in relation to situations of heightened risk such as drinking–driving), having conversations about drinking, and willingness to intervene with others who are seen as hazardous drinkers. Considering the small size and relative obscurity of the typical US warning label, it is surprising that any impacts have been observed. It is possible that the impact of warning labels can be enhanced by combining it with other strategies, such as community-based campaigns to change alcohol policies or enforce regulations.

11.2.3 Low-risk drinking guidelines

Epidemiological research on the effects of moderate drinking on cardiovascular problems (e.g., Marmot 2001) has created political pressures in some countries to provide the public with promotional and educational material about the benefits of moderate alcohol use. Surveys in several countries have noted an increase in the number of adults who are aware of these putative health benefits. For example, in New South Wales, Australia, the proportion identifying health benefits increased from 28% in 1990 to 46% in 1994, with relaxation (54%) and cardiovascular benefits (39%) most often mentioned (Hall 1995).

In this context, official or semi-official guidelines have been adopted in a number of countries on 'moderate' drinking or 'low-risk drinking' (Bondy *et al.* 1999). Given the complex considerations that underlie any such guidelines, it is not surprising that the guidelines vary considerably from one country to another (Stockwell 2001). There is at present little research on the impact of these messages (Walsh *et al.* 1998). Furthermore, it is unclear whether such messages should decrease or increase alcohol consumption and related problems (Casswell 1993).

11.3 **School-based programs**

The goal of most school-based **alcohol education programs** is to change the adolescent's drinking beliefs, attitudes, and behaviours, and to modify factors such as general social skills and self-esteem that are assumed to underlie adolescent drinking (Paglia and Room 1999). School-based interventions popular during the 1970s and 1980s relied solely on informational approaches and taught students about the dangers of drug use. Such programs have not been found to be effective (Tobler 1992; Hansen 1994; Botvin *et al.* 1995). Although they can increase knowledge and change attitudes toward alcohol, tobacco, and drug use, actual substance use remains largely unaffected. In addition, there is some evidence that providing information about the dangers of different psychoactive substances may, in some cases, actually increase use (Hansen 1980, 1982). In particular, such information may serve to arouse curiosity in those who are risk takers or who seek adventure (Norman *et al.* 1997). Affective approaches that address values clarification, self-esteem, general social skills, and 'alternatives' approaches that provide activities inconsistent with alcohol use (e.g., sports) are equally ineffective (Moskowitz 1989). Findings from evaluations of the most common school-based prevention programs are summarized in Box 11.1.

11.3.1 **Social influence programs**

Partly in response to the ineffectiveness of informational, affective, and alternatives approaches, social influence programs were developed from contemporary social psychological theory. These programs were based on the assumption that most adolescents are negatively predisposed toward alcohol and drug use, but rarely have to justify their unfavourable attitudes toward these behaviours. As a result, when challenged, their beliefs were easily undermined. These new programs attempted to 'inoculate' young people against such challenges to their beliefs by addressing resistance to social pressures to use drugs and by focusing on short-term and immediate social consequences (Evans *et al.* 1978). Early evaluations of these programs seemed promising, at

Box 11.1 **Evidence for effectiveness of school-based prevention programs**

Approach	Evidence
Information	Some evidence that strictly informational programs change attitudes and beliefs. No evidence that such programs reduce or prevent drinking by young people. Some evidence that these programs may be counterproductive and encourage drinking among some young people.
Affective education	No evidence that these programs reduce or prevent drinking by young people.
Alternatives	No evidence that these programs reduce or prevent drinking by young people.
Resistance skills	Behavioural changes may be small and short-lived without regular 'booster' sessions. Some conflicting evidence regarding effectiveness.
Normative education	Studies report significant changes in perceived norms and small to moderate behavioural changes.

least for tobacco, and they form the basis for many current school-based alcohol prevention efforts. More recently, it has been recognized that adolescent alcohol use results not so much from direct pressures to drink, but from more subtle social influences (Hansen 1993). It has even been suggested that **resistance skills training** may be counterproductive because it leads young people to conclude that drinking is prevalent among, and approved by, their peers (Hansen and Graham 1991; Donaldson *et al.* 1997). As a result, there has been a shift toward providing **normative education** that corrects adolescents' tendency to overestimate the number of their peers who drink and approve of drinking (Hansen 1992, 1993, 1994). Many contemporary school-based programs include both resistance skills training and normative education.

Scientific evaluations of school-based resistance and normative education interventions have produced mixed results with regard to alcohol. On the one hand, some researchers believe these interventions are effective in reducing drinking and alcohol-related problems (e.g., Botvin and Botvin 1992; Hansen 1993, 1994; Dielman 1995). On the other hand, others are critical of the research evidence for their effectiveness (e.g., Gorman 1996, 1998; Foxcroft *et al.* 1997; Brown and Kreft 1998; Paglia and Room 1999).

The Alcohol Misuse and Prevention Study (AMPS) is typical of the current generation of US school-based education programs focusing on pressures to use alcohol, risks of alcohol misuse, and ways to resist pressures to drink (Shope *et al.* 1996a, b). The AMPS program had positive effects on alcohol and resistance skills knowledge that persisted up to 26 months (Shope *et al.* 1992). Overall, there were few effects on actual drinking behaviour, except for some short-term changes for students in specific grades (Shope *et al.* 1996a). Other school-based alcohol resistance skills programs have produced similar modest results (Botvin *et al.* 1995; Klepp *et al.* 1995).

Normative education programs have two goals:

1. To correct the tendency for students to overestimate the amount of drinking in their peer group.

2. To change the acceptable level of peer drinking.

Within these programs, teachers provide information from survey data showing actual prevalence rates, and guide class discussions about appropriate and inappropriate alcohol use. Initial evaluations of normative education programs seemed promising. Hansen and Graham (1991) found an 8% decrease in reported drunkenness by eighth graders in these programs compared with eighth graders in information-only programs. Similar results have been reported for other normative education interventions (Graham *et al.* 1991; Hansen 1993), although some investigators have been critical of the research on these programs (e.g., Kreft 1997).

School-based educational interventions, even when using the most recent normative education and resistance skill training program innovations, generally produce modest effects that are short-lived unless accompanied by ongoing booster sessions. A recent review (Foxcroft *et al.*, in press) of 56 primary prevention studies found only two showing promise as effective interventions with young people over the long term, and only one was a school-based program. Although some evaluations have measured heavy drinking and self-reported problems, few have demonstrated substantive effects on rates of intoxication, drinking–driving, injury, and alcohol-related crashes. In most cases, such outcomes are not even reported. There is some evidence that certain sub-groups may be more affected by school-based interventions. For example, youth with previously unsupervised drinking experience may be more responsive to resistance skills training (Shope *et al.* 1994; Dielman 1995), while those who are more rebellious may be less responsive to normative education (Kreft 1997).

11.3.2 Comprehensive programs

Some programs include both individual-level education and family- or community-level interventions. One such program, Project Northland, was a school and community intervention designed to prevent or delay the onset of drinking among young adolescents in 10 communities in northeastern Minnesota (Perry *et al.* 1993, 1996). The primary school-based intervention was a series of resistance skills, media literacy, and normative education sessions. The program also provided parents with information on adolescent alcohol use. Task forces in some communities were involved in local policy actions such as the passage of local ordinances requiring responsible beverage service training. Other activities included the enlistment of local businesses to give discounts to students who promised to remain alcohol- and drug-free and sponsorship of alcohol-free activities for youth. Evaluation of Project Northland indicated that the program had a positive influence on alcohol knowledge and family communication about alcohol. Alcohol use, however, was not significantly reduced at the end of the sixth grade (Williams *et al.* 1995) or the seventh grade, with the program having no overall effect on drinking (Perry *et al.* 1996). Other analyses showed that those who were actively involved in peer-planned social activities were less likely to report using alcohol in the past month than those who attended the alcohol-free activities but were not actively involved in planning, and those who were non-participants (Komro *et al.* 1996). Participation in the parents' program in seventh grade was related to increases in parent communication about alcohol, especially in terms of family rules and the consequences of breaking those rules (Toomey *et al.* 1996). By eighth grade, additional differences emerged on program-related attitudes and beliefs (Perry *et al.* 1996). Students in the intervention schools scored lower on a measure of tendency to use alcohol than students in comparison schools. They also reported significantly less alcohol use in the past month. All of these differences dissipated after the intervention ended (Perry *et al.* 1998).

Another comprehensive program, the Midwestern Prevention Project, was implemented in 50 public schools in 15 communities in the state of Kansas (USA). A replication was conducted in 57 schools and 11 communities in another state. The intervention consisted of five components:

1. A 10–13 session school-based program with five booster sessions.

2. A mass media program.

3. A parent education and organization program.

4. Training of community leaders.

5. Local policy changes initiated by the community organization.

Monthly drinking was significantly lower in the intervention than in the comparison schools after one year (Pentz *et al.* 1989; MacKinnon *et al.* 1991), but it did not differ (34% vs. 33%) after three years (Johnson *et al.* 1990).

Effects on monthly intoxication were significant through the end of high school.

In summary, these well-designed evaluations suggest that even comprehensive school-based prevention programs may not be sufficient to delay the initiation of drinking, or to sustain a small reduction in drinking beyond the operation of the program. Reduced drinking was found when coupled with community interventions, especially those that were successful in reducing alcohol sales and provision of alcohol to youth. More research is needed to confirm the findings of these early studies, which couple school education with family and community interventions, including local policy initiatives. As noted elsewhere in this volume, community-based prevention programs are effective in curtailing drinking and alcohol-related problems (Hingson *et al.* 1996; Holder *et al.* 2000; Wagenaar *et al.* 2000). These initiatives primarily involve a combination of policy or regulatory changes, enforcement, and community organizing.

11.4 College and university programs

11.4.1 Rationale and models

Interventions directed at alcohol use in college and university settings have been developed in response to concerns about the extent of heavy drinking (Engs *et al.* 1994; Wechsler 1996), its relation to sexual assaults (Meilman *et al.* 1993; Meilman and Haygood-Jackson 1996; Schwartz and Kennedy 1997), and its impact on school performance, drinking–driving (Hingson *et al.* 2002), and other alcohol-related problems such as disorderly conduct. Large-scale surveys of college students in the US (Wechsler 1996) and Canada (Gliksman *et al.* 2000) have documented the extent of drinking and alcohol-related risks. Both abstinence and harm-reduction goals are reflected in college intervention programs. While the goal of abstinence from alcohol is consistent with the legal drinking age of 21 in the US, total abstinence may be unrealistic, even in that country, because the majority of underage students drink on a regular basis. In most other countries the legal drinking age is lower, and this may explain the relatively low number of university- or college-based prevention programs outside of North America. However, there is a growing interest by World Health Organization and European Union groups in alcohol-related problems among young people (Grube and Nygaard 2001).

Recent prevention efforts in the US have been oriented to local and state authorities, university administrators, heavy drinkers, their peers, and alcohol retailers and producers (DeJong and Langford 2002; Larimer and Cronce

2002; Perkins 2002). Typically, a combination of strategies is used, including persuasive measures, staff training, guidelines and regulations, voluntary arrangements pertaining to alcohol marketing, restrictions on location of outlets, and campus alcohol policies. Interventions that rely primarily on educational and informational strategies are influenced by several theoretical approaches (Gonzalez and Clement 1994; Werch *et al.* 1994), such as the **health belief model** (Broughton 1997), the **empowerment model** (Cummings 1997), and by social marketing strategies (Zimmerman 1997). The social marketing approach uses research to plan communications and is intended to change the environment as well as individual behaviour.

11.4.2 Specific programs

Evaluation of college and university prevention programs is uncommon. A survey by Wood (1994) of 360 four-year public colleges found that 81% of the responding institutions had never conducted an evaluation of their program. In cases where evaluation data are available, even with a relatively short follow-up period (e.g., three to six months), the results tend to be equivocal (e.g., Harrington *et al.* 1999).

Normative education is the organizing principle in several interventions. Steffian (1999) reports on an experimental program designed to challenge misperceptions of college drinking norms. Students assigned to an education group later demonstrated more accurate perceptions of campus drinking norms and showed a significant reduction in alcohol-related problems, in contrast to students in a control group. Robinson *et al.* (1993) studied the impact of a five week psycho-educational course. After five weeks subjects in the experimental module knew significantly more about substance abuse than did control subjects. But no effects on actual substance use were found. Cameron *et al.* (1993) explored the impact of a multi-media program directed at first year students. Participants experienced a 22% decline in alcohol consumption, whereas non-participants experienced a 50% increase.

In another study, Turner (1997) compared a 'Health Enhancement Led by Peers' (HELP) group with an academic control group. There were significant improvements in knowledge following exposure to the program, but no changes were found in attitudes or behaviour. A study of brief interventions with heavy and hazardous college drinkers (Dimeff 1998) found no differences on major alcohol consumption measures between experimental and control subjects at one month follow-up, although some improvement was observed for experimental group participants who had a longer exposure. A review of mass media (DeJong 2002) campaigns focusing on heavy and hazardous college drinkers found that while such campaigns were common, none were rigorously evaluated.

In summary, there is clear evidence of the increased awareness of risks of heavy drinking and alcohol problems among college students exposed to the aforementioned interventions. Alternatively, there is no convincing scientific support for the effectiveness of campus-wide educational programs or awareness campaigns (Larimer and Cronce 2002), in reducing heavy drinking or alcohol-related problems.

11.5 **Conclusion**

In recent years, the number of informational and educational programs has grown exponentially (see Foxcroft *et al.* 1997). Many of these programs have not been evaluated. Where evaluations have been conducted, they often do not meet the criteria of 'methodological soundness' (Foxcroft *et al.* 1997; White and Pitts 1998, p. 1477). The range of programs evaluated has been relatively narrow, and the results do not provide an adequate basis for recommending expansion of efforts or elaboration of strategies. The impact of these programs tends to be small at best and most effects do not persist (White and Pitts 1998). Compared to other interventions and strategies such as law enforcement initiatives, outlet zoning, pricing policies, and responsible serving practices, educational programs are expensive and appear to have little effect on alcohol consumption levels and drinking-related problems. Their hegemony and popularity seems not to be a function of either their demonstrated impact or their potential for reducing alcohol-related harms.

This chapter began with a declaration that the lesson from alcohol education programs lies in the value of reporting a negative case. It is tempting to lessen this conclusion by emphasizing the few positive findings emerging from one or another study. But the weight of the negative evidence is more convincing than any small positive findings.

It is likely that even with adequate resources, strategies that try to use only education to prevent alcohol-related harm are unlikely to deliver large or sustained benefits. Education alone may be too weak a strategy to counteract other forces that pervade the environment. An unanswered question, beyond the scope of this monograph, is why significant resources continue to be devoted to initiatives with limited potential for reducing or preventing alcohol-related problems.

References

Agostinelli G. and Grube J. (2002) Alcohol counter-advertising and the media: A review of recent research. *Alcohol Research and Health*, 26, 15–21.

Andrews J.C. (1995) Effectiveness of alcohol warning labels: A review and extension. *American Behavioral Scientist* 38, 622–32.

Austin E.W. and Johnson K.K. (1997) Immediate and delayed effects of media literacy training on third graders' decision making for alcohol. *Health Communication* 9, 323–49.

Bondy S.J., Rehm J., Ashley M.J., *et al.* (1999) Low-risk drinking guidelines: Scientific evidence. *Canadian Journal of Public Health* 90, 264–70.

Barlow T. and Wogalter M.S. (1993) Alcoholic beverage warnings in magazine and television advertisements. *Journal of Consumer Research* 20, 147–56.

Botvin G.J. and Botvin E.M. (1992) Adolescent tobacco, alcohol, and drug abuse: Prevention strategies, empirical findings, and assessment issues. *Developmental and Behavioral Pediatrics* 13, 290–301.

Botvin G.J., Baker E., Dusenbury L., *et al.* (1995) Long-term follow-up results of a randomized drug abuse prevention trial in a white middle-class population. *Journal of the American Medical Association* 273, 1106–12.

Broughton E.A. (1997) Impact of informational methods among drinking college students applying the Health Belief Model. *Dissertation Abstracts International* 57, 3839–40A.

Brown J.H. and Kreft I.G.G. (1998) Zero effects of drug prevention programs: Issues and solutions. *Evaluation Review* 22, 3–14

Cameron J., Whitehead P.C., and Hayes M.J. (1993) Evaluation of a program to modify alcohol-related knowledge, attitudes, intentions and behaviors among first-year university students. In: Greenfield T.K. and Zimmerman R. (eds.) *Second international research symposium on experiences with community action projects for the prevention of alcohol and other drug problems*, pp. 167–73. Washington, DC: US Department of Health and Human Services.

Canzer B. (1996) Social marketing approach to media intervention design in health and lifestyle education. *Dissertation Abstracts International* 57, 647A.

Casiro O.G., Stanwick R.S., Pelech A., *et al.* (1994) Public awareness of the risks of drinking alcohol during pregnancy: The effects of a television campaign. *Canadian Journal of Public Health* 85, 23–7.

Casswell S. (1993) Public discourse on the benefits of moderation: Implications for alcohol policy development. *Addiction* 88, 459–65.

Casswell S. (1997) Public discourse on alcohol. *Health Promotion International* 12, 251–7.

Connolly G.M., Casswell S., Zhang J.F., *et al.* (1994) Alcohol in the mass media and drinking by adolescents: A longitudinal study. *Addiction* 89, 1255–63.

Cummings S. (1997) Empowerment model for collegiate substance abuse prevention and education programs. *Journal of Alcohol and Drug Education* 43, 46–62.

DeJong W. (2002) The role of mass media campaigns in reducing high-risk drinking among college students. *Journal of Studies on Alcohol* (Suppl.) 14, 182–92.

DeJong W. and Langford L.M. (2002) A typology for campus-based alcohol prevention: Moving toward environmental management strategies. *Journal of Studies on Alcohol* (Suppl.) 14, 140–7.

Dielman T.E. (1995) School-based research on the prevention of adolescent alcohol use and misuse: Methodological issues and advances. In: Boyd G.M., Howard J., and Zucker R.A. (eds.) *Alcohol problems among adolescents: Current directions in prevention research*, pp. 125–46. Hillsdale, NJ: Lawrence Erlbaum.

Dimeff L.A. (1998) Brief intervention for heavy and hazardous college drinkers in a student primary health care setting. *Dissertation Abstracts International* **58**, 6805B.

Donaldson S.I., Graham J.W., Piccinin A.M., *et al.* (1997) Resistance-skills training and onset of alcohol use: Evidence for beneficial and potentially harmful effects in public schools and private Catholic schools. In: Marlatt G.A. and VandenBos G.R. (eds.) *Addictive behaviors: Readings on etiology, prevention, and treatment*, pp. 215–38. Washington, DC: American Psychological Association.

Edwards G., Anderson P., Babor T.F., *et al.* (1994) *Alcohol policy and the public good.* Oxford: Oxford University Press.

Engs R.C., Diebold B.A., and Hanson D.J. (1994) Drinking patterns and problems of a national sample of college students, 1994. *Journal of Alcohol and Drug Education* **41**, 13–33.

Evans R.I., Rozelle R.M., Mittlemark M.B., *et al.* (1978) Deterring the onset of smoking in children: Knowledge of immediate physiological effects and coping peer pressure, media pressure, and parental modeling. *Journal of Applied Social Psychology* **8**, 126–35.

Fedler F., Philips M., Raker P., *et al.* (1994) Network commercial promote legal drugs: Outnumber anti-drug PSAs 45-to-1. *Journal of Drug Education* **24**, 291–302.

Foxcroft D.R., Lister-Sharp D., and Lowe G. (1997) Alcohol misuse prevention for young people: A systematic review reveals methodological concerns and lack of reliable evidence of effectiveness. *Addiction* **92**, 531–7.

Foxcroft D.R., Ireland D., Lister-Sharp D.J., Lowe G., and Breen R. (2003) Longer-term primary prevention for alcohol misuse in young people: a systematic review. *Addiction* **98**, (Suppl. 4), 397–411.

Gerber G. (1995) Alcohol in American culture. In: Martin S.E. and Mail P. (eds.) *Effects of the mass media on the use and abuse of alcohol*, pp. 3–29. Bethesda, Maryland: National Institute on Alcohol Abuse and Alcoholism.

Giesbrecht N. (2000) Roles of commercial interests in alcohol policies: Recent developments in North America. *Addiction* **95** (Suppl. 4), 581–95S.

Giesbrecht N. and Greenfield T.K. (1999) Public opinions on alcohol policy issues: A comparison of American and Canadian surveys. *Addiction* **94**, 521–31.

Giesbrecht N., Conley P., Denniston R., *et al.* (eds.) (1990) *Research, action, and the community: Experiences in the prevention of alcohol and other drug problems.* Rockville, Maryland: Office for Substance Abuse Prevention.

Givel M.S. and Glantz S.A. (2000) Failure to defend a successful state tobacco control program: Policy lessons from Florida. *American Journal of Public Health* **90**, 762–7.

Gliksman L., Demers A., Adlaf E.M., *et al.* (2000) *Canadian campus survey, 1998.* Toronto: Centre for Addiction and Mental Health.

Gonzalez G.M. and Clement V.V. (eds.) (1994) *Research and intervention: Preventing substance abuse in higher education.* Washington, DC: US Department of Education.

Goodstadt M. and Flynn L. (1993) Protecting oneself and protecting others: Refusing service, providing warnings, and other strategies for alcohol warnings. *Contemporary Drug Problems* **20**, 277–91.

Gorman D.M. (1995) Are school-based resistance skills training programs effective in preventing alcohol abuse? *Journal of Alcohol and Drug Education* **41**, 74–98.

Gorman D.M. (1996) Do school-based social skills training programs prevent alcohol use among young people? *Addiction Research* **4**, 191–210.

Gorman D.M. (1998) The irrelevance of evidence in the development of school-based drug prevention policy, 1986–1996. *Evaluation Review* 22, 118–46.

Graham J.W., Collins L.M., Wulgalter S.E., *et al.* (1991) Modeling transitions in latent stage-sequential processes: A substance use prevention example. *Journal of Clinical and Consulting Psychology* 59, 48–57.

Graves K. (1993) Evaluation of the alcohol warning label: A comparison of the United States and Ontario, Canada in 1990 and 1991. *Journal of Public Policy and Marketing* 12, 19–29.

Greenfield T.K. (1997) Warning labels: Evidence of harm-reduction from long-term American surveys. In: Plant M., Single E., and Stockwell T. (eds.) *Alcohol: Minimizing the harm*, pp. 105–25. London: Free Association Books.

Greenfield T.K. and Kaskutas L.A. (1998) Five years' exposure to alcohol warning label messages and their impacts: Evidence from diffusion analysis. *Applied Behavioral Science Review* 6, 39–68.

Greenfield T.K. and Zimmerman R. (eds.) (1993) *Second international research symposium on experiences with community action projects for the prevention of alcohol and other drug problems*. Washington, DC: US Department of Health and Human Services.

Greenfield T.K., Graves K.L., and Kaskutas L.A. (1993) Alcohol warning labels for prevention: National survey results. *Alcohol, Health and Research World* 17, 67–75.

Greenfield T.K., Giesbrecht N., Johnson S.P., *et al.* (1999) *US federal alcohol control policy development: A manual*. Berkeley, California: Alcohol Research Group.

Grube J.W. and Nygaard P. (2001) Adolescent drinking and alcohol policy. *Contemporary Drug Problems* 28, 87–131.

Gusfield J. (1995) Meta-analytic perspective on 'alcohol in American culture'. In: Martin S.E. and Mail P. (eds.) *Effects of the mass media on the use and abuse of alcohol*, pp. 31–5. Bethesda, Maryland: National Institute on Alcohol Abuse and Alcoholism.

Hall W. (1995) Changes in public perceptions of the health benefits of alcohol use, 1989 to 1994. *Australian and New Zealand Journal of Public Health* 20, 93–5.

Hansen D.J. (1980) Drug education: Does it work? *Evaluation Studies Review Annual* 6, 572–603.

Hansen D.J. (1982) Effectiveness of alcohol and drug education. *Journal of Alcohol and Drug Education* 27, 1–13.

Hansen D.J. (1992) School-based substance abuse prevention: A review of the state of the art in curriculum, 1980–1990. *Health Education Research* 7, 403–30.

Hansen D.J. (1993) School-based alcohol prevention programmes. *Alcohol, Health and Research World* 17, 54–61.

Hansen D.J. (1994) Prevention of alcohol use and abuse. *Preventive Medicine* 23, 683–7.

Hansen D.J. and Graham J.W. (1991) Preventing alcohol, marijuana, and cigarette use among adolescents: Peer pressure resistance training versus establishing conservative norms. *Preventive Medicine* 20, 414–30.

Harrington N.G., Brighton N.L., and Clayton R.R. (1999) Alcohol risk reduction for fraternity and sorority members. *Journal of Studies on Alcohol* 60, 521–7.

Hingson R., McGovern T., Howland J., *et al.* (1996) Reducing alcohol-impaired driving in Massachusetts: The Saving Lives Program. *American Journal of Public Health*, 86 (6), 791–7.

Hingson R., Heeren T., Zakocs R., *et al.* (2002) Magnitude of alcohol-related morbidity, mortality, and alcohol dependence among US college students age 18–24. *Journal of Studies on Alcohol* 63, 136–44.

Holder H.D. (1994) Mass communication as an essential aspect of community prevention to reduce alcohol-involved traffic crashes. *Alcohol, Drugs and Driving* 10, 3–4.

Holder H.D., Gruenewald P.J., Ponicki W.R., *et al.* (2000) Effect of community-based interventions on high-risk drinking and alcohol-related injuries. *Journal of the American Medical Association* 284, 2341–7.

Johnson C.A., Pentz M.A., Weber M.D., *et al.* (1990) Relative effectiveness of comprehensive community programming for drug abuse prevention with high risk and low risk adolescents. *Journal of Consulting and Clinical Psychology* 58, 447–56.

Kaskutas L.A. (1995) Interpretations of risk: The use of scientific information in the development of the alcohol warning label policy. *International Journal of the Addictions* 30, 1519–48.

Kaskutas L.A. and Greenfield T.K. (1992) First effects of warning labels on alcoholic beverage containers. *Drug and Alcohol Dependence* 31, 1–14.

Kaskutas L.A. and Greenfield T.K. (1997) Behavior change: The role of health consciousness in predicting attention to health warning messages. *American Journal of Health Promotion* 11, 183–93.

Kaskutas L.A., Greenfield T.K., Lee M., *et al.* (1998) Reach and effects of health messages on drinking during pregnancy. *Journal of Health Education* 29, 11–17.

Klepp K.I., Kelder S.H., and Perry C.L. (1995) Alcohol and marijuana use among adolescents: Long-term outcomes of the Class of 1989 Study. *Annals of Behavioral Medicine* 17, 19–24.

Komro K.A., Perry C.L., Murray D.M., *et al.* (1996) Peer-planned social activities for preventing alcohol use among young adolescents. *Journal of School Health* 66, 328–34.

Kreft I.G.G. (1997) The interactive effect of alcohol prevention programs in high school classes: An illustration of item homogeneity scaling and multilevel analysis techniques. In: Bryant K.J., Windle M., and West S.G. (eds.) *The science of prevention: Methodological advances from alcohol and substance abuse research*, pp. 251–77. Washington, DC: American Psychological Association.

Larimer M.E. and Cronce J.M. (2002) Identification, prevention and treatment: A review of individual-focused strategies to reduce problematic alcohol consumption by college students. *Journal of Studies on Alcohol* (Suppl.) 14, 148–63.

Ludwig M.J. (1994) Mass media and health education: a critical analysis and reception study of a selected anti-drug campaign. *Dissertation Abstracts International* 55, 1479A.

MacKinnon D.P., Johnson C.A., Pentz M.A., *et al.* (1991) Mediating mechanisms in a school-based drug prevention program. First-year effects of the Midwestern Prevention Project. *Health Psychology* 10, 164–72.

MacKinnon D.P., Pentz M.A., and Stacy A.W. (1993) The alcohol warning label and adolescents: The first year. *American Journal of Public Health* 83, 585–7.

Marmot M.G. (2001) Alcohol and coronary heart disease. *International Journal of Epidemiology* 30, 724–9.

Martin S.E. (1995) Alcohol and the mass media: Issues, approaches, and research directions. In: Martin S. (ed.) *The effects of mass media on the use and abuse of alcohol*, pp. 277–95. Rockville, MD: National Institute on Alcohol Abuse and Alcoholism.

Meilman P.W. and Haygood-Jackson D. (1996) Data on sexual assault from the first 2 years of a comprehensive campus prevention program. *Journal of American College Health* 44, 157–65.

Meilman P.W., Burwell C., Smith K.E., *et al.* (1993) Using survey data to capture students' attention: Three institutions look at alcohol-induced sexual behavior. *Journal of College Student Development* 34, 72–3.

Moskowitz J.M. (1989) Primary prevention of alcohol problems: A critical review of the research literature. *Journal of Studies on Alcohol* 50, 54–88.

Murray J.P., Jr., Stam A., and Lastovicka J.L. (1996) Paid- versus donated-media strategies for public service announcement campaigns. *Public Opinion Quarterly* 60, 1–29.

Norman E., Turner S., Zunz S., *et al.* (1997) Prevention programs reviewed: What works? In: Norman E. (ed.) *Drug free youth: A compendium for prevention specialists*, pp. 22–46. New York: Garland.

Paglia A. and Room R. (1999) Preventing substance use problems among youth: A literature review and recommendations. *Journal of Primary Prevention* 20, 3–50.

Pentz M.A., Dwyer J.H., MacKinnon D.P., *et al.* (1989) A multi-community trial for primary prevention of drug abuse. Effects on drug use prevalence. *Journal of the American Medical Association* 261, 3259–66.

Perkins H.W. (2002) Social norms and the prevention of alcohol misuse in collegiate contexts. *Journal of Studies on Alcohol* (Suppl.) 14, 164–72.

Perry C.L., Williams C.L., Forster J.L., *et al.* (1993) Background, conceptualization and design of a community-wide research program on adolescent alcohol use: Project Northland. *Health Education Research: Theory and Practice* 8, 125–36.

Perry C.L., Williams C.L., Veblen-Mortenson S., *et al.* (1996) Project Northland: Outcomes of a community-wide alcohol use prevention program during early adolescence. *American Journal of Public Health* 86, 956–65.

Perry C.L., Williams C.L., Komro K.A., *et al.* (1998) Project Northland–phase II: Community action to reduce adolescent alcohol use. Paper presented at the Kettil Bruun Society Thematic Meeting, February, Russell, Bay of Islands, New Zealand.

Pissochet P., Biache P., and Paille F. (1999) Alcool, publicité et prévention: le régard des jeunes (Alcohol, advertising and prevention: young people's point of view). *Alcoologie* 21, 15–24.

Robinson S.E., Roth S.L., Gloria A.M., *et al.* (1993) Influence of substance abuse education on undergraduates' knowledge, attitudes and behaviors. *Journal of Alcohol and Drug Education* 39, 123–30.

Rohrbach L.A., Howard-Pitney B., Unger J.B., *et al.* (2002) Independent evaluation of the California Tobacco Control program: Relationships between program exposure and outcomes, 1996–1998. *American Journal of Public Health* 92, 975–83.

Saffer H. (1996) Studying the effects of alcohol advertising on consumption. *Alcohol, Health and Research World* 20, 266–72.

Saffer H. (2002) Alcohol advertising and youth. *Journal of Studies on Alcohol* (Suppl.) 14, 173–81.

Schwartz M.D. and Kennedy W.S. (1997) Factors associated with male peer support for sexual assault on the college campus. In: Schwartz M.D. and DeKeseredy W.S. (eds.) *Sexual assault on the college campus: The role of male peer support*, pp. 97–136. Thousand Oaks, California: Sage.

Shope J.T., Dielman T.E., Butchart A.T., *et al.* (1992) An elementary school-based alcohol misuse program: A follow-up evaluation. *Journal of Studies on Alcohol* 53, 106–21.

Shope J.T., Kloska D.D., Dielman T.E., *et al.* (1994) Longitudinal evaluation of an enhanced Alcohol Misuse Prevention Study (AMPS) curriculum for grades six–eight. *Journal of School Health* 64, 160–6.

Shope J.T., Copeland L.A., Maharg R., *et al.* (1996a) Effectiveness of a high school alcohol misuse prevention program. *Alcoholism: Clinical and Experimental Research* 20, 791–8.

Shope J.T., Copeland L.A., Marcoux B.C., *et al.* (1996b) Effectiveness of a school-based substance abuse prevention program. *Journal of Drug Education* 26, 323–37.

Slater M.D., Rouner D., Murphy K., *et al.* (1996) Adolescents counterarguing of TV beer advertisements: Evidence for effectiveness of alcohol education and critical viewing discussions. *Journal of Drug Education* 26, 143–58.

Sly D.F., Heald G.R., and Ray S. (2001) The Florida 'truth' anti-tobacco media evaluation: Design, first year results, and implications for planning future state media evaluations. *Tobacco Control* 10, 9–15.

Snyder L.B. and Blood D.J. (1992) Caution: Alcohol advertising and the Surgeon General's alcohol warning may have adverse effects on young adults. *Journal of Applied Communication Research* 20, 37–53.

Steffian G. (1999) Correction of normative misperception: An alcohol abuse prevention program. *Journal of Drug Education* 29, 115–38.

Stockwell T. (2001) Harm reduction, drinking patterns and the NHMRC drinking guidelines. *Drug and Alcohol Review* 20, 121–9.

Tobler N.S. (1992) Prevention programs can work: Research findings. *Journal of Addictive Diseases* 11, 1–28.

Toomey T.L., Williams C.L., Perry C.L., *et al.* (1996) An alcohol primary prevention program for parents of 7th graders: The amazing alternatives! Home program. *Journal of Child and Adolescent Substance Use* 5, 35–53.

Turner S.C. (1997) Effects of peer alcohol abuse education on college students' drinking behavior. *Dissertation Abstracts International* 57, 4276A.

Wagenaar A.C., Murray D.M., and Toomey T.L. (2000) Communities Mobilizing for Change on Alcohol (CMCA): Effects of a randomized trial on arrests and traffic crashes. *Addiction* 95, 209–17.

Walsh G.W., Bondy S.J., and Rehm J. (1998) Review of Canadian low-risk drinking guidelines and their effectiveness. *Canadian Journal of Public Health* 89, 241–7.

Wechsler H. (1996) Alcohol and the American college campus: A report from the Harvard School of Public Health. *Change* 28, 20–5 and 60.

Werch C.E., Lepper J.M., Pappas D.M., *et al.* (1994) Use of theoretical models in funded college drug prevention programs. *Journal of College Student Development* 35, 359–63.

White D. and Pitts M. (1998) Educating young people about drugs: A systematic review. *Addiction* 93, 1475–87.

Williams C.L., Perry C.L., Dudovitz B., *et al.* (1995) A home-based prevention program for sixth-grade alcohol use: Results from Project Northland. *Journal of Primary Prevention* 16, 125–47.

Wood B.A. (1994) Study to assist administrators of public, four-year colleges and universities in establishing alcohol and other drug abuse prevention and education programs. *Dissertation Abstracts International* 55, 55A.

Wyllie A., Waa A., and Zhang J.F. (1996) *Alcohol and moderation advertising expenditure and exposure: 1996.* Auckland, New Zealand: University of Auckland.

Zimmerman R. (1997) *Social marketing strategies for campus prevention of alcohol and other drug problems.* Newton, MA: Higher Education Center for Alcohol and other Drug Prevention.

Chapter 12

Treatment and early intervention services

12.1 Introduction

Alcohol policies are primarily the concern of local, regional, and national governments, which often view the provision of treatment as part of a comprehensive approach to alcohol-related problems. In addition to its value in the reduction of human suffering, treatment can be considered as a form of prevention. When it occurs soon after the onset of alcohol problems, it is called secondary prevention; when it is initiated to control the damage associated with chronic drinking, it is called tertiary prevention. As one of the first societal responses to alcohol problems, treatment interventions have not been critically examined as policy options, despite the resources they consume and the scientific evidence that is available concerning their effectiveness and costs. This chapter examines the scientific basis of alcohol treatment policies in terms of research on the effectiveness and costs of a wide range of treatment interventions.

12.2 Treatment services and systems of care

Treatment for alcohol problems typically involves a set of services, ranging from diagnostic assessment to therapeutic interventions and continuing care. Researchers have identified more than 40 therapeutic approaches, called treatment modalities, which have been evaluated by means of randomized clinical trials (Miller *et al.* 1995). Examples include motivational counselling, marital and family therapy, cognitive-behavioural therapy, relapse prevention training, aversion therapy, pharmacotherapy, and interventions based on the Twelve Steps of Alcoholics Anonymous. These modalities are delivered in a variety of settings, including freestanding residential facilities, psychiatric and general hospital settings, outpatient programs, and primary care. More recently, treatment services in some countries have been organized into systems that are defined by linkages between different facilities and levels of care, and by the extent of integration with other types of services, such as mental health, drug dependence treatment, and mutual help organizations (Klingemann *et al.* 1993; Klingemann and Klingemann 1999).

Several international comparative studies have been conducted to monitor developments in alcohol treatment systems during the last quarter of the 20th century. The first (Klingemann *et al.* 1992, 1993) was conducted in 16 countries chosen for their geographical, cultural, and economic diversity. The study found that since the end of the Second World War most countries have experienced significant growth in their alcohol treatment services along with changes in how alcohol problems are conceptualized and administered. Alcoholism is now viewed more as a disease or illness than a criminal offence, with increasing decentralization, deinstitutionalization, and diversification of available treatment. Outpatient treatment predominates, offering more choices to a wider variety of people with drinking problems. Treatment has become more a part of the mainstream health care system, and community-level administration has been replacing federal and national controls. However, large differences exist among the treatment systems in different countries. Economic resources and treatment need play less of a role than cultural and political traditions in determining the resources devoted to alcohol treatment. And during periods of economic retrenchment, governments tend to neglect their treatment services.

In a study of drug and alcohol treatment services in 23 countries, Gossop (1995) found that most countries have a scarcity of resources for these kinds of services, and many report an inadequate level of professional training. In countries such as Congo, there are no specialist services for alcohol problems; native healers provide the majority of treatment. In many countries the disparity between supply and demand for treatment is compounded by the maldistribution of services, which tend to be concentrated in large cities. Although 70% of countries surveyed deliver treatment primarily in non-residential settings, Ghana, Norway, Nigeria, Spain, and Pakistan were found to favour residential settings (Gossup 1995). Little information exists at the program level about the effectiveness of particular treatment interventions. In Peru, Japan, Poland, and Germany, drug and alcohol services are provided separately, but in most countries they are integrated. In some countries mutual help organizations such as Alcoholics Anonymous (AA) and Croix Bleu are sufficiently well established to provide a substantial contribution to the national system of treatment services (Gossop 1995).

In another international study, Grant and Ritson (1990) evaluated trends in national treatment policies in a wide variety of countries (Australia, Bulgaria, Costa Rica, Kenya, Mexico, Norway, the United Kingdom, the USSR, and Zimbabwe). The study found that in many of the countries the concept of alcohol-related problems was not just limited to alcoholism but also included problem drinking. Because of this broader concept of alcohol-related problems, a wider array of services was favoured, including early recognition of hazardous drinking, low cost interventions in primary care, and more effective ways to match patients' needs with appropriate programs. It was also concluded that national alcohol policies provide a stimulus to new developments in many countries, but that treatment policy needed to be integrated within a broader preventive strategy that enabled ministerial support and intersectoral collaboration.

Mäkelä *et al.* (1996) surveyed the activities of AA and other mutual help organizations in eight countries, noting wide variation in the proportions of recovering persons who affiliate with these community-based organizations. In North America, for example, AA operates more than 50 000 groups. In Italy, Clubs for Alcoholics in Treatment (CATs) account for 86% of the mutual help services provided (Room 1998). These groups serve as adjuncts to professional treatment in some countries, but in other countries, such as Croatia, they represent the major resource for managing persons with alcohol-related problems.

This brief overview of the emerging systems of specialized services and policies provides only a suggestion of the broad array of programs, treatments, and settings that have been developed in the past 25 years to manage persons with various kinds of alcohol-related problems. The remainder of this chapter concentrates on three types of intervention within the emerging treatment systems of countries where information on efficacy and effectiveness is available:

1. Interventions for non-dependent high-risk drinkers.

2. Formal treatment for problem drinkers and alcoholics.

3. Mutual help interventions.

The final section considers how evidence-based treatment interventions might be implemented cost-effectively and on a systematic basis in communities and nation states.

12.3 **Interventions directed at high-risk drinkers**

In 1980, a World Health Organization (WHO) Expert Committee called for the development of efficient methods to detect persons with harmful alcohol consumption before the onset of pronounced health and social consequences (WHO 1980). Since then, the concepts of early identification and brief intervention have attracted widespread attention from researchers and policy makers, as indicated by the growing amount of clinical and applied research being conducted throughout the world. In the 1990s, the development of effective, inexpensive screening and brief interventions for alcohol misuse (Babor *et al.* 2001) moved beyond the stage of clinical trials to the point where national dissemination plans started to be considered (Babor and Higgins-Biddle 2000).

Brief interventions are characterized by their low intensity and short duration. They typically consist of one to three sessions of counselling and education. They are intended to provide early intervention, before or soon after the onset of alcohol-related problems. Most programs are designed to motivate high-risk drinkers to moderate their alcohol consumption, rather than to promote total abstinence with specialized treatment techniques.

Since the 1980s, numerous randomized controlled trials were conducted to evaluate the efficacy of brief interventions. The results of these trials have been summarized in several integrative literature reviews and meta-analyses (Bien *et al.* 1993; Babor 1994; Kahan *et al.* 1995; Wilk *et al.* 1997; Poikolainen 1999). Figure 12.1 shows the results of a secondary analysis of research data from seven random assignment studies having quantitative estimates of alcohol consumption before and after exposure to a brief intervention. The figure also presents comparable information from untreated control groups that did not receive an intervention (Higgins-Biddle and Babor 1996). The results show a net reduction in the intervention groups (minus reductions in controls) of 22%.

The cumulative evidence of randomized controlled trials (conducted in a variety of settings) indicates that clinically significant changes in drinking behaviour and related problems can follow from brief interventions. Nevertheless, the

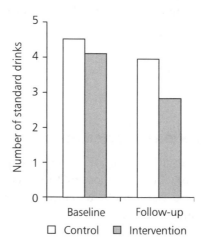

Fig. 12.1 Effects of brief intervention on drinks per day. Weighted average of seven studies comparing intervention group with control group male drinkers, 12 month follow-up. Source: Higgins-Biddle and Babor (1996).

results were not always consistent across studies (Poikolainen 1999), the duration of effect remains unknown, and there is little evidence that these interventions are beneficial for alcohol-dependent individuals (Mattick and Jarvis 1994). An important consideration is the degree to which implementation can be achieved in routine clinical practice. Persuading family physicians, for instance, to use the methods on a sustained basis has often proved difficult (Richmond *et al.* 1998).

12.4 **Specialist treatment**

The range of agencies and individuals involved in specialist treatment of alcohol-related problems is extensive. In addition to the medical sector, which encompasses psychiatric services and specialist treatment units, treatment is also delivered by social and welfare agencies, workplace programs, and court-mandated programs for persons convicted of drinking–driving. Some of the key issues that treatment research addressed with increasing scientific rigor over the last decade include therapeutic effectiveness, the effects of treatment intensity, and modality patient/treatment matching.

There is no consistent evidence that intensive inpatient treatment provides more benefit than less intensive outpatient treatment. Nevertheless, residential treatment may be indicated for patients who:

1. Are highly resistant to treatment.
2. Have few financial resources.
3. Come from environments that are not conducive to recovery.
4. Have more serious, coexisting medical or psychiatric conditions (Finney *et al.* 1996).

A study of the long-term outcomes of treated and untreated alcoholics (Timko *et al.* 2000) indicates that individuals who obtain help for a drinking problem, especially in a timely manner, have better outcomes over eight years than those who do not receive help. The type of help they receive (e.g., self-help or formal treatment) makes little difference in long-term outcomes.

Regarding specific treatment modalities, the weight of evidence suggests that behavioural treatments are likely to be more effective than insight-oriented therapies (Miller and Hester 1986). Recent research (Ouimette *et al.* 1999; Babor and Del Boca 2002) also indicates that Twelve Step Facilitation, which is based on the principles of Alcoholics Anonymous, is as effective as more theory-based therapies. In general, when patients enter treatment, exposure to any treatment is associated with significant reductions in alcohol use and related problems, regardless of the type of intervention used.

Interest on the part of the pharmaceutical industry in medications to treat alcohol dependence has increased in the past decade, and a variety of compounds for alcoholism treatment are now available in the US and Europe. Until recently, the aversive agent disulfiram was the main drug used to treat alcohol dependence, but its efficacy has been questioned by the results of controlled trials (Fuller *et al.* 1986). In the 1990s, naltrexone, an opioid antagonist, became available for medical management of alcohol dependence, following positive studies showing incremental benefits of psychotherapy combined with this medication (O'Malley *et al.* 1992). Acamprosate (calcium acetylhomotaurinate), an amino acid derivative, has been studied in countries throughout Europe and is now in widespread clinical use (Kranzler and Van Kirk 2001). Although cost and efficacy questions remain prior to the widespread clinical application of these treatments, these medication developments open the way to pharmacological strategies for treatment of alcohol dependence.

The possibility of rational treatment/patient matching continues to attract interest, and there is some evidence to suggest that patients with certain characteristics (e.g., severe dependence, high levels of anger, social networks that support drinking) respond marginally better to certain types of therapy (e.g., Twelve Step Facilitation, motivational enhancement, cognitive behavioural) (Project MATCH Research Group 1997a, b, 1998; Ouimette *et al.* 1999). Beyond therapy, treatment matching may be more effective when specific services are provided to address the psychological and social needs of the patient, such as employment counselling and psychiatric services (McClellan *et al.* 1997).

Despite advances in the identification and treatment of alcohol problems, there are impediments to be overcome in providing access to these services, including reluctance on the part of physicians and other health professionals to ask about their patients' drinking habits. Given the scarcity of specialized treatment services in most countries (Klingemann *et al.* 1992), they are not likely to have an impact on morbidity and mortality at the level of communities and nation states. Nevertheless, there is some evidence that treatment has the potential to produce aggregate impact in countries where the treatment system is relatively well developed (Smart and Mann 2000). Several researchers have identified associations between declining liver cirrhosis rates and the growth of specialized treatment. Mann *et al.* (1988) found that decreased hospital discharges for liver cirrhosis were associated with increased treatment in Ontario, Canada. Romelsjö (1987) suggested that in addition to decreased *per capita* consumption, the growth of outpatient treatment may have accounted for the reduction in liver cirrhosis rates in Stockholm, Sweden. Holder and

Parker (1992) found that increased alcohol treatment admissions (both in- and outpatient) over a 20-year period in North Carolina were related to a significant reduction in cirrhosis mortality. Although these three studies from three different countries provide promising support for the aggregate-level impact of treatment systems, the evidence of impact would be strengthened by replication in other countries.

12.5 Alcoholics Anonymous and other mutual help societies

Although mutual help societies composed of recovering alcoholics are not considered to be formal treatment, they are often used as substitutes, alternatives, and as adjuncts to treatment (McCrady and Miller 1993). Mutual help groups based on the Twelve Steps of AA have proliferated throughout the world (Mäkelä 1993). Related organizations have been developed within a number of other countries, such as Danshukai in Japan, Krcuzbund in Germany, Croix d'Or and Vie Libre in France, Abstainers Clubs in Poland, and Links in the Scandinavian countries (Room 1998). According to AA World Services, Inc. (2002), the world-wide membership of AA is estimated to be approximately 2.2 million. To the extent that AA and other mutual help groups outnumber outpatient treatment programs, they may constitute a significant resource for problem drinkers who are attempting to reduce or stop drinking.

It is difficult to assess the efficacy of AA or other mutual help groups using controlled research designs because of methodological challenges such as self-selection and ethical concerns about random assignment to an untreated control condition. However, the effects of referral to AA from a treatment or other agency can be studied, and several large-scale, well-designed studies of this nature (Walsh *et al.* 1991; McCrady and Miller 1993; Ouimette *et al.* 1999; Babor and Del Boca 2002) suggest that AA can have an incremental effect when combined with formal treatment, and that AA attendance alone may be better than no intervention at all.

If AA were effective in reducing alcohol dependence and chronic drinking, then its impact on population rates of alcohol-related problems and mortality would depend on the number of problem drinkers actively involved in its programs. Researchers at the Addiction Research Foundation of Ontario (Smart *et al.* 1989; Smart and Mann 1990, 1993; Mann *et al.* 1991) have reported an inverse relationship over time between AA membership and alcohol-related problems, including cirrhosis rates. They argue that in the US and Canada the large reductions in liver cirrhosis rates and alcohol-related hospital discharges in the last three decades are in part attributable to increased levels of AA membership. Mann *et al.* (1991) estimated that a 1% increase in AA membership would be associated with a 0.06% decrease in cirrhosis mortality. According to these estimates, large increases in AA membership would be necessary to substantially reduce cirrhosis deaths. Although these North American studies do not establish causality, they do provide correlational evidence to suggest the potential of AA membership to affect cirrhosis and possibly other alcohol-related problems at an aggregate level. If these relationships are in some degree causal, the implication is that with greater availability of AA, alcoholic cirrhosis could be reduced significantly.

12.6 **Cost considerations**

A major issue with regard to the feasibility and extensiveness of specialist treatment approaches is cost. Little research has been conducted on the cost of services for alcohol treatment, but in recent years there have been significant improvements in the methodological tools used and a better formulation of policy questions. One policy question is whether individuals who undergo treatment for alcohol dependence have lower health care expenditures afterwards (i.e., cost offsets). Another question is whether some settings or treatment modalities are more cost-effective than others, i.e., they deliver similar outcomes for lower costs. Still other questions concern whether shorter or longer periods of inpatient treatment are more cost-effective.

Cost offset studies (Holder 1987; Goodman *et al.* 1997) conducted primarily in the United States have shown that:

1. Alcoholics and their family members are heavier users of health care services than are non-alcoholics of the same age and gender.

2. Prior to entering treatment, general medical care costs for those who eventually seek treatment tend to increase.

3. Following treatment, the demand for health services by alcoholics and their families declines. In some cases these savings are large enough to compensate for the expense of treatment.

Regarding cost-effective alternatives to inpatient alcoholism treatment, reviews of this literature (Finney *et al.* 1996) conclude that:

1. Inpatient alcoholism programs lasting from four weeks to several months do not have higher success rates than periods of brief hospitalization.

2. Some patients can be safely detoxified without pharmacotherapy and in non-hospital-based environments.

3. Partial hospitalization programs ('day hospitalization' with no overnight stays) have results equal or superior to inpatient hospitalization, at one-half to one-third the cost.

4. In some populations, outpatient programs produce results comparable to those of inpatient programs.

An obvious question is whether some treatment modalities and treatment settings are more cost-effective than the others. In one analysis of treatment modalities used in the US, the range of treatment costs across settings was enormous, with a high of US $585 per day for hospital-based care and a low of US $6 per visit at social model, non-residential programs. Nevertheless, the research evidence did not show that more expensive treatment was more effective (Holder *et al.* 1991; Goodman *et al.* 1997).

12.7 **Treatment and the public's health**

It has become axiomatic in public health practice that population approaches using individually-directed interventions should not be initiated unless:

1. There is a clear consensus about the definition of the condition or disease.

2. The natural history of the condition is understood.

3. Accurate screening tests have been developed to identify persons with the condition.

4. There is good evidence for intervention effectiveness to manage persons with the condition.

5. The cost and potential benefits of implementing a state-of-the-art approach have been considered (Babor and Kadden 1985; Thompson *et al.* 1995).

During the past fifteen years the first three prerequisites for a public health approach based on individually-directed interventions to alcohol problems have been advanced on an international level through improvements in screening, diagnosis, and nomenclature (Saunders *et al.* 1993; WHO 1993).

Considerable progress has also been made in the development of cost-effective treatments, including brief interventions and more intensive therapies, to manage persons whose drinking places them at risk (Institute of Medicine 1990). To the extent that the prerequisites for a public health approach have been established, it is important to consider strategies designed to disseminate cost-effective intervention strategies so that appropriate treatment will be available to those who need it. But the dissemination of individual-level interventions needs to be considered in the context of a population approach that goes beyond the traditional model of acute care focused on specific disease entities. If treatment is to be integrated into the overall policy response to alcohol, there are a number of requirements that treatment planning in the public health arena will need to meet. These requirements are identified in Box 12.1.

Box 12.1 **Conditions for a population approach to health services for alcohol-related problems**[a]

1. Attention to definition of cases

The national planning of any treatment response should start with a definition of suitable cases for treatment. The following behaviours and conditions must be included when defining the types of care with which alcohol treatment services should be concerned:

1. Personal alcohol consumption at a level likely to threaten or impair health.

2. Alcohol dependence.

3. Alcohol-related health or social impairments.

4. Drinking–driving, where drinking causes damage to others.

2. Determination of the prevalence of cases within the population

In most developed countries survey data are available that can provide this kind of information about the extent of alcohol problems.

3. Determination of the proportion of cases, which will at any time seek and engage in treatment

Many people with drinking problems may be unwilling to become involved in treatment. Encouragement of help-seeking should be part of the strategy.

4. Treatment planning needs to take cognisance of natural history

Many seemingly troublesome alcohol-related problems are likely to remit spontaneously, while an individual who is a habitual heavy drinker may have much less likelihood of spontaneous remission. These considerations may speak to targeting of resources.

5. The treatment effectiveness question

This question relates not only to modality, but also to the duration and intensity of treatment and to the duration of any beneficial changes achieved. Alcohol problems are characterized by high relapse rates.

6. Economic benefits

Treatment policies need to be informed by awareness of costs and benefits in economic terms. In most countries the treatment response to alcohol

Conditions for a population approach to health services for alcohol-related problems[a] *(continued)*

problems has up to now more often developed from the compassionate effort to help individuals, rather than from a consideration of the characteristics of a treatment system that would be needed to fit the kinds of criteria defined above. If in the future the treatment effort is more fully to achieve its public health potential, it will need to be based on objective performance criteria.

[a] Adapted from World Health Organization (1993).

Treatment and prevention are traditionally conceived, implemented, and evaluated as largely unrelated activities. A more holistic vision is needed if alcohol policies are to address the complete spectrum of alcohol problems. Despite evidence of the effectiveness of treatment interventions, little attention has been paid to the mechanisms of action that would translate individual benefits to the population. Treatment interventions are primarily designed to serve the needs of individual patients and clients, but there are a number of ways that these interventions may have an impact at community and population levels: by raising public awareness of alcohol problems, influencing national and community agendas, involving health professionals in advocacy for prevention, and providing secondary benefits to families, employers, and automobile drivers. The effect of treatment interventions can also be manifested more directly by not only reducing the amount of alcohol consumed by the drinker (and his or her associated risks), but also influencing the social milieu of the drinker. By removing a source of reciprocal influence that is likely to contribute to the maintenance of heavy drinking subcultures (Skog 1985), treatment may diminish the alcohol-related problem rates of an entire society.

References

Alcoholics Anonymous World Services, Inc. (2002) AA Fact File: Membership. Website: www.alcoholics-anonymous.org

Babor T.F. (1994) Avoiding the 'horrid and beastly sin of drunkenness': Does dissuasion make a difference? *Journal of Consulting and Clinical Psychology* 62, 1127–40.

Babor T.F. and Del Boca F.K. (eds.) (2002) *Treatment matching in alcoholism.* Cambridge, UK: Cambridge University Press.

Babor T.F. and Higgins-Biddle J.C. (2000) Alcohol screening and brief intervention: Dissemination strategies for medical practice and public health. *Addiction* 95, 677–86.

Babor T.F. and Kadden R. (1985) Screening for alcohol problems: Conceptual issues and practical considerations. In: Change N.C. and Chao H.M. (eds.) *Research monograph No. 17: Early identification of alcohol abuse*, pp.1–30. Washington, DC: US Government Printing Office.

Babor T.F., Higgins-Biddle J., Saunders J.B., *et al.* (2001) *AUDIT The alcohol use disorders identification test: Guidelines for use in primary care*, 2nd edn. Geneva, Switzerland: World Health Organization.

Bien T.H., Miller W.R., and Tonigan S. (1993) Brief intervention for alcohol problems: A review. *Addiction* 88, 315–36.

Finney J.W., Hahn A.C., and Moos R.H. (1996) The effectiveness of inpatient and outpatient treatment for alcohol abuse: The need to focus on mediators and moderators of setting effects. *Addiction* 91, 1773–96.

Fuller R.K., Branchey L., Brightwell D.R., *et al.* (1986) Disulfiram treatment of alcoholism: A veterans administration cooperative study. *Journal of the American Medical Association* 256, 1449–55.

Goodman A.C., Nishiura E., and Humphreys R.S. (1997) Cost and usage impacts of treatment initiation: A comparison of alcoholism and drug abuse treatments. *Alcoholism: Clinical and Experimental Research* 21, 931–8.

Gossop M. (1995) The treatment mapping survey; a descriptive study of drug and alcohol treatment responses in 23 countries. *Drug and Alcohol Dependence* 39, 7–14.

Grant M. and Ritson B. (1990) International review of treatment and rehabilitation services for alcoholism and alcohol abuse. In: Institute of Medicine (ed.) *Broadening the base of treatment for alcohol problems*, pp. 550–78. Washington, DC: National Academy Press.

Higgins-Biddle J.C. and Babor T.F. (1996) *Reducing risky drinking*. Report prepared for the Robert Wood Johnson Foundation, Farmington, University of Connecticut Health Center.

Holder H.D. (1987) Alcoholism treatment and potential health care cost saving. *Medical Care* 25, 52–71.

Holder H. and Parker R.N. (1992) Effect of alcoholism treatment on cirrhosis mortality: A 20-year multivariate time series analysis. *British Journal of Addiction* 87, 1263–74.

Holder H., Longabaugh R., Miller W.R., *et al.* (1991) The cost of effectiveness of treatment of alcoholism. A first approximation. *Journal of Studies on Alcohol* 52, 517–40.

Institute of Medicine (1990) *Broadening the base of treatment for alcohol problems*. Washington, DC: National Academy Press.

Kahan M., Wilson L., and Becker L. (1995) Effectiveness of physician-based interventions with problem drinkers: A review. *Canadian Medical Association Journal* 152, 851–9.

Klingemann H. and Klingemann H.D. (1999) National treatment systems in global perspective. *European Addiction Research* 5, 109–17.

Klingemann H., Takala J.P., and Hunt G. (1992) *Cure, care or control: Alcoholism treatment in sixteen countries*. Albany, New York: State University of New York Press.

Klingemann H., Takala J.P., and Hunt G. (1993) The development of alcohol treatment systems: An international perspective. *Alcohol Health and Research World* 3, 221–7.

Kranzler H.R. and Van Kirk J. (2001) Naltrexone and acamprosate in the treatment of alcoholism: A meta-analysis. *Alcoholism: Clinical and Experimental Research* 25, 1335–41.

Mäkelä K. (1993) International comparisons of Alcoholics Anonymous. *Alcohol Health and Research World* 17, 228–34.

Mäkelä K., Arminen I., Bloomfield K., *et al.* (1996) *Alcoholics Anonymous as a mutual-help movement: A study in eight societies.* Madison: University of Wisconsin Press.

Mann R.E., Smart R., Anglin L., *et al.* (1988) Are decreases in liver cirrhosis rates a result of increased treatment for alcoholism. *British Journal of Addiction* 83, 683–8.

Mann R.E., Smart R., Anglin L., *et al.* (1991) Reduction in cirrhosis deaths in the United States: Associations with *per capita* consumption and AA membership. *Journal of Studies on Alcohol* 52, 361–5.

Mattick R.P. and Jarvis T. (1994) Brief or minimal intervention for 'alcoholics'? The evidence suggests otherwise. *Drug and Alcohol Review* 13, 137–44.

McClellan A.T., Grant G.R., Zanis D., *et al.* (1997) Problem-service 'matching' in addiction treatment. *Archives of General Psychiatry* 54, 730–5.

McCrady B.S. and Miller W.R. (eds.) (1993) *Research on Alcoholics Anonymous: Opportunities and alternatives*, pp. 41–78. New Brunswick, NJ: Rutgers Center of Alcohol Studies.

Miller W.R. and Hester R. (1986) Inpatient alcoholism treatment. Who benefits? *American Psychologist* 41, 794–805.

Miller W.R., Brown J.M., Simpson T.L., *et al.* (1995) What works? A methodological analysis of the alcohol treatment outcome literature. In: Hester R.K. and Miller W.R. (eds.) *Handbook of alcoholism treatment approaches: Effective alternatives*, 2nd edn., pp. 12–44. Boston, MA: Allyn and Bacon.

O'Malley S.S., Jaffe A.J., Chang G., *et al.* (1992) Naltrexone and coping skills therapy for alcohol dependence: A controlled study. *Archives of General Psychiatry* 49, 894–8.

Ouimette P.C., Finney J.W., Gima K., *et al.* (1999) A comparative evaluation of substance abuse treatment: examining mechanisms underlying patient-treatment matching hypotheses for 12-step and cognitive-behavioral treatments for substance abuse. *Alcoholism: Clinical and Experimental Research* 23, 545–51.

Poikolainen K. (1999) Effectiveness of brief interventions to reduce alcohol intake in primary health care populations: A meta-analysis. *Preventive Medicine* 28, 503–9.

Project MATCH Research Group (1997a) Matching alcoholism treatments to client heterogeneity: Project MATCH posttreatment drinking outcomes. *Journal of Studies on Alcohol* 58, 7–29.

Project MATCH Research Group (1997b) Project MATCH secondary a priori hypotheses. *Addiction* 92, 1671–98.

Project MATCH Research Group (1998) Matching patients with alcohol disorders to treatments: Clinical implications from Project MATCH. *Journal of Mental Health* 7, 589–602.

Richmond R.L., Novak K.G., Kehoe L., *et al.* (1998) Effect of training on general practitioners' use of a brief intervention for excessive drinkers. *Australian and New Zealand Journal of Public Health* 22, 206–9.

Romelsjö A. (1987) Decline in alcohol-related in-patient care and mortality in Stockholm County. *British Journal of Addiction* 82, 653–63.

Room R. (1998) Mutual help movements for alcohol problems in an international perspective. *Addiction Research* 6, 131–45.

Saunders J.B., Aasland O.G., Babor T.F., *et al.* (1993) Development of the alcohol use disorders identification test (AUDIT): WHO collaborative project on early detection of persons with harmful alcohol consumption. Part II. *Addiction* 88, 791–804.

Skog O.-J. (1985) The collectivity of drinking cultures: A theory of the distribution of alcohol consumption. *British Journal of Addiction* 80, 83–99.

Smart R.G. and Mann R.E. (1990) Are increased levels of treatment and Alcoholics Anonymous membership large enough to create the recent reauditions in liver cirrhosis? *British Journal of Addiction* 85, 1385–7.

Smart R.G. and Mann R.E. (1993) Recent liver cirrhosis declines: estimates of the impact of alcohol abuse treatment and Alcoholics Anonymous. *Addiction* 88, 193–8.

Smart R.G. and Mann R.E. (2000) The impact of programs for high-risk drinkers on population levels of alcohol problems. *Addiction* 95, 37–52.

Smart R.G., Mann R.E., and Anglin L. (1989) Decrease in alcohol problems and increased Alcoholics Anonymous membership. *British Journal of Addiction* 54, 507–13.

Thompson R.S., Taplin S.H., McAfee T.A., *et al.* (1995) Primary and secondary prevention services in clinical practice, twenty years' experience in development, implementation, and evaluation. *Journal of the American Medical Association* 273, 1130–5.

Timko C., Moos R.H., Finney J.W., *et al.* (2000) Long-term outcomes of alcohol use disorders: comparing untreated individuals with those in Alcoholics Anonymous and formal treatment. *Journal of Studies on Alcohol* 61, 529–38.

Walsh D.C., Hingson R.W., Merrigan D.M., *et al.* (1991) A randomized trial of treatment options for alcohol-abusing workers. *New England Journal of Medicine* 325, 775–81.

Wilk A.I., Jensen N.M., and Havighurst T.C. (1997) Meta-analysis of randomized control trials addressing brief interventions in heavy alcohol drinkers. *Journal of General Internal Medicine* 12, 274–83.

WHO. See World Health Organization.

World Health Organization (1980) *Problems related to alcohol consumption: Report of a WHO expert committee.* Technical Report Series 650. Geneva: World Health Organization.

World Health Organization (1993) *Assessing the standards of care in substance abuse treatment.* Geneva: WHO.

The process: formation of effective alcohol policy

Chapter 13

Alcohol policymaking: putting the strategies into effect

13.1 The scope of alcohol policies

The previous section of this book provided a critical review of a wide range of intervention strategies designed to prevent or minimize alcohol-related problems. If an understanding of the evidence were all that were necessary to put an effective range of strategies into practice, the world would undoubtedly experience far fewer alcohol-related problems. But there is a gap between the possible and the practical, which is linked by the process of alcohol policy-making. That process is the concern of this and the next two chapters.

At its broadest meaning, alcohol policy refers to any measure that affects the market in alcohol, the level and patterning of alcohol consumption, or the occurrence of alcohol-related problems. In this sense, policy can include a whole range of governmental actions that have little to do with alcohol specifically (such as mandating seat-belts in cars), or which have little connection to social and health problems from drinking (such as beer bottle recycling programs). From a public health perspective, there is a smaller but still broad range of policies that affect rates of social and health problems from drinking, including policies controlling the production, distribution, and marketing of alcoholic beverages, policies affecting drinking patterns and rates of alcohol-related problems, and policies on social responses to drinking problems such as treatment and other interventions.

Governing agencies at all levels—international, national, provincial, regional, and local—make decisions on such policies every day, although they often do not recognize or account for the decision's potential to affect rates of alcohol-related problems in the population. Some governments also have an overall alcohol policy or strategy, considering some or all of the policy actions in a coordinated frame. In some places, such an orientation is longstanding, while in others it is a new idea (Room 1999).

13.2 Trends in alcohol policies

Measures affecting alcohol consumption are a common feature of legal and regulatory systems throughout the world. All governments have to deal with alcohol or alcoholic beverages as consumer goods in one way or another. Public policy that regards alcohol as a special social or health problem, or as a subject for comprehensive regulation, has been less common, however. In earlier times, alcoholic beverages were recognized as special commodities. This was done, for example, by giving monopoly control to trade in alcoholic beverages in a certain area to some company, or by using alcoholic beverages as a tax base for the state (see Österberg 1985; Room 1993). In the 19th century, the temperance movement gave rise to national, regional, and local alcohol policies, especially in the Anglo-Saxon and Nordic countries. In many countries, popular pressure from these movements ultimately led to laws prohibiting all sales and production of alcoholic beverages. This happened, for instance, in the United States and Canada, in Finland, Iceland, and Norway, and in Russia. All of these countries abolished their prohibition laws on alcohol before the Second World War. However, total alcohol prohibition still remains a crucial part of some government policies, mostly in Islamic countries and states of India.

In Europe, the last fifty years have seen a convergence in alcohol policies. In the early 1950s, alcohol policy in the Nordic countries was based on social policy and public health considerations, and included high excise duties on alcoholic beverages, comprehensive state alcohol monopoly systems for production and trade, and strict controls on alcohol availability (Karlsson and Österberg 2001). In the Mediterranean wine-producing countries there were very few alcohol control measures in force in the early 1950s, and most of them were motivated by industrial or commercial interests. Some countries between the Nordic and Mediterranean areas, like Ireland and the United Kingdom, developed a strict licensing system, especially for on-premise sales of alcoholic beverages. Other countries, like Belgium and the Netherlands, still have in force leftovers of former alcohol control systems.

The convergence of alcohol policies in the present European Union (EU) member states during the second half of the 20th century can be best understood by looking separately at different areas of alcohol controls. On the one hand, the control of alcohol production, distribution, and sales has decreased in the EU member states (see Box 13.1). On the other hand, measures targeted at alcohol demand, like alcohol education and controls on alcohol advertising, as well as measures targeted directly at a few alcohol-related problems like drinking–driving, have become more prevalent and harsher during the last fifty years. In the present EU member states there have also been converging trends with regard to taxing alcoholic beverages, although the convergence has been rather weak. In the year 2000, alcohol excise duties were still clearly lowest in wine-producing countries, and highest among the Nordic countries, Ireland, and the United Kingdom (Karlsson and Österberg 2001).

Box 13.1 **Public policies are not always public health policies**

In the Nordic countries, the influence of the commercial policies of the European Union has undermined previously strong national alcohol policies (Holder *et al.* 1998; Sulkunen *et al.* 2000). As a consequence, there is now much greater interest in the local arena for handling alcohol-related problems (Larsson and Hanson 1999). For example, in Sweden, the Alcohol Act of 1995 not only disestablished the state monopoly for import, export, distribution, and production of alcohol, but also shifted responsibility for the licensing of on-premise sales and control of licensed establishments to a more local level, from the 25 counties to the 272 municipalities (Romelsjö and Andersson 1999). Similarly, in a number of North American contexts there has been a move away from government involvement in alcohol management as exemplified by full or partial privatization of retail monopolies (Her *et al.* 1999), and increasing emphasis by government-run monopolies on commercial issues at the expense of control mandates.

In North America there has been a gradual decline in alcohol control in most jurisdictions in recent decades, with more dramatic changes such as privatization of alcohol retail sales in several US states and one Canadian province. In the last two decades, divergent trends were evident with regard to alcohol prices: in Canada, alcohol prices tended to parallel changes in the Consumer Price Index, whereas in the US a general decline in real prices was evident in many jurisdictions. Alcohol taxes have not been raised to match inflation. Both countries have lax controls on alcohol advertising, especially in the United States. In contrast, there are extensive education and law enforcement efforts to control drinking–driving.

Similar developments have taken place in other parts of the world. For instance, the collapse of the communist system in the former Soviet Union (see Box 13.2) and many Eastern European countries has meant that alcohol control, especially the control of alcohol availability, has lost much of its effect in these countries (Moskalewicz 2000; Reitan 2000). On the other hand, in the 1990s, under the impetus of the European Alcohol Action Plan, many Eastern European countries have adopted national alcohol programs or participated in projects aimed at strengthening local alcohol control.

In many developed countries, general alcohol policies affecting the whole population and oriented to the collective good have been under sustained

Box 13.2 **Alcohol policies in transition**

A large vacuum in alcohol policy was created by the breakup of the Soviet Union, after which public administration and political authority became less unified within each of the countries in transition. Whereas it was possible to talk of a national policy before the breakup of the Soviet Union, after 1991 it was more appropriate to describe the situation in the Russian Federation as a national framework within which an assortment of local alcohol policies existed (Nemtsov and Krasovsky 1996; Reitan 2000). Furthermore, the weakness of the central governments in Eastern Europe following the fall of communism was a serious obstacle for preventive alcohol policies (Simpura 1995). The limited capacity of public authorities to control the alcohol trade and the opposition of the alcoholic beverage industry to state measures made it very difficult to bring public control and order to the alcohol trade.

attack. Policies remaining from the past have been gradually eroded (e.g., privatization of monopolies, erosion of taxes by inflation, extension of closing hours). At the same time, however, popular concern about alcohol-related problems has risen, although it has only fitfully found political expression, for example, in concerns about drinking–driving, or about public intoxication at football matches. The rise in public concern partly reflects an increase in the rates of alcohol-related problems. Public health advocacy, as well as scientific documentation of the hidden ways in which social and health harms often result from drinking, have also contributed to this growing concern.

In general, there has been a decline in alcohol control policies on several fronts, including those interventions that have the greatest and broadest potential for curtailing alcohol-related harms. Ironically, many of the studies that have documented the effectiveness of such interventions have only been possible because the strategies were being weakened or dismantled.

Trends in the developing world have been less well documented (Room *et al.* 2002). In some parts of the world, such as Papua New Guinea, prohibitions imposed by colonial powers lasted until the 1960s, provoking an association of drinking and Western-style beverages with autonomy and prestige. Some forms of alcohol control, such as municipally-owned beer halls in southern Africa, have in many places been weakened or dismantled, often under pressure from the 'structural adjustment' programs of international development agencies. The control of alcohol advertising, alcohol education, and driving under the influence of alcohol have also become issues in developing countries. In many countries there has been an increase in educational programs, despite research on their lack of effect, along with some interventions to curtail drinking–driving.

13.3 Section overview: the process of policymaking

The international context for alcohol policymaking, including international action in the public health interest, is described in Chapter 14. One factor behind the weakening of national and local alcohol policies has been the impact of international trade agreements and common markets. While alcohol policy used to be essentially a national or sub-national matter, nowadays it can be strongly affected by international treaties and commitments. In the context of industry globalization and the growing influence of market ideology (Castells 1996), the ability of national-level decision-makers to determine alcohol policies has been weakened. Two trends have become apparent. Regional and international responses have evolved, and there has been a shift of emphasis towards local-level responses in a number of jurisdictions. The globalization of alcohol production and promotion, and the growth of trade and common market agreements, means that attention to the international level must now be part of a national alcohol policy.

In Chapter 15 we consider the following question: Who makes alcohol policy? The answer is not simple and it differs across countries and between different levels of government within countries. The goal of this chapter is to describe the policymaking arena at the local and national levels. Implicit in our review is a model of the policymaking process that comprises the institutions, stakeholders, and the environment within which policy decisions are made. Ideally, the policy process forms a cycle, beginning with an assessment of alcohol-related problems, followed by implementation of evidence-based interventions and systematic evaluation. But the reality of the policymaking process is rarely that simple or straightforward.

References

Castells M. (1996) *The rise of the network society (The information age: Economy, society and culture)*, Vol. 1. Malden: Blackwell Publishers.

Her M., Giesbrecht N., Room R., *et al.* (1999) Privatizing alcohol sales and alcohol consumption: Evidence and implications. *Addiction* **94**, 1125–39.

Holder H., Kühlhorn E., Nordlund S., *et al.* (1998) *European integration and Nordic alcohol policies*. Aldershot, Hants, UK: Ashgate.

Karlsson T. and Österberg E. (2001) A scale of formal alcohol control policy in 15 European countries. *Nordic Studies on Alcohol and Drugs* **18** (English Suppl.), 117–31.

Larsson S. and Hanson B.S. (1999) Prevent alcohol problems in Europe by community actions: Various national and regional contexts. In: Larsson S. and Hanson B.S. (eds.) *Community-based alcohol prevention in Europe: Research and evaluations*, pp. 220–39. Lund: Lunds Universitet.

Moskalewicz J. (2000) Alcohol in the countries in transition: The Polish experience and the wider context. *Contemporary Drug Problems* 27, 561–92.

Nemtsov A.V. and Krasovsky C.S. (1996) An overview of national and local alcohol-related problems in the CIS. *Drugs: Education, Prevention and Policy* 3, 21–8.

Österberg E. (1985) From home distillation to the state alcohol monopoly. *Contemporary Drug Problems* 12, 31–51.

Reitan T.C. (2000) Does alcohol matter? Public health in Russia and the Baltic countries before, during, and after the transition. *Contemporary Drug Problems* 27, 511–60.

Romelsjö A. and Andersson T. (1999) Emergence of community alcohol and drug prevention programs in municipalities and communities during a transition phase for alcohol policy in Sweden. In: Larsson S. and Hanson B.S. (eds.) *Community-based alcohol prevention in Europe: Research and evaluations*, pp. 208–19. Lund: Lunds Universitet.

Room R. (1993) Evolution of alcohol monopolies and their relevance for public health. *Contemporary Drug Problems* 20, 169–87.

Room R. (1999) The idea of alcohol policy. *Nordic Studies on Alcohol and Drugs* 16 (English Suppl.), 7–20.

Room R., Jernigan J., Carlini Marlatt B., *et al.* (2002) *Alcohol in developing societies: A public health approach.* Helsinki: Finnish Foundation for Alcohol Studies.

Simpura J. (1995) Alcohol in Eastern Europe: Market prospects, prevention puzzles. *Addiction* 90, 467–70.

Sulkunen P., Sutton C., Togerstedt C., *et al.* (eds.) (2000) *Broken spirits: Power and ideas in Nordic alcohol control.* NAD Publication No. 39. Helsinki: Nordic Council for Alcohol and Drug Research.

Chapter 14

The international context of alcohol policy

14.1 Introduction

The basic premise of this book, as laid out in Chapter 2, is that alcohol is no ordinary commodity. There was a moment in history, a century ago, when this was recognized at the international level. A series of agreements between the European colonial powers effectively controlled the market in 'trade spirits' by forbidding exports to Africa (Bruun *et al.* 1975). In recent decades, however, the operating assumption in international agreements has often been to treat alcoholic beverages as an ordinary commodity. In a world of increasing trade globalization, this operating assumption has meant that national and local alcohol policies, predicated on the extraordinary nature of alcohol, have increasingly come under pressure at the international level. This chapter describes how these pressures have arisen, and how they affect national alcohol policies and the prospects for **alcohol control** at an international level. It is argued that the current assumption in international trade and market regimes that alcohol is an ordinary commodity is not irreversible, and can be changed by purposive action in the interests of public health.

14.2 International trade agreements and economic treaties

Many international trade agreements and economic treaties have been drafted and signed since the Second World War to promote free movement of goods, services, people, and capital (see Box 14.1 for a list of organizations and trade agreements discussed in this chapter). At a global level, multilateral trade agreements are now the business of the World Trade Organization (WTO), which in 1995 succeeded the General Agreement on Tariffs and Trade (GATT). In the decades after GATT was signed in 1947, there were several rounds of negotiation that strengthened the international control of trade matters. At the beginning of the 1990s, GATT was subscribed to by more than 100 governments, which together accounted for nearly 90% of world trade.

Box 14.1 **List of economic organizations and related agreements**

CMEA	Council for Mutual Economic Assistance
EEA	European Economic Area
EFTA	European Free Trade Association
EU	European Union
GATS	General Agreement on Trade in Services
GATT	General Agreement on Tariffs and Trade
ILO	International Labour Organization
IMF	International Monetary Fund
NAFTA	North American Free Trade Agreement
WTO	World Trade Organization

The WTO's principal objective is to liberalize and stabilize international trade, in the interest of stimulating economic growth and development. The WTO acts both as a code of rules, enforced through mechanisms for resolving trade disputes, and as a forum in which countries can discuss solutions to their trade problems and negotiate the reduction of various national restrictions and market controls that affect international trade.

There are also a number of important multinational economic agreements operating at a regional level. In some respects the European Union (EU) is the clearest example. Agreements in Europe developed beyond their original focus on a common market, so that the control of trade within the region became part of a more comprehensive international structure. The EU, the European Free Trade Association (EFTA), and the Council for Mutual Economic Assistance (CMEA) have been the most important multinational economic agreements in Europe since the Second World War. The fall of the Soviet Union put an end to the CMEA. In the 1990s, most EFTA countries signed an agreement with the EU. Concurrently most former CMEA countries, as well as some parts of the former Soviet Union, applied for membership in the EU. As the number of the EU member states has grown from six to 15, the EU treaties are affecting alcohol control policies in large parts of Europe.

Although there are free trade agreements in other parts of the world, many of them only exist on paper, and have not developed into structures able to influence alcohol policies. The most economically important regional trade agreement outside Europe is the North American Free Trade Agreement

(NAFTA) between the United States, Canada, and Mexico, which went into effect in 1994. Other regional trade associations and agreements include the Common Market of Eastern and Southern Africa (COMESA), the Economic Community of West African States (ECOWAS), and the Association of Southeast Asian Nations Free Trade Agreement (AFTA). As of May 2000, there were altogether 127 regional and other trade agreements registered at the World Trade Organization (Andriamananjara 2001). Besides trade in commodities, international and multinational economic agreements have also begun to affect other spheres of life in the participating countries. At the same time, the number of participating countries in these agreements and treaties has greatly increased.

14.3 **Effects on alcohol policies**

One of the core principles of the GATT and WTO is that participating countries have to extend the most favoured treatment that is afforded to domestic buyers and sellers to buyers and sellers from foreign signatories. This ensures that internal tax and regulatory measures are applied equally to imported and domestic products, so there is no protection for domestic production. Other international commercial agreements have extended this 'national treatment' principle beyond goods. NAFTA, for example, applies the best national treatment principle to international trade in goods, services, and investments (though with some exceptions for alcoholic beverages). In the EU, the single European market is built on 'the four freedoms', which refers to the free flow of goods, services, labour, and capital across the national borders of the member states. How do these economic principles affect alcohol policies? One example is the French and Swedish restrictions on alcohol advertising, which have come under increasing criticism because they are considered counter to the principles of the single market. Another example is the General Agreement on Trade in Services (GATS), whose implications for alcohol policy are reviewed in Box 14.2.

The treatment of foreign and domestic goods on equal terms brings up the question of what should be construed as 'like commodities'. The European Court of Justice has dealt with this question several times as it relates to alcoholic beverages (Lubkin 1996). We give two examples in Boxes 14.3 and 14.4. The issue of whether beverages are 'like commodities', and thus need to be treated the same in terms of taxation, has also arisen under the GATT and WTO, usually in terms of the equitability of the tax treatment of different imported and local alcoholic beverages. In 1996, the traditional Japanese liquor *shochu* was deemed to be a like product to vodka, and subsequently also

Box 14.2 General Agreement on Trade in Services (GATS)

1. **Purpose:** To promote free movement of services world-wide.

2. **Services included:** All aspects of international services that are provided, traded, and shared between countries.

3. **Examples of alcohol-related services:** Alcohol production, distribution, and marketing; grain production; transportation of grain to breweries and distilleries; marketing and serving alcohol products; investments in alcohol production facilities.

4. **Implications for alcohol policies:** The GATS does not distinguish between alcohol-related services, which may have important public health consequences, and any other service. Although the treaty contains exceptions and exclusions, they may be interpreted narrowly and may not provide significant and lasting protection for preventive alcohol control measures. And like other international treaties, the GATS effectively restricts future possibilities for certain alcohol policy measures. For example, rules on alcohol monopolies must conform to the most-favoured nation rule.

Box 14.3 Aquavit and pickled herring sandwiches

Case 171/78, 'European Commission versus Denmark', dealt with the Danish rules according to which the excise duty for Danish aquavit was 35% lower than the excise duty for other distilled spirits like gin and whiskey. The Danish government argued that Danish drinking habits provided adequate cause for distinguishing aquavit from other distilled alcoholic beverages, as aquavit was consumed mainly at meals as an accompaniment to certain typical Danish dishes like pickled herring sandwiches. Therefore, aquavit could not, according to the Danish government, be placed on the same footing as other distilled spirits, as the real consumer choice was between aquavit and beer or aquavit and wine, and not between aquavit and other distilled spirits. In other words, aquavit and distilled spirits were not substitutes or like products. The court, however, did not accept this interpretation. In the court's view, aquavit could well serve as a substitute for other distilled beverages in some cases and could therefore be classified as a product competing with other distilled spirits (Germer 1990, p. 482).

Box 14.4 **Can wine be taxed more than beer?**

Case 170/78, 'European Commission versus the United Kingdom', examined whether the United Kingdom could tax wine more than beer. In this case the UK government denied the existence of a competitive relationship between wine and beer, and thus the possibility of substitution, whereas the Commission argued that wine and beer were at least potential substitutes for each other. Both could be used for thirst-quenching and to accompany meals, and both also belonged to the same category of alcoholic beverages, i.e., products of natural fermentation (cf. Germer 1990, p. 485). The European Court of Justice decided that the argument of the Commission was well founded. It stated, furthermore, that 'the tax policy of a member state must not crystallize existing consumer habits so as to be biased in favor of the relevant national industries' (Germer 1990, p. 485). On the other hand, the court did not accept the Commission's proposal for a single criterion for comparison in setting beer and wine excise duties. It stated that no matter which guideline for comparison was used, the United Kingdom's tax system protected domestic beer production from imported wines, and had to be altered.

to other imported distilled spirits like gin, rum, brandy, and whiskey. As a result, equal tax treatment was given to all of these beverages. In a similar case, the EU successfully used the WTO rules in 1999 to overturn South Korea's tax system for distilled spirits. The WTO Appellate Body ruled that imported spirits and locally produced *soju* were directly competitive or substitutable products. Therefore, Korea's differential tax system violated the GATT rules (Grieshaber-Otto *et al.* 2000). In a case against Chile, the WTO panel ruled that imported spirits with higher alcohol content than the Chilean liquor *pisco* could not be taxed at higher rates because this had the effect of protecting domestic liquor production. Given the political dynamics following such decisions, the result is usually a lowering of the net tax rate on the affected group of beverages.

There is great variation in alcohol excise levels across EU member states, with no tax on wine in six countries in southern and central Europe, and relatively high taxes in the United Kingdom, Ireland, and the Nordic countries. This is the situation, despite the fact that the EU has made repeated attempts in the last thirty years to harmonize the alcohol taxes of its member states, on the grounds that different taxes in member states interfere with the efficient operation of the single market (Österberg and Karlsson 2002). In 1987, the EU Commission proposed that uniform alcohol excise duties should be adopted in all member states. In 1992, a target rate was adopted for distilled spirits, and minimum rates were fixed for all alcoholic beverages. The minimum rate for wine was, however, set at zero. By accepting a wide divergence in taxes, the directive has effectively put pressure on high-tax jurisdictions to lower their alcohol excise duties, but does not pressure low-tax jurisdictions to raise them. A common structure for excise duties in the EU, adopted in 1993, also means that it is impossible to put a special tax on a beverage causing special harm. Beverages within each of the four alcoholic beverage categories—beer, wine, 'intermediate products', and spirits—are treated the same.

When the harmonization of alcohol excise duties seemed to be impossible through administrative decisions, the EU Commission tried to let market forces harmonize alcohol excise duties by increasing the rights of travellers to take alcoholic beverages across borders within the EU, thereby putting pressure on countries with higher-tax neighbours to lower their excise duty levels. As a general rule, EU citizens are allowed to take with them up to 10 litres of spirits, 20 litres of intermediate products, 90 litres of wine, and 110 litres of beer from other EU member countries without paying tax on them when entering the home country. This liberal allowance has exerted a downward pressure on excise tax levels (Österberg 1993).

When market forces put pressure on neighbouring countries to harmonize their alcohol excise duties in order to decrease the border trade in alcoholic beverages, taxes tend to gravitate towards the lowest levels of excise duties. For instance, to counter the effects of the low excise taxes in Germany, Denmark decreased excise duties on beer and wine by half in the early 1990s. As a consequence, Sweden decreased its excise duties on beer to counter the pressure from Danish prices (Holder *et al.* 1998).

A number of international trade agreements and economic treaties have been designed expressly to constrain the activities of state enterprises and monopolies. While most such agreements recognize the right of participating countries to run monopolies, their activity is restricted. This is because monopolies, by definition, reduce competitive opportunities for private international traders. Finland, Sweden, and Norway were thus compelled to abandon their import, export, wholesale, and production monopolies for alcoholic beverages when they entered the EEA, although they have managed to retain their off-premise alcohol retail monopolies (Holder *et al.* 1998). While in the WTO complaints must be brought by national governments, in the EU context they are often brought by commercial enterprises. Two cases that were instrumental in settling the status of the Nordic alcohol monopolies are described in Boxes 14.5 and 14.6. As these examples indicate, the principles of free market competition, and the free flow of goods, services, labour, and capital, affect

Box 14.5 **The Restamark case**

This case played an important role in the partial de-monopolization of the alcohol market in Finland, Norway, and Sweden (Ugland 1996; Lund 1997; Holder *et al.* 1998). In January 1994, a Finnish enterprise, Restamark, which was owned by the Finnish Restaurant and Cafeteria Association, tried to import a shipment of alcoholic beverages into Finland. This was not allowed, as it was against the current Finnish Alcohol Act. But the importer claimed that it was justified according to the EEA Agreement, which had been in force since the beginning of 1994. The case was bought to the Court of the European Free Trade Area (EFTA). The Court concluded in December 1994 that the Finnish import monopoly on alcoholic beverages was not compatible with the EEA Agreement, and had to be abolished (Alavaikko and Österberg 2000). This ruling also doomed the Norwegian and Swedish alcohol import monopolies. Finland and Sweden abolished their monopolies on production, imports, exports, and wholesale in 1995, and Norway followed suit in 1996.

Box 14.6 **The Franzén case**

On January 1, 1994, a Swedish shopkeeper, Harry Franzén, tried to sell wine in his store. In a chaotic situation, he ended up donating the bottles to his customers without being able to collect payment for them. As Franzén's aim was to be prosecuted, he tried to break the law again on April 7, 1994, and on January 1, 1995. On these two occasions Franzén sold wine in his grocery store, was stopped by the police, and was prosecuted in the district court of Landskrona. In court Franzén claimed that he could not be convicted because the prevailing Swedish Alcohol Act was contrary to the EU Treaty. Consequently, the Landskrona court asked the European Court of Justice for a preliminary ruling. In this case the European Court found that the operation of the Swedish off-premise retail alcohol monopoly, Systembolaget, was organized in a non-discriminatory manner and was not against the EU treaties (Holder *et al.* 1998). The Franzén case's effect on the Nordic alcohol control system was very important because it ended the legal struggle to try to prove that the off-premise retail alcohol monopolies were in conflict with the EU treaties.

major elements of national alcohol policies, such as the possibility to use alcohol monopoly systems as an instrument for public health and social welfare policy.

Thus far, many alcohol control measures, such as minimum age limits, public information campaigns, school-based alcohol education programs, and blood alcohol limits for driving, have not been affected by international trade or common market agreements. But some of the most powerful alcohol control measures, such as tax rates and public monopolization of the alcohol market, are threatened by international trade agreements. Thus US and EU trade complaints under GATT about the operation of Canadian provincial alcohol monopolies resulted in a weakening of the Ontario monopoly and a decrease in the minimum price for beer (Ferris *et al.* 1993). EU oversight of retail licensing procedures has also weakened the control of private retail sales outlets for alcoholic beverages. In most EU countries, licensing policy has become a formal procedure whereby every applicant fulfilling some basic requirements (e.g., no criminal record) automatically receives a license.

'National treatment' obligations force countries to treat foreign products on a basis equal to domestic products. This obligation constrains government measures developed to control alcohol as a special commodity. From a public health perspective, it may be eminently sensible to freeze preferences for traditional commodities and to discourage consumers from developing a taste for new types of beverages. But increasingly, the WTO and EU consider such measures illegal protectionism. The increasing application of the 'national treatment' standard to services and investments, combined with the doctrine of effective equality opportunities for foreign investments or service producers, could prove especially problematic for alcohol control in the future. The basic problem is the tendency for decisions under such trade agreements to treat alcoholic beverages as an ordinary commodity. On an *ad hoc* basis, decisions such as those described in the Franzén case (Box 14.6) may recognize the public health aims of the measure, but there is no guarantee that this perspective will be taken into account.

14.4 International financial organizations and national alcohol policies

Until recently, relatively little attention was paid by alcohol policy analysts to the intersection between alcohol issues and the operations of international development and financial agencies. However, the actions of such bodies as the International Monetary Fund (IMF) and the World Bank have often had major effects on alcohol policies in developing societies. Many developing countries have had alcohol production, such as brewing lager beer, organized as a state-owned concern. State monopolies of alcoholic beverages at the wholesale and retail levels have also been common, for instance in Indian states (Kortteinen 1989). In a number of places, particularly in southern Africa, municipally-owned beer halls have been the main retail outlet for some alcoholic beverages. International agencies concerned with economic functioning and development have had a strong ideological bias against government ownership of production or distribution functions. They have often encouraged dismantling or sale of government monopoly agencies as a condition of development grants, particularly in 'structural adjustment' programs for countries with financial difficulties. There has been no differentiation of alcoholic beverages from other commodities, with the result that many government ownership arrangements have been dismantled in recent years.

Government monopolization of the alcohol market in developing countries has often served other interests than public health, including revenue generation, protectionist interests, and employment. But a public health interest has also been served, even when not stated explicitly. For instance, a municipal monopoly on beer halls tends to keep the number down. Privatization of beer halls in Zimbabwe resulted very quickly in an increase in the number of outlets (Jernigan 1999).

To a limited extent, international financial bodies have also intervened in the alcohol market by financing new or modernized alcohol production plants as part of a general strategy to promote economic development. For instance, the World Bank Group once financed breweries and wineries, though not distilled beverage production. In an important precedent, in 2000 the Group adopted a policy recognizing that investment in alcoholic beverage production was 'highly sensitive'. World Bank staff were mandated to be 'highly selective' in supporting only those projects 'with strong developmental impacts which are consistent with public health issues and social policy concerns' (World Bank Group 2000). This precedent could be expanded across the board to influence the activities of international and financial agencies.

14.5 Alcohol control at the international level

Since the colonial agreements prohibiting African trade in spirits, which fell into disuse by the 1940s, there have been almost no international-level agreements that seek to limit alcohol-related harms. An exception to this is the Convention Concerning the Protection of Wages of the International Labour Organization (ILO), which forbids 'the payment of wages in the form of liquor of high alcoholic content' (Article 4, Section 1) and the 'payment of wages in taverns', except for a tavern's employees (Article 13, Section 2; ILO 1949). It is clear that public policies at the international level have considerably limited the ability of nations and local governments to control alcohol consumption and related problems, and virtually nothing has been done at the international level that would enhance the ability of governments to control alcohol problems.

The situation for alcohol is quite different from other commodities that have implications for public health. A series of international agreements, dating back to the European colonial era at the beginning of the 20th century, have established a common system for the control of opiates, cocaine, and marijuana. Since 1971, the market in common psychoactive pharmaceuticals such as benzodiazepines and amphetamines has also been controlled internationally, with nations pledging to support control efforts at national and local levels. Since 1988, the control regime has been progressively extended to cover also chemical precursors to controlled psychoactive drugs (Room and Paglia 1999).

The path forward for alcohol at the international level is unlikely to include an International Alcohol Control Board modelled on the International Narcotics Control Board. However, the contrast between alcohol and controlled drugs is stark, particularly when WHO's Global Burden of Disease estimate for alcohol is five times greater than the drugs under international control, taken together (Ezzati *et al.* 2002).

A more likely model for future international agreements on alcohol is the Framework Convention on Tobacco, which has been negotiated under World Health Organization auspices (Joossens 2000; WHO 2003). There are several similarities between the situations of alcohol and tobacco. Both are widely available and commonly used psychoactive substances, with substantial dependence potential and devastating effects on health. For both, the present customary levels of consumption will be difficult to change. And many of the issues that have been on the agenda in the Framework Convention on Tobacco also apply to problems in regulating the alcohol market. These issues include:

1. International harmonization of taxes in a direction that will promote public health.

2. Provisions to reduce smuggling, including expectations of comity between nations in enforcing anti-smuggling laws.

3. Agreement on abolishing duty-free travellers' allowances for alcohol.

4. Restrictions on advertising and sponsorship by alcoholic beverage brands and companies.

5. International standards for testing alcoholic beverages for purity, and for warning labels and controls on alcohol packaging.

6. A shift away from agricultural subsidies for raw materials for alcoholic beverages.

At the international level of alcohol policy issues, the prime mover up to this point has been the World Health Organization, a division of the United Nations. While the WHO's role in alcohol issues has been limited in the past (Room 1984), the WHO Regional Office for Europe was particularly active in the 1990s in its promotion of the European Alcohol Action Plan (see Box 14.7; Gual and Colom 2001; WHO 2000), which provides an example of a coordinated effort to develop national alcohol policies through international collaboration between WHO and its member states. There are also signs that effort levels may be increasing at the WHO's global headquarters in Geneva. In 2001, the Director General named an Alcohol Policy Strategy Advisory Committee to aid in the development of the WHO's work in this area. It is hoped that new developments will follow from this. As previously noted, however, many alcohol-related problems do not commonly fall under the rubric of health, but are concerns of other governmental agencies such as law enforcement and social welfare agencies. There is thus a need to expand the scope of international collaborative action on alcohol problems beyond the World Health Organization.

In the European context, EU attention to the public health aspects of alcohol has increased. In fact, in 2001 the EU adopted a ministerial resolution concerning the promotion of alcohol to youth (WHO 2001). The resolution noted that 'public health policies concerning alcohol need to be formulated by public health interests, without interference from commercial interests', and added that 'one source of major concern is the efforts made by the alcohol beverage industry and the hospitality sector to commercialize sport and youth culture by extensive promotion and sponsorship'. This kind of attention to alcohol reflects the fact that, under the Amsterdam Treaty enlarging the responsibilities of the EU, public health has now become an official EU concern.

14.6 Conclusion: alcohol and trade agreements

Most international trade agreements and economic treaties since the Second World War have been built on the idea of free trade and a global free market economy. They aim to increase the division of labour between participating countries, the economic efficiency of the world economy, and ultimately the prosperity and well-being of the participating countries and their citizens. On a global level, it is thought that this increase in wealth will be achieved

Box 14.7 **The European Alcohol Action Plan**

Since 1992, the European Alcohol Action Plan (EAAP) has provided a basis for alcohol policy development and implementation in WHO member states throughout the European Region. The objectives of this initiative are to generate greater awareness of the harm caused by alcohol, reduce the risk of alcohol-related problems, provide accessible and effective treatment for people with alcohol problems, and protect young people from pressures to drink (World Health Organization 2000; Gual and Colom 2001).

The EAAP was officially inaugurated in 1995 with the adoption of the European Charter on Alcohol, which sets out ethical principles and goals that countries can use to develop comprehensive alcohol policies. Two main strategies were proposed to achieve a significant reduction in the health-damaging consumption of alcohol:

1. A population-based approach to reduce overall alcohol consumption by the targeted amount of 25%.

2. A harm reduction approach aimed at high-risk groups and behaviours.

The strategies are linked to specific actions in the areas of drinking–driving, alcohol education, alcohol availability, treatment for alcohol problems, and regulation of alcohol advertising.

In 1998 the WHO Regional Office for Europe surveyed its member states to evaluate the implementation of EAAP. The following findings were reported (WHO 2000):

1. Over half of the 33 countries responding to the survey had developed a national alcohol plan and had a coordinating body responsible for its implementation.

2. A number of new legislative measures were reported in some countries, including alcohol tax increases, more rigorous rules governing the marketing of alcohol, and stricter drinking–driving regulations.

Although the impact of EAAP is difficult to evaluate without more systematic study and a longer time period to observe changes, it is clear that the Action Plan has the potential to serve as a catalyst to the development of evidence-based alcohol policy. Based in part on the initial success of the EAAP, WHO European member states agreed in 1999 that the Action Plan should continue for the period 2000–2005.

by agreements promoting the freer flow of goods, services, labour, and investments, especially through the reduction of obstacles to free trade and production like tariff barriers, quantitative trade restrictions, state or private monopoly arrangements, and state subsidies to domestic industries.

In these international trade agreements and economic treaties, alcoholic beverages are almost always treated like normal consumer goods. Even when alcoholic beverages like wine are treated as special commodities, this is usually because they fall within the category of important agricultural products, not because they are harmful to health.

As Section II of this book has shown, alcohol is a commodity that causes social, health, and economic problems to the drinker and to society as a whole. Because of these problems, many countries and smaller communities have implemented a wide variety of policies to decrease problems caused by alcohol consumption, as discussed in Section III. The most effective strategies include raising the prices of alcoholic beverages with special alcohol taxes, as well as restricting the physical availability of alcohol by controlling the market, by either maintaining state monopolies or licensing the production and trade of alcoholic beverages. These 'more effective' strategies are also those most likely to be threatened or weakened by international trade agreement disputes. To the extent that alcohol is considered to be an ordinary commodity, these agreements and treaties often become severe obstacles for conducting purposeful and efficient alcohol control policies.

References

Alavaikko M. and Österberg E. (2000) The influence of economic interests on alcohol control policy: a case study from Finland. *Addiction* 95 (Suppl. 4), 565–79.

Andriamananjara S. (2001) Preferential trade agreements and the multilateral trading system. *International economic review*, January/February, pp. 1–4. Washington, DC: United States International Trade Commission, Publication 3402.

Bruun K., Pan L., and Rexed I. (1975) *The gentlemen's club: International control of drugs and alcohol.* Chicago IL: University of Chicago Press.

Ezzati M., *et al.* and the **Comparative Risk Assessment Collaborative Group** (2002) Selected major risk factors and global and regional burden of disease. *Lancet* 360, 1347–60.

Ferris J., Room R., and Giesbrecht N. (1993) Public health interests in trade agreements in alcoholic beverages in North America. *Alcohol Health and Research World* 17, 235–41.

Grieshaber-Otto J., Sinclair S., and Schacter N. (2000) Impacts of international trade, services and investment treaties on alcohol regulation. *Addiction* 95 (Suppl. 4), 491–504S.

Gual A. and Colom J. (2001) From Paris to Stockholm: where does the European Alcohol Action Plan lead to? *Addiction* 96, 1093–6.

Germer P. (1990) Alcohol and the single market: juridical aspects. *Contemporary Drug Problems* 17, 461–79.

Holder H.D., Kühlhorn E., Nordlund S., *et al.* (1998) *European integration and Nordic alcohol policies: Changes in alcohol controls and consequences in Finland, Norway and Sweden, 1980–1997.* Aldershot: Ashgate.

International Labour Organization (ILO) (1949) *Protection of wages convention, C95.* Geneva: ILO. Web address: http://ilolex.ilo.ch:1567/scripts/convd.pl?C95

Jernigan D.H. (1999) Country profile on alcohol in Zimbabwe. In: Riley L. and Marshall M. (eds.) *Alcohol and public health in 8 developing countries*, pp. 157–75. WHO/HSC/SAB/99.9. Geneva: WHO Substance Abuse Department.

Joossens L. (2000) From public health to international law: possible protocols for inclusion in the Framework Convention on Tobacco Control. *Bulletin of the World Health Organization* 78, 930–7.

Kortteinen T. (ed.) (1989) *State monopolies and alcohol prevention.* Report No. 181. Helsinki: Social Research Institute of Alcohol Studies.

Lubkin G. (1996) *Is Europe's glass half-full or half-empty? The taxation of alcohol and the development of a European identity.* Jean Monnet Center, Working Paper 96/7. Cambridge, MA: Harvard University. http://www.jeanmonnetprogram/papers/papers96.html

Lund I. (1997) *Alkohol og Marked. Nye Utfordringer i Kjølvannet av EØS-avtalen*, SIFA-rapport Nr. 2/97. Oslo: Statens institutt for alkohol- og narkotikaforskning.

Österberg E. (1993) Implications for monopolies of the European integration. *Contemporary Drug Problems* 20, 203–27.

Österberg E. and Karlsson T. (eds.) (2002) *Alcohol policies in EU member states and Norway: A collection of country reports.* Helsinki: STAKES.

Room R. (1984) The World Health Organization and alcohol control. *British Journal of Addiction* 79, 85–92.

Room R. and Paglia A. (1999) The international drug control system in the post-Cold War era: managing markets or fighting a war? *Drug and Alcohol Review* 18, 305–15.

Ugland T. (1996) EØS, EU og *Alkoholmonopolene: En Komparativ Studie av de Nordiske Lands Respons og Strategivalg.* SIFA-rapport Nr. 4/96. Oslo: Statens institutt for alkohol- og narkotikaforskning.

World Bank Group (2000) *World bank note on alcoholic beverages.* Washington, DC: World Bank Group. http://www.ifc.org/policies/arp.pdf

WHO. See World Health Organization.

World Health Organization (2000) *European alcohol action plan 2000–2005.* Copenhagen: World Health Organization, available from URL: http://www.who.dk/adt/aaction.htm.

World Health Organization (2001) *Declaration on young people and alcohol, 2001.* Copenhagen: WHO. http://www.who.dk/eprise/main/WHO/aboutWHO/Policy/20010927_1

World Health Organization (2003) Agreement reached on global framework convention on tobacco control, press release, 1 March. http://www.who.int/mediacentre/releases/2003/pr21/en/

Chapter 15

The policy arena

15.1 **Introduction**

An arena is a place where contests, and at times conflicts, take place. When applied to policy, the word takes on the connotation of a sphere of action for opposing views, contending groups, and competing interests. In Section III (Chapters 5–12), we examined the evidence with regard to a wide range of prevention and treatment strategies that could serve as instruments of alcohol policies. While there is now a growing scientific basis to support alcohol policy initiatives, there is much less understanding of the way in which different countries and communities operate within the policy arena. In this chapter, we move from the economic context of alcohol policy (Chapter 14) to the process through which policy is implemented by governments and other players at the national and local levels. This chapter also considers the constituency groups, stakeholders, and social forces that affect both the development and maintenance of effective policy as it is formulated by national and local governments. Although private organizations have policies, our analysis here applies primarily to government actions in the areas of public health, public safety, and social welfare.

This chapter focuses primarily on the following question: Who makes alcohol policy? The answer is not simple, and it differs across countries and between different levels of government within countries. But alcohol policies have been implemented at the national and local levels for more than a century, and much has been learned about the process. In addition to government, the formation of alcohol policy increasingly involves commercial interests, the media, public interest groups, the scientific community, and the general public.

15.2 **Commercial interests**

As discussed in Chapter 2, alcohol is a commodity, and there are significant commercial interests involved in promoting its manufacture, distribution, pricing, and sale. In most industrialized countries and increasingly in other parts of the world, the market system consists of relatively large-scale producers and wholesalers who market alcoholic beverages to retailers who then distribute them for sale through bars, restaurants, and off-premise establishments (Jernigan 1997). For the purposes of this discussion, this is what is labelled the 'alcoholic beverage industry'. In developing countries, an organized industry is a relatively new phenomenon, taking its place in the national economy along with smaller producers and suppliers.

Although the alcoholic beverage industry is not monolithic in terms of its motives, power, or operations, its commercial interests often come into conflict with public health measures. The elimination of restrictions on hours of sale, for example, can lead to an increase in alcohol consumption and related problems (Chapter 7). Media advertising is considered by health advocates to pose risks for vulnerable populations like adolescents (see Chapter 10), but restrictions on advertising are often opposed by industry. The introduction of new products and marketing schemes is considered a right of the free market, but some products, variously called '**alcopops**', 'malternatives', and 'designer drinks', have been associated with problem drinking by adolescents. Supported by free market values and concepts, the alcoholic beverage industry has become increasingly involved in the policy arena in order to protect its commercial interests. In some countries, the industry is the dominant non-governmental presence at the policymaking table. A common claim among public health advocates is that industry representatives are influential in setting the policy agenda, shaping the perspectives of legislators on policy issues, and determining the outcome of policy debates (e.g., Cahalan 1987; Baggott 1990; Hawks 1993).

The relative scale of industry vested interests is illustrated by the situation in the UK, where the amount spent on health education and the support of voluntary organizations in the alcohol field in 1984 represented less than 1% of the expenditure by the alcohol industry on advertising in the same year (Baggott 1986b). The alcohol industry's combined wealth exceeds the GNP of most non-industrialized countries, and its capacity to influence the public policy arena is significant (Edwards 1998; Room 1998). In many countries, large sums of money are spent on marketing, thus making the advertising industry, the communications media, and even some parts of the sports industry interested in alcohol policy, especially when restrictions on alcohol sponsorship and advertising are proposed.

With these kinds of vested interests in the promotion of alcohol use, it is not surprising that the alcohol industry should be actively involved in the policy-making process. In 1990, an attempt to increase the excise tax in California was successfully opposed by a media campaign funded by the alcohol industry costing in excess of US $30 million (Advocacy Institute 1992). Similarly, excise taxation was opposed in Australia by industry interests during the drafting of a National Alcohol Policy (Hawks 1993). In France, the alcohol industry opposed the Loi Evin, which introduced strong controls over advertising on television, in movies, and at sporting events (Craplet 1997).

To promote their interests and maintain their influence on policy decisions, industry sources have funded a network of national, regional, and now global 'social aspects' organizations that sponsor selected 'prevention initiatives' and industry-friendly views on alcohol problems and policies (Rae 1991; Sheldon 1996; McCreanor *et al.* 2000; Anderson 2002). One consequence of these prevention initiatives is that the industry perspective is present in the policy debates of many of the major producer and consumer nations (Hawks 1990; Casswell *et al.* 1993; Portman Group 1994; Simpura 1995; Babor *et al.* 1996; Raistrick *et al.* 1999; Jernigan *et al.* 2000).

15.3 **The mass media**

The mass media can have a significant influence on the policy debate at the national and local levels, given their dominant role in contemporary culture (Milio 1988). Media coverage influences whether policy-makers perceive a problem and how salient that problem is. This is an 'agenda-setting' function (McCombs and Shaw 1972; Erbring *et al.* 1980). For example, the media's interest in UK alcohol issues in the 1970s (and the impact of this interest on parliamentary questions) was followed by an unprecedented interest in alcohol issues by the UK health sector (Baggott 1986a). The media influences policy by framing the issue, defining the problem, and suggesting possible solutions. The media can also establish the credibility of commentators on current issues (Flora *et al.* 1989).

The importance of the media in shaping the policy debate has led to an increasing interest in media advocacy among public health advocates engaged in national and local policy debates (Wallack and Dorfman 1992; Chapman and Lupton 1994; Jernigan and Wright 1996). 'Media advocacy' refers to the strategic use of the media to advance policy goals (Wallack 1990; Holder and Treno 1997). The aim of media advocacy is to move public discourse from a focus on the individual person to an appreciation of the social, economic, and political influences on alcohol problems. Media advocacy is usually undertaken as a component of a multi-faceted community action initiative (Stewart and Casswell 1993), or in connection with regulatory changes, law enforcement, community mobilization, and monitoring of high-risk behaviour (Treno *et al.* 1996; Holder and Treno 1997; Treno and Holder 1997). As noted by Wallack and DeJong (1995), media advocacy is used to gain access to the media and to frame stories so that they focus on policy issues rather than on the unhealthy behaviour of individuals. By having newspaper or television reporters 'tell the story', alcohol policy supporters can avoid having to purchase media services for counter-advertising, and thus save valuable resources (Jernigan and Wright 1996). The results of the New Zealand Community Action Project (Stewart and Casswell 1993), for example, showed that media advocacy could produce a significant increase in media coverage of alcohol-related material focusing on moderation and informed alcohol policy.

15.4 **The scientific community**

Policy debate often relies on research findings to bolster a point of view (Moskalewicz 1993). However, there is no simple relation between scientific findings and policymaking. Bruun's (1973) conclusion that research 'produces arguments rather than logical conclusions regarding policy and action' remains valid.

Researchers often provide the raw material for policy decisions, measuring trends in alcohol consumption and related harms by monitoring social indicator statistics and social survey data. These data can play an important role in evaluating the need for alcohol policy. The absence of such data in Eastern Europe and most developing countries has made it difficult for public interest groups to challenge the view that alcohol should be treated as an ordinary commodity with no special controls on its marketing, price, or availability.

Researchers also play an important role evaluating the effectiveness of particular programs or policies. Our knowledge of the effectiveness of brief interventions (Chapter 12) and alcohol control measures (Chapter 7), and of the general ineffectiveness of school-based alcohol education (Chapter 11), for instance, is based on the accumulation of evaluation studies in each of these areas.

One of the clearest examples of research contributing to an effective policy was the debate over random breath testing (RBT) legislation in New South Wales, Australia (Homel 1993). Research findings that suggested the effectiveness of RBT were disseminated widely in a context of high public concern over drinking–driving statistics. Another policy initiative in which research played a key role was United States federal and state legislation that raised the minimum alcohol purchasing age to 21, after it had been lowered in many states in the 1970s. The process of communicating key research findings to policy-makers influenced the adoption of an effective policy (Wagenaar 1993), which was later confirmed by further research.

An important long-term contribution of research is to provide new ways of thinking about old issues. The broad perspective on 'alcohol problems' in which this book is written, for instance, can be seen as having first emerged in the course of epidemiological alcohol research (Room 1984). For another example, biomedical research on dopamine and other pathways through which alcohol acts in the brain has led us to understand the commonalities which drinking shares with other sources of pleasure—not only illicit drugs and tobacco, but also eating and sexual behaviour.

Research is not value-free, in the sense that the framing and choice of research topics inevitably reflects judgements and choices between competing priorities. However, investigators have a duty to be faithful to the research evidence, wherever it may lead. This inevitably means that the findings of researchers will sometimes conflict with conventional beliefs and fixed policy positions.

In an applied field such as the alcohol studies, scientific investigators should be attuned to the potential utility of their research. To be useful, research evidence must be simply communicated and give meaning to current issues. To contribute constructively to policy debates, researchers need to frame policy-relevant research questions and generate the data to answer them (Bucuvalas and Weiss 1980). Such contributions may only be possible in the context of a long-term publicly funded research programme designed to engage members of the scientific community in each country in the collection, evaluation, and interpretation of research data that is relevant to a country's alcohol policy needs.

15.5 Public interest groups and non-governmental organizations

Public interest groups, often represented by non-governmental organizations, also contribute to the policymaking process. In the early part of the 20th century, the temperance movement was a major stakeholder in the alcohol policy arena in a number of countries, and it still contributes to the policy process in some of them (Sulkunen 1997). More recently, alcohol issues have increasingly become the concern of health professionals, mirrored by a change in the organization of health and welfare services as well as increasing professionalization in the 'caring' occupations (Raistrick *et al.* 1999). The public health policy developments in France in the 1980s, for example, were initiated by the efforts of a group of medical specialists, 'the five sages' (Craplet 1997), who employed traditional welfare state arguments (Sulkunen 1997).

Professionals concerned with law and order have also played a role in the policymaking process in some countries (Baggott 1986b).

In many nations there is a vacuum in advocacy for the public interest. It is difficult for state employees to engage in political activity and policy advocacy, leaving members of non-governmental organizations as the most likely candidates to represent the public interest (Craplet 1997). These have occasionally involved interest groups representing victims of alcohol-related harm, Mothers Against Drunk Driving being a notable US example (DeJong and Russell 1995).

15.6 Public opinion and related activities

In many countries, public concern about alcohol-related problems only occasionally finds political expression. For example, concerns about drinking–driving, or about drunken disorders in central cities or among football supporters, have periodically resulted in changes in public opinion about the need for a particular alcohol policy. In some countries there is public support for a number of alcohol policies (Room *et al.* 1995; Giesbrecht and Greenfield 1999; Giesbrecht and Kavanagh 1999), although actual policy changes in recent years seem to reflect the views of heavier drinkers rather than the majority of adults in the jurisdictions surveyed. Rising popular concern reflects both a real increase in the rates of alcohol-related problems, and greater attention by the media and scientific community to alcohol-related issues. Unfortunately, the general public has relatively limited opportunities to influence alcohol policy in most countries. In Canada, for example, the general public is considerably more concerned and cautious about such issues as alcohol availability than those involved in the public discourse and political debate (Giesbrecht *et al.* 2001).

Consumers of alcoholic beverages can exert a negative influence on policies dealing with pricing, taxation, hours of sale, and other control measures if these measures are perceived by the public as being irrelevant to the prevention of alcohol-related problems. For example, in countries with a tradition of non-commercial production, tax increases on commercial alcoholic beverages may be seen as a potential stimulus to the illicit trade.

Public activities that bring attention to alcohol problems have a valuable place in the policy process, but they are never sufficient. Campaigns such as an 'Alcohol Awareness Week' produce personally satisfying experiences for citizens and leaders, but are unlikely to have an impact on alcohol-related problems. Such programs generate enthusiasm and public recognition, and may give the appearance that something is being done, without providing substantive and effective interventions.

15.7 **National governments**

Alcohol policies can be developed and implemented at many different levels of government. Nevertheless, federal and national laws often establish the legislative framework pertaining to alcohol. Examples include national legislation of state control over the production, export, and import of commercial alcohol products; control of wholesaling and retailing; legal minimum purchase ages for alcoholic beverages; apprehension of drivers with specified blood alcohol levels; alcohol advertising restrictions; and prohibition of service to intoxicated and underage persons. Furthermore, special taxes on alcoholic beverages are also subject to a regulatory framework that is enacted at a federal or national level.

Many different decision-making authorities are involved in the formulation and implementation of alcohol policy. Policy systems at the national level are rarely dominated by one decision-making authority, but tend rather to be decentralized and delegated to a variety of different and sometimes competing decision-making entities, such as the health ministry, the transportation authority, and the taxation agency (Bruun 1982). Countries vary tremendously, making it difficult to generalize about the policymaking process.

Civil servants are the only 'permanent' players within government. Some of these individuals may be responsible for the process of alcohol policy development and implementation, although some policy development tasks can be contracted out to consultants. *Ad hoc* committees and quasi-permanent advisory groups are sometimes appointed by governments to advise on alcohol policy, and independent research or policy institutes have sometimes become important sources of policy analysis and advice.

Recent policy development history in many countries has been one of public health advocates unsuccessfully opposing policy moves that were not supported by the research evidence (Mäkelä *et al.* 1981; Casswell 1993; Hawks 1993; Moskalewicz 1993). In a few nations, most noticeably France and the US, the past decade has seen a policy debate driven by health sector stakeholders (Dubois *et al.* 1989). This has resulted in a number of effective policies being introduced (Craplet 1997).

In some countries, the health and welfare sectors have attempted to establish broader national alcohol policies, which encompass a number of policy issues within an overall government philosophy and approach to alcohol issues (Room 1999). This was an approach strongly promoted by the World Health Organization in the 1980s. A number of alcohol policy reviews have been published to provide a basis for such policy development (Farrell 1985), including the precursors to this book (Bruun *et al.* 1975; Edwards *et al.* 1994).

Establishing a national policy entails the appointment of an organizational entity that represents the views of a number of sectors. Although the goal is to reach consensus, the diverse interests represented by these sectors makes agreement on any but the least contentious (and often least effective) policies impossible (Christie and Bruun 1969). In light of the strong positions of the vested interest groups, national alcohol policy is not likely to become a strong tool for public health advancement (Hawks 1990).

A national-level legislative and regulatory framework remains essential to the promotion of effective measures that curtail alcohol-related health and safety problems. Market liberalization and privatization has frequently been associated with increased regulation, albeit of a decentralized, less interventionist kind (Ayres and Braithwaite 1992). This offers the opportunity for 'responsive regulation', in which less prescriptive laws can enable a more negotiated process between commercial interests, regulators, and the community to increase both compliance and community satisfaction. Liquor licensing lends itself well to this model.

Another approach to national alcohol policy is to delegate or share responsibility within a state-level framework. In the United States, alcohol legislation is promulgated at the state level, with licensing controlled by Alcohol Beverage Control agencies. Local enforcement of controls on alcohol availability (shown by the extent of the budgets, the number of workers, and the citations issued) across different US states tends to be higher in states that have enacted formal laws and regulations controlling the marketplace, particularly with regard to price restrictions (Gruenewald et al. 1992).

National and regional jurisdictions have taken an active stance on some specific policy issues, such as drinking–driving. For example, the raising of the alcohol purchasing age in the United States was encouraged by a federal bill that provided highway development funds to those states that raised the age to 21. Currently US highway federal funding is only allotted to states that establish a blood alcohol concentration (**BAC**) level of 0.08 on drinking–driving. A number of other countries also have extensive national policies when it comes to drinking–driving, as discussed in Chapter 10.

National control and influence also remains paramount in the key alcohol policy area of taxation. As a result of the relationship between the real price of alcohol and levels of consumption and alcohol-related harms, taxation is central to alcohol policy (see Chapter 6). Taxation has a major influence on the real price of commercially-produced alcohol in all jurisdictions. Industry sectors are opposed to taxation because of the deflating effect it has on alcohol sales and consumption (Hawks 1990; Advocacy Institute 1992). However, alcohol taxation provides an important revenue stream for both national and sub-national governments, and it is relatively easy to collect. In industrialized countries such as the UK, governments obtain about 5% of their revenue from alcohol taxes (Raistrick *et al.* 1999). In contrast, the proportion of alcohol tax revenue in developing countries can be as much as 20% (WHO 1999).

15.8 **Community coalitions**

Many alcohol policy approaches that have demonstrated evidence of effectiveness at the national or regional level can also be enacted at the community level. This approach has a number of advantages. Local communities must personally deal with injuries and deaths from crashes involving alcohol-impaired drivers. They must provide hospital and emergency medical services, conduct autopsies, and deal with rehabilitation and recovery. Alcohol problems are often personal experiences for community members, who are motivated to take local action. Parent groups, for example, have been formed around a concern for underage drinking. Such groups can create public pressure against retail alcohol sales to underage persons and against access to alcohol at youth social events. The consequences of community-level involvement are experienced locally. Examples of two comprehensive community action projects are provided in Boxes 15.1 and 15.2.

Box 15.1 **The COMPARI project—Australia (1992–1995)**

University researchers initiated the Community Mobilisation for the Prevention of Alcohol Related Injury (COMPARI) project in the Western Australian regional city of Geraldton. The project was designed to reduce alcohol-related injury by focusing on the general context of alcohol use in the community and not solely on alcoholics or heavy drinkers. Project activities addressed five areas:

1. Networking and support (e.g., coordinating a local committee on domestic violence).

2. Community development (e.g., giving presentations to community service groups related to the prevention of alcohol-related injury).

3. Alternative non-drinking activities (e.g., underage youth disco).

4. Social marketing (e.g., media campaign presenting safe partying tips).

5. Policy institutionalization (e.g., implementation of guidelines for licensing applications to serve liquor on council property, and the development and delivery of a training package in responsible beverage service) (Midford *et al.* 1999).

Box 15.2 **Community trials project—USA (1992–1996)**

The Community Trials Project (Holder *et al.* 1997) was a five component community-level intervention conducted in three experimental communities matched to three comparison communities selected for geographical and cultural diversity. The five interacting components included:

1. A 'Community Knowledge, Values, and Mobilization' component to develop community organization and support for the goals and strategies of the project.

2. A 'Responsible Beverage Service Practices' component to reduce the risk of intoxicated as well as underage customers in bars and restaurants.

3. A 'Reduction Of Underage Drinking' component to reduce underage access.

4. A 'Risk Of Drinking and Driving' component to increase enforcement of drinking–driving.

5. An 'Access to Alcohol' component to reduce overall availability of alcohol.

The program evaluation showed a statistically significant increase in coverage of alcohol issues in local newspapers and on local TV in the experimental communities, a significant reduction in alcohol sales to minors, increased adoption of responsible alcohol serving policies, and a statistically significant reduction in alcohol-involved traffic crashes over the initial 28-month intervention period (see Voas *et al.* 1997), largely due to the introduction of special and highly visible drinking–driving enforcement and support from increased news coverage.

While it is relatively easy locally to introduce educational or informational campaigns, challenges are quick to emerge against the actual implementation of policies that are directed to law enforcement, drinking environments, access to alcohol, and regulation changes. Such controversies occurred in the US Community Trials Project (see Box 15.2). Unless the citizens who support efforts to implement special policies are prepared for opposition, the enthusiasm and effectiveness of local groups can be reduced. Unfortunately, in some communities the prevailing local efforts are devoted to initiatives that have a high profile (e.g., providing free coffee to drivers on New Year's Eve) but little or no impact on alcohol-related problems. These programs are popular and relatively uncontroversial, but may channel resources away from strategies with a much higher potential for impacting alcohol-related problems.

Some of the earliest attempts to develop, implement, and evaluate local-level strategies (Casswell and Gilmore 1989; Casswell and Stewart 1989; Casswell *et al.* 1989; Duignan *et al.* 1993) took place in New Zealand in the 1980s and 1990s following considerable liberalization of alcohol licensing laws (Stewart *et al.* 1993). Administration of licensing monitoring and enforcement was delegated to the local level, while licensing decisions and appeals were retained at the national level. Community action projects conducted during this period resulted in the establishment of local partnerships, which included a public health perspective, as well as the increased compliance and responsible management of local licensed premises to reduce alcohol-related harm (Hill and Stewart 1996; Stewart *et al.* 1997). Despite some limitations, New Zealand's two-tier decision-making structure provides a model of increasing community control over alcohol outlets within a national-level legislative framework. In contrast, UK alcohol licensing occurs entirely at the local level, where there is little national oversight. A disadvantage to the latter approach has been the absence of a clear framework of decision-making. Licensing authorities vary in the extent to which they use their authority to prevent alcohol-related problems (Raistrick *et al.* 1999).

15.9 **Conclusion**

Ideally, the policy process forms a cycle, beginning with a systematic assessment of alcohol-related problems, followed by the implementation of intervention policies, and ending with an objective evaluation of their effects. As this chapter has suggested, however, the reality of the policymaking process is rarely so simple or straightforward. Within each jurisdiction of the policy arena, there is an interplay of different interest groups. Groups involved in for-profit production and sales are always key players in policy debates. The media also play an important role, and those who communicate research findings are often drawn into the policy arena. Addiction professionals and non-governmental organizations often represent the public interest in many jurisdictions.

An appreciation of the various players in the alcohol policy arena can heighten our understanding of the following fundamental conclusion: alcohol policy is often the product of competing interests, values, and ideologies. Like any other commodity, alcohol is a good that is exchanged for economic or social capital, but it is also a product that requires an extraordinary amount of public policy attention in the form of regulation, taxation, and human services to address the damage it causes.

The process of alcohol policy creation needs to be more transparent and more responsive to the needs of the citizens who are the end consumers of emerging policies. Too much of the action in the alcohol arena is conducted behind the scenes, subject to political considerations or vested interests. Uninformed by science, and insufficiently monitored in its outcomes, alcohol policy is often neither evidence-based nor effective. If alcohol-related problems are to be minimized, mechanisms are needed at the international, national, and local levels to ensure that alcohol policies serve the public good.

References

Advocacy Institute (1992) *Taking initiative: The 1990 citizen's movement to raise California alcohol excise taxes to save lives.* Washington, DC: Advocacy Institute.

Anderson P. (2002) The beverage alcohol industry's social aspects organizations: a public health warning. *The Globe* 3, 3–30.

Ayres I. and Braithwaite J. (1992) *Responsive regulation: Transcending the deregulation debate.* Oxford: Oxford University Press.

Babor T.F., Edwards G., and Stockwell T. (1996) Science and the drinks industry: cause for concern [editorial]. *Addiction* 91, 5–9.

Baggott R. (1986a) Alcohol, politics and social policy. *Journal of Social Policy* 15, 467–88.

Baggott R. (1986b) By voluntary agreement: the politics of instrument selection. *Public Administration* 64, 51–67.

Baggott R. (1990) *Alcohol, politics and social policy.* Aldershot, UK: Avebury.

Bruun K. (1973) Social research, social policy and action. *The epidemiology of drug dependence: Report on a conference,* London 25–29 September 1972, pp. 115–19. Copenhagen: World Health Organization, Regional Office for Europe, EURO 5436 IV.

Bruun K. (ed.) (1982) *Alcohol policies in the United Kingdom* (Suppressed report of the UK Central Policy Review Staff). Stockholm: Sociology Department, Stockholm University.

Bruun K., Edwards G., Lumio M., *et al.* (1975) *Alcohol control policies in public health perspective.* Helsinki: Finnish Foundation for Alcohol Studies.

Bucuvalas M. and Weiss C. (1980) Truth tests and utility tests: decision makers' frames of reference for social science research. *American Sociological Review* 45, 302–13.

Cahalan D. (1987) *Understanding America's drinking problem: How to combat the hazards of alcohol.* San Francisco, CA: Jossey-Bass.

Casswell S. (1985) The organisational politics of alcohol control policy. *British Journal of Addiction* 80, 357–62.

Casswell S. (1993) Public discourse on the benefits of moderation: implications for alcohol policy development. *Addiction* 88, 459–65.

Casswell S. and Gilmore L. (1989) An evaluated community action project on alcohol. *Journal of Studies on Alcohol* 50, 339–46.

Casswell S. and Stewart L. (1989) A community action project on alcohol: community organisation and its evaluation. *Community Health Studies* 13, 39–48.

Casswell S., Gilmore L., Maguire V., *et al.* (1989) Changes in public support for alcohol policies following a community-based campaign. *British Journal of Addiction* 84, 515–22.

Casswell S., Stewart L., and Duignan P. (1993) The negotiation of New Zealand alcohol policy in a decade of stabilized consumption and political change: the role of research. *Addiction* 88 (Suppl.), 9–17S.

Chapman S. and Lupton D. (1994) *The fight for public health: Principles and practice of media advocacy.* London: BMJ.

Christie N. and Bruun K. (1969) Alcohol problems: the conceptual framework. In: Keller M. and Coffey T. (eds.) *Proceedings of the 28th International Congress on Alcohol and Alcoholism,* Vol. 2, pp. 65–73. Highland Park, NJ: Hillhouse Press.

Craplet M. (1997) Alcohol advertising: The need for European regulation. *Commercial Communications: The Journal of Advertising and Marketing Policy and Practice in the European Community* 9, 1–3.

DeJong W. and Russell A. (1995) MADD's position on alcohol advertising: a response to Marshall and Oleson. *Journal of Public Health Policy* 16, 231–8.

Dubois G., Got C., Gremy F., *et al.* (1989) Non au ministere de la maladie! *Le Monde* 15 November.

Duignan P., Casswell S., and Stewart L. (1993) Evaluating community projects: conceptual and methodological issues illustrated from the community action project and the liquor licensing project in New Zealand. In: Greenfield T. and Zimmerman R. (eds.) *Experiences with community action projects: new research in the prevention of alcohol and other drug problems.* Rockville, MD: US Department of Health and Human Services.

Edwards G. (1998) Should the drinks industry sponsor research? If the drinks industry does not clean up its act, pariah status in inevitable. *British Medical Journal* 317, 336.

Edwards G., Anderson P., Babor T.F., *et al.* (1994) *Alcohol policy and the public good.* Oxford: Oxford University Press.

Erbring L., Goldenberg E., and Miller A. (1980) Front page news and real world cues: a new look at agenda setting by the media. *American Journal of Political Science* 24, 16–49.

Farrell S. (1985) *Review of national policy measures to prevent alcohol-related problems.* Geneva: World Health Organization.

Flora J., Maibach E., and Maccoby N. (1989) The role of the media across four levels of health promotion intervention. *Annual Review of Public Health* 10, 181–201.

Giesbrecht N. and Greenfield T. (1999) Public opinions on alcohol policy issues: a comparison of American and Canadian surveys. *Addiction* 94, 521–31.

Giesbrecht N. and Kavanagh L. (1999) Public opinion and alcohol policy: comparison of two Canadian general population surveys. *Drug and Alcohol Review* 18, 7–19.

Giesbrecht N., Ialomiteanu A., Room R., and Anglin L. (2001) Trends in public opinion on alcohol policy measures: Ontario 1989–1998. *Journal of Studies on Alcohol* 62, 142–9.

Gruenewald P.J., Madden P., and Janes K. (1992) Alcohol availability and the formal power and resources of state alcohol beverage control agencies. *Alcoholism: Clinical and Experimental Research* 16, 591–7.

Hawks D. (1990) The watering down of Australia's health policy on alcohol. *Drug and Alcohol Review* 9, 91–5.

Hawks D. (1993) The formulation of Australia's National Health Policy on Alcohol. *Addiction* 88 (Suppl.), 19–26S.

Hill L. and Stewart L. (1996) The Sale of Liquor Act 1989: reviewing regulatory practices. *Social Policy Journal of New Zealand* 7, 174–90.

Holder H.D. and Treno A.J. (1997) Media advocacy in community prevention: news as a means to advance policy change. *Addiction* 92 (Suppl. 2), 189–99S.

Holder H.D, Saltz R.F., Grube J.W., *et al.* (1997) Summing up: lessons from a comprehensive community prevention trial. *Addiction* 92 (Suppl. 2), 293–301S.

Homel R. (1993) Random breath testing in Australia: getting it to work according to specifications. *Addiction* 88, 27–33S.

Jernigan D. (1997) *Thirsting for markets: The global impact of corporate alcohol.* California: The Marin Institute for the Prevention of Alcohol and Other Drug Problems.

Jernigan D. and Wright P. (1996) Media advocacy: lessons from community experiences. *Journal of Public Health Policy* 17, 306–30.

Jernigan D., Monteiro M., Room R., *et al.* (2000) Towards a global alcohol policy: alcohol, public health and the role of WHO. *Bulletin of the World Health Organization* 78, 491–9.

Mäkelä K., Österberg E., and Sulkunen P. (1981) Drink in Finland: increasing alcohol availability in a monopoly state. In: Single E., Morgan P., and deLint J. (eds.) *Alcohol, society and the state II: The social history of control policy in seven countries.* Toronto: Addiction Research Foundation.

McCombs M. and Shaw D. (1972) The agenda-setting function of the mass media. *Public Opinion Quarterly* 36, 176–87.

McCreanor T., Casswell S., and Hill L. (2000) ICAP and the perils of partnership. *Addiction* 95, 179–85.

Midford R., Boots K., Masters L., *et al.* (1999) COMPARI: A three year community based alcohol harm reduction project in Australia. In: *Community action to prevent alcohol problems*, pp. 215–26. Copenhagen: World Health Organization.

Milio N. (1988) Making healthy public policy; developing the science by learning the art: an ecological framework for policy studies. *Health Promotion* 2, 263–74.

Moskalewicz J. (1993) Lessons to be learnt from Poland's attempt at moderating its consumption of alcohol. *Addiction* 88 (Suppl.), 135–42S.

Portman Group (1994) *A commentary on the European Alcohol Action Plan.* London: Portman Group.

Rae J. (1991) Too many ifs and buts on alcohol [letter]. *The Times* 26 December.

Raistrick D., Hodgson R., and Ritson B. (eds.) (1999) *Tackling alcohol together: The evidence base for a UK alcohol policy.* London: Free Association Books.

Room R. (1984) Alcohol control and public health. *Annual Review of Public Health* 5, 293–317.

Room R. (1998) Thirsting for attention [editorial]. *Addiction* 93, 797–8.

Room R. (1999) The idea of alcohol policy. *Nordic Studies on Alcohol and Drugs* 16, 7–20.

Room R., Graves K., Giesbrecht N., *et al.* (1995) Trends in public opinion about alcohol policy initiatives in Ontario and the US: 1989–91. *Drug and Alcohol Review* 14, 35–47.

Sheldon T. (1996) Dutch anti-alcohol campaign is under attack [news]. *British Medical Journal* 313, 1349.

Simpura J. (1995) Alcohol in Eastern Europe: market prospects, prevention puzzles. *Addiction* 90, 467–70.

Stewart L. and Casswell S. (1993) Media advocacy for alcohol policy support: results from the New Zealand Community Action Project. *Health Promotion International* 8, 167–75.

Stewart L., Casswell S., and Duignan P. (1993) Using evaluation resources in a community action project: formative evaluation of public health input into the implementation of the New Zealand Sale of Liquor Act. *Contemporary Drug Problems* 20, 681–704.

Stewart L., Casswell S., and Thomson A. (1997) Promoting public health in liquor licensing: perceptions of the role of alcohol community workers. *Contemporary Drug Problems* 24, 1–37.

Sulkunen P. (1997) Logics of prevention: mundane speech and expert discourse on alcohol policy. In: Sulkunen P., Holmwood J., Radner H., *et al.* (eds.) *Constructing the new consumer society*. New York: St. Martins Press.

Treno A.J. and Holder H.D. (1997) Community mobilization, organizing, and media advocacy. A discussion of methodological issues. *Evaluation Review* 21, 166–90.

Treno A.J., Breed L., Holder H.D., *et al.* (1996) Evaluation of media advocacy efforts within a community trail to reduce alcohol-involved injury: Preliminary newspaper results. *Evaluation Review* 20, 404–23.

Voas R.B., Holder H.D., and Gruenewald P.J. (1997) The effect of drinking and driving interventions on alcohol-involved traffic crashes within a comprehensive community trial. *Addiction* 92 (Suppl. 2), 221–36S.

Wagenaar A. (1993) Research affects public policy: the case of the legal drinking age in the United States. *Addiction* 88 (Suppl. 2), 75–81S.

Wallack L.M. (1990) Social marketing and media advocacy: two approaches to health promotion. *World Health Forum* 11, 143–54.

Wallack L. and DeJong W. (1995) Mass media and public health: Moving the focus from the individual to the environment. In: Martin, S. (ed.) *The effects of the mass media on the use and abuse of alcohol*. Bethesda, MD: National Institute on Alcohol Abuse and Alcoholism, Research Monograph No. 28.

Wallack L. and Dorfman L. (1992) Television news, hegemony and health. *American Journal of Public Health* 82, 125–6.

WHO. See World Health Organization.

World Health Organization (1999) *Global status report on alcohol*. Geneva: World Health Organization.

Section V

Conclusion

Chapter 16

Alcohol policies: a consumer's guide

16.1 Alcohol policy-makers are answerable to the policy consumers

People consume not only goods, but also services, and alcohol policy is one such service. In any jurisdiction alcohol policy serves two purposes: to enhance the benefits resulting from the use of beverage alcohol, and to contain and reduce alcohol-related harms. Citizens have the right to assess and audit policies on health care provision, education, and crime prevention. They also deserve to know whether enacted alcohol policies are apt and well chosen. Alcohol policy issues overlap with almost every aspect of the public policy domain. Alcohol-related issues are pervasively important for the state at both central and local levels; they cannot be minimized or ignored. In an age of consumerism, it behoves policy-makers to ensure that alcohol policies are fashioned with public health interests in mind.

High quality policies will be those that are evidence-based. The preceding chapters have provided critical and detailed reviews of the relevant science base. We will now try to make explicit the connection between the research and the practical needs of the policymaker who wants to implement evidence-based responses. Our intention is to make science useful at the real world front lines of policy. The difference between good and bad alcohol policy is not an abstraction, but very often a matter of life and death. We believe that it is right to ask for the science to be taken seriously. Research has the capacity to indicate which strategies are likely to succeed in their public health intentions, and which are likely to be less effective or even useless, diversionary, and a waste of resources. Table 16.1 shows very clearly the imbalance among different strategies, both in the effectiveness findings and in the breadth of the literature.

16.2 Choosing effective strategies

With an ever-expanding research output, the need increases for a systematic procedure to evaluate the evidence, compare alternative interventions, and assess the benefits to society of different approaches. To that end, several attempts have been made in the addiction field to synthesize information

Table 16.1 Ratings of policy-relevant strategies and interventions

Strategy or intervention	Effectiveness	Breadth of research support	Cross-cultural testing	Cost to implement	Target group[a] (TG) and comments
Regulating physical availability					
Total ban on sales	+++	+++	++	High	TG = GP; Substantial adverse side-effects from black market, which is expensive to suppress. Ineffective without enforcement.
Minimum legal purchase age	+++	+++	++	Low	TG = HR; Reduces hazardous drinking, but does not eliminate drinking. Effective with minimal enforcement but enforcement substantially increases effectiveness.
Rationing	++	++	++	High	TG = GP; Particularly affects heavy drinkers; difficult to implement.
Government monopoly of retail sales	+++	+++	++	Low	TG = GP; Effective only if operated with public health and public order goals.
Hours and days of sale restrictions	++	++	++	Low	TG = GP; Effective in certain circumstances.
Restrictions on density of outlets	++	+++	++	Low	TG = GP; Requires a longer time course for implementation when drinking establishments have become concentrated because of vested economic interests.
Server liability	+++	+	+	Low	TG = HR; Required legal definition of liability mostly limited to North America.
Different availability by alcohol strength	++	++	+	Low	TG = GP; Mostly tested for strengths of beer.
Taxation and pricing					
Alcohol taxes	+++	+++	+++	Low	TG = GP; Effectiveness depends on government oversight and control of alcohol production and distribution. High taxes can increase smuggling and illicit production.

Altering the drinking context

Strategy					Comments
Outlet policy to not serve intoxicated patrons	+	+++	++	Moderate	TG = HR; Training alone is insufficient. Outside enforcement essential to effectiveness.
Training bar staff and managers to prevent and better manage aggression	+	+	+	Moderate	TG = HR
Voluntary codes of bar practice	0	+	+	Low	TG = HR; Ineffective without enforcement.
Enforcement of on-premise regulations and legal requirements	++	+	++	High	TG = HR; Compliance depends on perceived likelihood of enforcement.
Promoting alcohol-free activities and events	0	++	+	High	TG = GP; Evidence mostly from youth alternative programs.
Community mobilization	++	++	+	High	TG = GP; Sustainability of changes has not been demonstrated.

Education and persuasion

Strategy					Comments
Alcohol education in schools	0[b]	+++	++	High	TG = HR; May increase knowledge and change attitudes but has no sustained effect on drinking.
College student education	0	+	+	High	TG = HR; May increase knowledge and change attitudes but has no effect on drinking.
Public service messages	0	++−	++	Moderate	TG = GP; Refers to messages to the drinker about limiting drinking; messages to strengthen policy support untested.
Warning labels	0	+	+	Low	TG = GP; Raise awareness, but do not change behaviour.

Regulating alcohol promotion

Strategy					Comments
Advertising bans	+[c]	++	++	Low	TG = GP; Strongly opposed by alcoholic beverage industry; can be circumvented by product placements on TV and in movies.
Advertising content controls	?	0	0	Moderate	TG = GP; Often subject to industry self-regulation agreements, which are rarely enforced or monitored.

Table 16.1 (Continued)

Strategy or intervention	Effectiveness	Breadth of research support	Cross-cultural testing	Cost to implement	Target group[a] (TG) and comments
Drinking–driving countermeasures					
Sobriety check points	++	+++	+++	Moderate	TG = GP; Effects of police campaigns typically short-term.
Random breath testing (RBT)	+++	++	+	Moderate	TG = GP; Somewhat expensive to implement. Effectiveness depends on number of drivers directly affected.
Lowered BAC Limits	+++	+++	++	Low	TG = GP; Diminishing returns at lower levels (e.g., 0.05–0.02%), but still significant.
Administrative license suspension	++	++	++	Moderate	TG = HD
Low BAC for young drivers ('zero tolerance')	+++	++	+	Low	TG = HR
Graduated licensing for novice drivers	++	++	++	Low	TG = HR; Some studies note that 'zero tolerance' provisions are responsible for this effect.
Designated drivers and ride services	0	+	+	Moderate	TG = HR; Effective in getting drunk people not to drive but do not affect alcohol-related accidents.
Treatment and early intervention					
Brief intervention with at-risk drinkers	++	+++	+++	Moderate	TG = HR; Primary care practitioners lack training and time to conduct screening and brief interventions.
Alcohol problems treatment	+	+++	+++	High	TG = HD; Population reach is low because most countries have limited treatment facilities.
Mutual help/self-help attendance	+	+	++	Low	TG = HD: A feasible, cost-effective complement or alternative to formal treatment in many countries.
Mandatory treatment of repeat drinking–drivers	+	++	+	Moderate	TG = HD: Punitive and coercive approaches have time-limited effects, and sometimes distract attention from more effective interventions.

[a] Each strategy applies to one of the following three target groups (TG): GP, the general population of drinkers; HR, high-risk drinkers or groups considered to be particularly vulnerable to the adverse effects of alcohol (e.g., adolescents); HD, persons already manifesting harmful drinking and alcohol dependence.

[b] Among the hundreds of studies, only two show significant lasting effects (after 3 years), and the significance of these is questionable when reanalyzed (Foxcroft et al. 2003). A few more studies show shorter-term effects, and in this frame the rating could be +.

[c] Econometric studies find effects of bans but direct studies of short-term impacts have generally found no effect on total alcohol consumption. Policy here might well be guided by the precautionary principle (sec 16.5).

from a wide variety of perspectives, using consensus panels, expert committee ratings, and objective decision models (Babor *et al.* 1999; Coffield *et al.* 2001; Karlsson and Österberg 2001; Shults *et al.* 2001).

Building on previous work in this area, we have developed a relatively simple method to synthesize the results of our review. Table 16.1 provides qualitative ratings for each of the interventions reviewed in Chapters 6 through 12. The ratings reflect the consensus views of the authors and are designed to serve as a guide to policy consumers who would like to evaluate the strengths and weaknesses of different policy options. The table is organized according to four major criteria:

1. Evidence of effectiveness.

2. Breadth of research support.

3. Extent of testing across diverse countries and cultures.

4. Relative cost of the intervention in terms of time, resources, and money.

Box 16.1 explains the four evaluation criteria and the scales used to rate them.

Evidence of effectiveness refers to the quality of scientific information about the effectiveness of the particular intervention. Judgement here was influenced by whether experimental studies show that a particular intervention produces a measurable and significant change in alcohol consumption or related outcomes. In addition, the raters took into consideration research conducted under real life circumstances, such as 'natural experiments', that suggest the intervention produces a significant change.

Breadth of research support goes beyond quality of the science to look at the quantity and consistency of the evidence available. Ratings were influenced by the quality of available integrative reviews or meta-analyses.

Cross-cultural testing means that the evidence for a particular intervention applies equally well to different countries, regions, sub-groups, and social classes. In evaluating the evidence, we were particularly interested in the extent to which interventions developed for and evaluated in the established market economies can be transferred to developing societies.

Cost to implement and sustain refers to the monetary and other costs associated with an intervention, regardless of its effectiveness.

Other policy-relevant considerations that are evaluated in the Comments section of the table include the target group for the intervention, adverse side-effects, population reach, and feasibility. Target group (TG) refers to the population most likely to be affected by the strategy:

1. The general population of drinkers.

2. High-risk drinkers or groups considered to be particularly vulnerable to the adverse effects of alcohol (e.g., adolescents).

3. Persons already manifesting harmful drinking and alcohol dependence.

Box 16.1 **Standards of evidence for evaluating prevention strategies and interventions**

Evidence of effectiveness

This criterion refers the scientific evidence demonstrating whether a particular strategy is effective in reducing alcohol consumption, alcohol-related problems, or their costs to society. Here we are concerned with the overall conclusion that a reasonable person can draw based on the quality of research and the strength of effect both under idealized research conditions (efficacy studies) and real world settings (effectiveness studies). To be considered in this compendium, strategies had to be carefully investigated in at least one well designed study, which accounted for alternative and competing explanations. Only studies that met minimum scientific standards were used in these evaluations. Particular attention was given to the rules of evidence (Chapter 5) and the studies cited in Section III. The following rating scale was used:

0	Evidence indicates a lack of effectiveness.
+	Evidence for limited effectiveness.
++	Evidence for moderate effectiveness.
+++	Evidence of a high degree of effectiveness.
?	No studies have been undertaken or there is insufficient evidence upon which to make a judgement.

Breadth of research support

Here we are concerned with the number of scientific studies and the consistency of the results, whereas the effectiveness criterion is concerned with the direction of the evidence independent of the number of studies undertaken. The highest rating was influenced by the availability of integrative reviews and meta-analyses by experts in their respective fields of study. Breadth of research support was evaluated independent of the effectiveness rating (i.e., it is possible for a strategy to be rated low in effectiveness but to also have a high rating on the breadth of research supporting this evaluation). We used the following scale:

0	No studies of effectiveness have been undertaken.
+	Only one well designed study of effectiveness completed.
++	Two to four studies of effectiveness have been completed.
+++	Five or more studies of effectiveness have been completed.

Standards of evidence for evaluating prevention strategies and interventions *(continued)*

Tested across cultures

This criterion is concerned with the diversity of geography and cultures within which each strategy has been applied and tested. It refers to the robustness of international or multinational testing of a strategy as well as the extent to which a strategy applies to multiple countries and cultures. The following scale was used:

0	The strategy has not been tested adequately.
+	The strategy has been studied in only one country.
++	The strategy has been studied in two to four countries.
+++	The strategy has been studied in five or more countries.

Cost to implement and sustain

This criterion seeks to estimate the relative monetary cost to the state to implement, operate, and sustain a strategy, regardless of its effectiveness. For instance, increasing alcohol excise duties does not cost much to the state but may be costly to alcohol consumers. As a guide, we used the following scale:

Low	Low cost to implement and sustain.
Moderate	Moderate cost to implement and sustain.
High	High cost to implement and sustain.

Side-effects include the tendency for some interventions to stimulate criminal activity such as tax evasion or illicit production of alcohol. The population reach refers to the number of people in the target group that can be reached or served when an intervention is provided under real world conditions. Finally, to be translated into effective policies, interventions need to be evaluated in terms of their feasibility. Feasibility can be assessed in terms of political considerations (leadership, opposition from industry, public support), economic implications (cost-effectiveness and cost-benefit analysis), and the presence or absence of adverse side-effects.

16.3 Policy options considered

The left-hand column of Table 16.1 lists a wide array of possible policy choices that were reviewed in Section III. Each strategy has at some point in time been employed as an instrument of alcohol policy in some part of the world. The list's extensiveness shows that alcohol policy-makers are not short of experience or choices.

16.3.1 The strong strategies: availability restrictions, taxation, and enforcement

In general, effectiveness is strong for the regulation of physical availability and the use of alcohol taxes. Given the broad reach of these strategies, and the relatively low expense of implementing them, the expected impact of these measures on public health is relatively high. Most drinking–driving countermeasures received high ratings on effectiveness as well. Not only is there good research support for these programs, they also seem to be applicable in most countries, and are relatively inexpensive to implement and sustain. If two or more pluses on effectiveness, breadth support, and cross-cultural testing, as well as the absence of high cost, can be considered an indication of a consistently good performance, the following 10 policy options stand out as 'best practices': minimum legal purchase age, government monopoly of retail sales, restrictions on hours or days of sale, outlet density restrictions, alcohol taxes, sobriety check points, lowered BAC limits, administrative license suspension, graduated licensing for novice drivers, and brief interventions for hazardous drinkers.

16.3.2 Education and public service messages

The expected impact is low for education and for public service messages about drinking. The education strategies have been coded at a relatively high cost, to reflect the expense of training and implementation for a full education program. From the viewpoint of a state or local government, the costs may be lower than this, because the teaching costs are charged locally, or because the education program is viewed as a low-cost add-on to existing commitments. But in terms of impact or value-for-money, the cost hardly matters: education strategies have shown little or no effect, regardless of the investment. Although the reach of educational programs is thought to be excellent (because of the availability of captive audiences in schools), the population impact of these programs is poor. Similarly, while feasibility is good, cost-effectiveness and cost-benefit are poor.

16.3.3 Treatment and early intervention strategies

Treatment and early intervention strategies have, at best, medium effectiveness. At the population level, their impact is limited, since full treatment for alcohol problems can only benefit the relatively small fraction of the population who come to treatment. Even brief interventions are restricted to those who use the services within which they are offered, and who are willing to accept the intervention. While providing treatment is an obligation of a humane society, its effect on the actual drinking problem rates of the population at large is necessarily limited.

16.3.4 Altering the drinking context

The relatively sparse amount of evidence on the effects of altering the drinking context reflects the fact that research in this area is only now getting under way. Nevertheless, it seems likely that strategies in this area will have some impact without being too costly. However, these strategies are primarily applicable to on-premise drinking in bars and restaurants, which somewhat limits their public health significance. In most developed countries, only a minority of drinking is done on-premise, although frequently this drinking is trouble-prone. One recurring theme in this literature is the importance of enforcement to strategies that alter the context of drinking. This theme also applies to strategies regulating physical availability. Passing a minimum purchasing age law, for instance, will have rather little effect if it is not reinforced with a credible threat to cancel the licenses of outlets that repeatedly sell to minors. Likewise, server training in responsible beverage service is unlikely to have an effect, unless it is backed by a threat to suspend the licenses of those who continue to serve already intoxicated patrons. Enforcement as a condition of licensing has some costs, of course, but the governmental costs are frequently defrayed by such means as license fees on bars and restaurants.

16.3.5 Enhancing the likelihood of effectiveness

Alcohol policies rarely operate independently or in isolation from other measures, as might be implied by the listing of individual strategies in Table 16.1. Research on local prevention efforts suggests that alcohol problems are best considered in terms of the community systems that produce them. Local strategies have the greatest potential to be effective when prior scientific evidence is utilized and multiple policies are implemented in a systematic way. Thus, complementary system strategies that seek to restructure the total drinking environment are more likely to be effective than single strategies. Finally, prevention strategies with a natural capacity for long-term institutionalization should be favoured over those that are only in place for the life of the project. This line of reasoning suggests that full-spectrum interventions are needed to achieve the greatest population impact.

16.3.6 Target groups

Table 16.1 provides information about three groups that alcohol policy interventions have been directed at:

1. The general population of a state or a community.
2. High-risk drinkers (e.g., adolescents or pregnant women, thought to be particularly vulnerable to the adverse effects of alcohol).
3. Harmful drinkers (i.e., persons already beginning to experience alcohol-related problems).

Of the 32 interventions and strategies evaluated, one-half (16) are targeted at the general population, 12 at high-risk drinkers, and four at harmful drinkers. Interventions directed at the general population have higher effectiveness ratings, on average, than those targeted at high-risk groups and harmful drinkers (1.8 vs. 1.4 and 1.3, respectively). And interventions directed at the general population and high-risk groups tend to be less costly to implement and maintain than interventions with harmful drinkers (average ratings, 2.2, 2.2, and 1.8, respectively). These are important considerations when weighing the relative advantages of population-based and harm reduction approaches.

Consistent with the notion of integrated alcohol policies, our ratings suggest that a combination of physical availability limits at the general population level, certain drinking–driving countermeasures directed at all three target groups, and brief interventions directed at high-risk drinkers, will offer the best value as the foundation for a comprehensive alcohol policy approach.

16.4 The need to make science more accessible to policy-makers

Because alcohol availability and control occur in a complex cultural, social, and political environment, policy changes should be made with caution and with a sense of experimentation to determine whether they have their intended effects. The knowledge needed to address health and social problems is unlikely to reside in a single discipline or research methodology. Interdisciplinary research is capable of playing a critical role in the progress of public health by applying the methodologies of the medical, behavioural, social, and population sciences to an understanding of alcohol-related problems and their prevention.

Policy-makers have neither the time nor the training to read, digest, and base their decisions on the research findings reported in the scientific literature. Responsibility for translating scientific research into effective policy is distributed across a wide variety of government agencies and public interest groups. As described in Chapter 15, this process rarely follows a rational plan of action. If the public's health is to be served, it will be necessary to strengthen the links between science and policy through an innovative strategy in which promising research findings are identified, synthesized, and effectively communicated to both the policy-makers and the public. In this book we have tried to illustrate such an approach by identifying what the critical health needs are in the alcohol field, describing the principal factors responsible for alcohol problems, integrating the disparate findings that point to causal mechanisms, identifying what is known (and unknown) about the prevention and management of alcohol-related problems, and describing critical barriers to effective public health policy. We do not claim this text to be the final and exemplary model of its kind, but we do believe that it shows how science can be made more useful in this arena.

Alcohol policies will, of course, always be based on more than pure science. They are likely to arise from a combination of political expediency, commercial interests, common sense, and public safety. But that realization should not discourage governments from giving much closer attention to ways in which the scientific asset can be intelligently used.

16.5 The 'precautionary principle'

The 'precautionary principle' is a general public health concept that we believe should be put to use in the alcohol policy arena (Kriebel and Tickner 2001). The main tenets of this principle are to take preventive action even in the face of uncertainty; to shift the burden of proof to the proponents of a potentially harmful activity; to offer alternatives to harmful actions; and to increase public involvement in decision-making.

When applied to alcohol policy, the precautionary principle implies that decision-making in areas like international trade agreements, the introduction of new alcohol products (high alcohol content malt beverages, for instance), removal of restrictions on hours of sale, and the promotion of alcohol through advertising, should be guided by the likelihood of risk, rather than the potential for profit. The application of the precautionary principle to alcohol policy will help to increase both public participation in the policymaking process and the transparency of decision-making, currently guided too often by economic considerations of the few, rather than public health concerns of the many.

16.6 Alcohol policy and alcohol science in developing societies

This book is largely based on research conducted in developed societies. Although the burden of illness attributable to alcohol is smaller in most developing regions, it nonetheless accounts for a considerable amount of premature death and disability, especially in Latin America (see Chapter 4 and Room *et al.* 2002). Despite relatively low levels of aggregate consumption, a pattern of occasional heavy drinking in many developing nations is associated with injuries and other acute alcohol problems. The findings suggest that as economic development occurs, alcohol consumption is likely to increase with rising incomes, confronting developing nations with greater levels of alcohol-related problems, and new challenges to fashion effective alcohol policies. Global trade agreements are also likely to have an adverse influence on developing nations. With the growing emphasis on free trade and free markets, international institutions such as the World Trade Organization have pushed to dismantle effective alcohol control measures, such as state alcohol monopolies and other restrictions on the supply of alcoholic beverages.

Despite the relative weaknesses in the alcohol policy research base in developing countries, many of the strategies recommended by the analysis offered in this book are applicable with due modification (Room *et al.* 2002). But we would caution against any assumption that policies found to be good for the developed world are automatically best for the developing world.

Developing countries need individual assessments of their own alcohol policy experiences and their own alcohol science. The scarcity of indigenous health science is a very general handicap affecting policy formulation in less developed countries, and goes beyond the alcohol arena. The world research community, in partnership with international agencies, has a special responsibility to rectify this situation.

16.7 Extraordinary opportunities

Alcohol is no ordinary commodity, but on the basis of the evidence arrayed in this book, extraordinary opportunities exist to strengthen the policy response to alcohol-related problems. The following considerations support this conclusion:

1. **Multiple opportunities**. The policy options listed along the left-hand column of Table 16.1 speak to the extraordinary range of available strategies from which policy-makers can choose. Each of those entries deserves separate scrutiny as we have argued above, but the extensiveness of the list carries its own message.

2. **Opportunity to make choices rationally**. The compendium of intervention strategies should not be read as an invitation to apply the listed approaches randomly and at whim. On the contrary, the research enables an informed and discriminating choice based on multiple lines of evidence.

3. **Opportunity to combine rationally selected strategies into an integrated overall policy.** Table 16.1 provides a basis for the selection of a set of integrated and mutually supportive strategies. Alcohol policy is likely to be most effective when a variety of complementary strategies are used, such as the combination of graduated licensing, lower BAC limits, and minimum legal purchasing age restrictions in order to prevent alcohol problems among youth. We strongly recommend the creation of such broadly based alcohol policies.

4. **The research base is strong.** Research technologies are now available to monitor policy effectiveness. Rather than viewing alcohol interventions as certain solutions or hopeful 'shots in the dark', it is now possible and highly desirable that outcomes be measured and policies be self-correcting. There are numerous and evolving opportunities for further application of prevention science to policy questions.

5. **Opportunities to implement policies at multiple levels.** Alcohol policies can be effective at both the community level and the national level. Within each of these levels, policies can be targeted at the general population, at high-risk drinkers, and at people already experiencing alcohol-related problems. Synergistic types of activity are likely to obtain the best results. International policies provide the third level. When responding to alcohol problems, there is thus always somewhere to start, always a layer to be strengthened.

6. **Opportunities to strengthen public awareness and support.** The consumers of the research reported in this book should be in part the general public. Significant, but so far largely neglected opportunities exist to translate the scientific evidence into plain language for the media, opinion leaders, community groups, and the man and woman in the street. An informed public climate can help build support for public policies on alcohol.

7. **Enhancing international collaboration in the response to alcohol.** This book has taken an international perspective throughout. The research we have presented and the policy experience we have described come from many different countries. International tariff agreements and the activities of the alcoholic beverage industry make an international view of alcohol-related problems mandatory. There are considerable opportunities to strengthen international collaboration and the sharing of experiences in this arena. The role of the World Health Organization (WHO) is paramount. In our view, the findings assembled in this book make a strong case for strengthened WHO initiatives on alcohol and public health.

In summary, opportunities for evidence-based alcohol policies that better serve the public good are more available than ever before, as a result of accumulating knowledge on which strategies work and how to make them work. This conclusion provides ample cause for optimism. However, this book must also be seen as carrying another well-evidenced and not so cheerful message. It provides the world community with new documentation that alcohol problems are inflicting, on a global scale, vast damage to the public health. But the policies to address these problems are too seldom informed by science, and there are still too many instances of policy vacuums filled by unevaluated or ineffective strategies and interventions.

Optimism or pessimism, which is it to be? The answer to that question must depend entirely on whether the future brings increased use of evidence-based alcohol policies. That is what the consumers of policy have a right to expect. After all, alcohol is no ordinary commodity.

References

Babor T.F., Aguirre-Molina M., Marlatt A., *et al.* (1999) Managing alcohol problems and risky drinking. *American Journal of Health Promotion* 14, 98–103.

Coffield A., Maciosek M.V., McGinnis J.M., *et al.* (2001) Priorities among recommended clinical preventive services. *American Journal of Preventive Medicine* 21, 1–9.

Foxcroft D.R., Ireland D., Lister-Sharp D.J., and Breen R. (2003) Longer-term primary prevention for alcohol misuse in young people: A systematic review. *Addiction* 98, 4, 397–411.

Karlsson T. and Österberg E. (2001) A scale of formal alcohol control policy in 15 European countries. *Nordisk Alkohol & Narkotikatidskrift* 18, 117–31.

Kriebel D. and Tickner J. (2001) Reenergizing public health through precaution. *American Journal of Public Health* 91, 1351–5.

Room R., Jernigan D., Carlini-Cotrim B., *et al.* (2002) *Alcohol in developing societies: A public health approach.* Helsinki: Finnish Foundation for Alcohol Studies.

Shults R.A., Elder R.W., Sleet D.A., *et al.*, and the Task Force on Community Preventive Services (2001) Reviews of evidence regarding interventions to reduce alcohol-impaired driving. *American Journal of Preventive Medicine* 21, 66–88

Glossary of terms*

Administrative license suspension Drivers license is suspended administratively, without the need of a judicial process, in the event of drinking–driving.

Advertising ban A total or partial legal prohibition of advertising for alcoholic beverages. Partial bans may relate to a particular type of alcoholic beverage, or a type of media, or may limit broadcast advertising to certain hours of the day.

Advertising codes Self-regulation of advertising standards by the alcohol and/or other industries, usually by specifying the content of alcohol advertisements, and the populations exposed to it.

Affective education Programs that address self-esteem, general social skills, values clarification, or similar factors assumed to underlie underage drinking.

Aggregate Population level; summary data representing a collection of individuals.

Alcohol control Any government measure that relates to the purchase, production, or trade in alcoholic beverages, regardless of the aims of such measures.

Alcohol dependence syndrome Term used in psychiatric classifications to identify the co-occurrence of at least three of six drinking-related behaviours (see Table 2.1) associated with dependence to alcohol.

Alcohol education programs Programs implemented in school settings with the aim of teaching students about the dangers of alcohol and ultimately preventing underage drinking.

Alcohol intoxication A more or less short-term state of functional impairment in psychological and psychomotor performance induced by the presence of alcohol in the body.

* Most definitions in this Glossary were adapted from:

Keller, M., McCormick, H., and Efron, V. (1982) *A dictionary of words about alcohol.* Rutgers Center of Alcohol Studies, New Brunswick, NJ.

Babor, T.F., Campbell, R., Room, R., *et al.* (1994) *Lexicon of alcohol and drug terms.* Geneva: World Health Organization.

Alcohol policy Measures designed to control the supply of and/or affect the demand for alcoholic beverages in a population (usually national), including education and treatment programs, alcohol control, and harm-reduction strategies. The term originated in the Scandinavian countries implying the need for a coordination of governmental efforts from a public health and/or public order perspective.

Alcohol taxes The part of the total cost of an alcoholic beverage paid by consumers that goes to one or another level of government. In case of a state alcohol monopoly (see below), this revenue may have a name other than tax (e.g., mark-up).

Alcoholism Term traditionally used to identify chronic excessive drinking by individuals who are physically dependent on alcohol.

Alcohol-related problems Any of the range of adverse accompaniments of drinking alcohol, including medical, social, and psychological consequences. It is important to note that 'related' does not necessarily imply causality.

Alcopops A relatively new form of alcoholic beverage characterized by carbonation, artificial colouring, sweetness, and sale by the 300 ml bottle. More formal names for alcopops are 'pre-mixed spirits', 'flavoured alcoholic beverages', and 'designer drinks'. With an alcohol content (approximately 5%) that is often slightly higher than beer, the marketing of alcopops has been criticized because of its potential attractiveness to children and young adults.

All-cause mortality Number of deaths in a population resulting from all possible causes.

Alternatives to drinking Programs that provide minors with alternative activities (e.g., sports, meditation) presumed to be incompatible with underage drinking.

Aquavit Scandinavian forms of *aqua vitae* or vodka flavoured with caraway seed.

Arrack A distillate from the fermented product of local vegetation in many parts of the world, often variously flavoured. Palm toddy or other juices, rice and molasses, are chiefly used in the East Indies and in India; grapes and other fruit in the Balkans; dates and other produce in the Middle East.

BAC Abbreviation for blood alcohol concentration, sometimes called BAL (blood alcohol level). This is the concentration of alcohol present in blood. In this book, the North American usage of percentage by volume is used (e.g., 0.10% BAC). Multiplying it by 10 gives the equivalent in European nomenclature (1.0 per mille or 1.0 g/ml).

Binge drinking A pattern of heavy drinking that occurs over an extended period of time. In earlier population surveys, the period was usually defined as more than one day of drinking at a time. More recently the term has been applied to drinking by young adults and has been defined by the number of alcoholic drinks (usually five or six) consumed on a single occasion.

Bratt rationing system A system of liquor control (named after a Swedish physician) incorporated into Swedish law in 1917, designed to discourage misuse of spirits by establishing individual alcohol rations for adult citizens. The system was abolished in 1955.

Chibuku Indigenous alcoholic beverage of southern Africa; also known as opaque beer.

Chicha A fermented drink made in Latin America mostly from maize but also from a great variety of juices.

Community mobilization Increasing public awareness of a particular problem and public support for policies directed at preventing the problem.

Confounding A distortion of results that occurs when the apparent effects of a variable of interest actually result entirely or in part from an extraneous variable that is associated with the factor under investigation.

Counter-advertising Actions involving the use of advertising-styled messages about the risks and negative consequences of drinking. Counter-advertising is used to balance the effects of alcohol advertising on alcohol consumption. Such measures can take the form of print or broadcast advertisements (e.g., public service announcements) as well as product warning labels.

Countries in transition As used in this book: countries whose economies are in transition from a centralized socialist or communist structure to a more market driven capitalist one.

Developing countries Countries in the Americas south of the United States, all countries in Asia except Japan and Russia, all countries in Africa, and the island states of Oceania except for New Zealand. Also included within this frame is what has sometimes been called the 'fourth world'—the partially autonomous societies of indigenous peoples that are located within developed countries or societies.

Different availability by alcohol strength Differential legal limitation on the availability of different types of alcoholic beverages based on their alcohol content.

Disability adjusted life years (DALYs) A composite health summary measure that combines years of life lost to premature death with years of life lost due to disability.

Disaggregate The process of breaking down population-level data into constituent parts, for example, by gender, age group, or nationality.

Econometric methods Statistical methods used by economists to investigate the association between economic factors and alcohol use or alcohol-related problems.

Empowerment model A strategy that attempts to solve problems by 'empowering' those most affected by a problem to use their knowledge, experience, and local resources instead of expert opinion or external resources.

Full price Term used by economists; includes not only the listed retail price but also other costs of obtaining the commodity (e.g., travel costs to and from the place of sale).

Graduated licensing Process by which drivers' licenses are issued with initial limitations on driving privileges.

Harm reduction/harm minimization Policies or programs designed to reduce the harm resulting from the use of alcohol, without necessarily reducing alcohol use *per se*. Examples include programs that offer free rides home to persons who are too intoxicated to drive their own cars.

Hazardous drinking A pattern or amount of alcohol consumption that poses risks to the drinker or others.

Health belief model A theoretical model developed in the 1950s, which states that the perception of a personal health behaviour threat is itself influenced by three factors: general health values, which include interest and concern about health; specific health beliefs about vulnerability to a particular health threat; and beliefs about the consequences of the health problem.

Hours and days of sale Days of the week and hours of the day in which it is legal to sell alcoholic beverages for consumption on- or off-premises.

House rules/policies Policies and procedures that are adopted by individual drinking establishments to guide their staff in dealing with such matters as intoxicated patrons and alcohol-related problems.

International classification of diseases and related health problems (ICD) The standard system used to classify, define, and report disease conditions and related health problems within health systems throughout the world. Published and revised periodically by the World Health Organization.

International classification of function, disability, and health (ICF) A standard system intended for use in classifying and recording different types of disability within health systems throughout the world. It was developed by the World Health Organization to facilitate standard record keeping on an international level.

Licensed premises A house or building equipped with a legal permit from the governing authority for the retail sale and consumption of alcoholic beverages.

Lower BAC limits Application to a geographical area or a population group of a lower blood alcohol concentration (BAC) under which it is legal to drive a vehicle.

Media advocacy Use of mass media to place or frame stories from a public health perspective.

Mediator An intervening or intermediate factor (e.g., intoxication) that occurs in a causal pathway from a risk factor (e.g., alcohol consumption) and a health (or social) problem (e.g., an accidental injury). It causes variation in the problem indicator, and variation within itself is caused by the risk factor.

Meta-analytic reviews (e.g., meta-analysis) Statistical analyses in which data from several different studies are culled and re-analysed together; the approach is particularly useful when there is a specific question to answer and at least a few relatively strong studies that come to different conclusions.

Minimum alcohol purchasing age The minimum age at which it becomes legal for someone to purchase alcoholic beverages. Depending on the country, it usually ranges from 16 to 21 years old. In some countries, there are different minimum ages for different beverages or circumstances of drinking.

Natural experiments The investigation of change within and in relation to its naturally occurring context, as when a policy is implemented in one community but not in a comparable community. Implies that the researcher had no influence on the occurrence of the change.

Normative education Classroom lectures, discussions, and exercises designed to provide objective information (often obtained from school surveys) about the extent of alcohol and drug use in the school-age population. The extent of substance use is generally over-estimated by students. This information is thought to reduce the pressure to imitate or conform to the perceived norm.

Number of outlets The number of establishments selling alcoholic beverages for consumption on- or off-premises in a particular geographical area.

Pattern of drinking Implies attention both to the number of drinks consumed per occasion and to the frequency, timing, and context of drinking occasions.

Per capita **consumption** The average amount of pure alcohol (usually estimated in litres) consumed during a given time period (e.g., one year), calculated by dividing the total amount of pure alcohol consumed during that time by the total number of people in the population, including children and abstainers. Adult *per capita* consumption (or per adult consumption) is the total amount of alcohol consumed divided by the number of adults, sometimes defined as persons over the age of 15.

Per se **laws** Laws that define drinking–driving as an offense in terms of driving with a BAC at or above a prescribed level.

Pisco A brandy made in South America (Chilean liquor).

Prevention paradox The notion that the majority of the alcohol-related problems in a population are not associated with drinking by alcoholics but rather with drinking by a larger number of non-alcoholic 'social' drinkers.

Price elastic The per cent change in the amount of alcohol consumed (or quantity demanded) is greater than the per cent change in price.

Price elasticity of demand The term 'elasticity' is used by economists to describe the responsiveness of one variable to changes in another variable. Price elasticity of demand measures the responsiveness of demand for alcoholic beverages to changes in price. It involves comparing the proportional changes in price with the proportional changes in the quantity demanded. The relationship is expressed in the form of a ratio or coefficient.

Price inelastic The per cent change in price is greater than the per cent change in the amount of alcohol consumed (or quantity demanded).

Public service announcements (PSAs) Messages prepared by non-governmental organizations, health agencies, and media organizations for the purpose of providing important information for the benefit of a particular audience. When applied to alcohol, they usually deal with 'responsible drinking', the hazards of driving under the influence of alcohol, and related topics.

Pulque Indigenous alcoholic beverage of Mexico. It is made out of juice from the maguey cactus that goes through a fermentation process (similar to beer's).

Quasi-experimental Lacking complete control over the scheduling of experimental stimuli that makes true experiments possible (see natural experiment). A quasi-experimental design does not include random assignment. The causal certainty of a quasi-experimental design is lower than that of a true experimental design.

Random breath testing (RBT) Roadside checks of randomly selected drivers to assess blood alcohol level based on breath alcohol content. Also called 'compulsory breath testing' in some countries.

Randomized clinical trial A study design in which research participants are randomly allocated to one or more intervention conditions to determine which one would be of greatest benefit. Randomization is done to eliminate error from self-selection or other kinds of systematic bias.

Rationing The sale of alcoholic beverages is limited to a certain amount (usually determined by government authorities) per person. The most notable example of rationing as a way to discourage alcohol misuse is the Bratt system, a form of legal control over alcohol availability in Sweden between 1917 and 1955.

Resistance skills training Classroom exercises designed to provide the social and verbal skills necessary to refuse peer pressure to consume alcohol or drugs.

Responsible beverage service (RBS) An education program that trains managers of alcohol outlets and alcohol servers or sellers how to avoid illegally selling alcohol to intoxicated or underage patrons. Training includes educating servers regarding state-, community-, and establishment-level alcohol policies, describing potential consequences for failing to comply with such policies (e.g., criminal or civil liability, job loss), and development of the necessary skills to comply with these policies.

Responsible drinking A term used by some governments for the drinking of alcoholic beverages in moderation; drinking that does not lead to loss of health or other harm to the drinker or to others.

Server training Servers of alcoholic beverages are taught about local drinking laws, how to handle sales to already intoxicated patrons, and how to prevent intoxication and underage drinking.

Shochu A low priced Japanese spirit having an alcohol content of about 25%.

Sick-quitter effect The fact that many people abstain from alcohol because they are already sick, thereby making abstainers look less healthy as a group than moderate drinkers.

Sobriety checkpoints Places where roadside tests, designed to evaluate whether an individual is driving under the influence of alcohol, are administered.

Social marketing An approach to health communications that applies standard marketing principles to 'sell' ideas, attitudes, and health behaviours.

Social marketing seeks to influence social behaviours in order to benefit the target audience and the general society.

Soju Traditional Korean liquor distilled from rice, barley, and sweet potatoes.

(State) alcohol monopoly Government ownership and management of some or all elements of the alcohol market. This can be at the production, wholesale, and/or retail level, and may be for some or all alcoholic beverages and for on- or off-premise sales or both. Current state monopolies in North American and Nordic countries are limited to the wholesale and/or retail level. In many (but not all) countries or states, the monopoly system attempts to reduce alcohol consumption through the elimination of private profit and limits on availability.

Time–series analysis A statistical procedure that allows inferences to be drawn from two series of repeated measurements made on the same individuals or organization over time. Where the emphasis is on understanding causal relations, the key question is how a change on one series correlates with a change on the other (with other factors controlled).

Total ban on sales A law or regulation making the sale of all or a specific type of alcoholic beverage illegal.

Unit price elastic The per cent change in price is equal to the per cent change in alcohol consumed (or quantity demanded).

Universal strategy A prevention strategy directed at the entire population, rather than high-risk drinkers.

Victim impact panels Restorative justice conferences where several people representing victims of drinking–driving meet with the offender in a structured situation controlled by a trained facilitator. These conferences collectively determine a penalty.

Warning labels Messages printed on alcoholic beverage containers warning drinkers about the harmful effects of alcohol on health.

World Health Organization (WHO) A United Nations agency established in 1948 to protect and promote the health of member states through public health measures and relevant policy research. In addition to the WHO's headquarters in Geneva, there are seven regional offices.

Zero tolerance Loss of driving license if BAC tested positive or if arrested in possession of alcohol for any person under legal drinking age.

Index